Christian Fasting:

A Theological Approach

Kent D. Berghuis, Ph.D.

About the Author

Kent D. Berghuis holds a B.A. from Faith Baptist Bible College, a Th.M. from Dallas Theological Seminary, and a Ph.D. from Trinity International University, Deerfield, Illinois. This book is his doctoral dissertation with only minor corrections, as accepted by the Trinity Evangelical Divinity School. He has previously served in several pastoral ministries, as well as Assistant Professor of Theological Studies at Dallas Theological Seminary. Kent is currently Senior Pastor of First Baptist Church of Lansdale, Pennsylvania, and Adjunct Professor at Palmer Theological Seminary and Biblical Theological Seminary.

Table of Contents

Acknowledgements

So many have encouraged me through the doctoral process that it will not be possible to adequately thank everyone. Yet I would like to acknowledge my debt here, with the hope that their efforts on my behalf will prove worthwhile.

The years spent on this project span two eras of my life, three years each at Trinity and Dallas. The time at Trinity was made possible by the support and love of the Clearview Baptist congregation in Round Lake Beach, who allowed their pastor to study and serve the kingdom of God in a generous way that reached beyond the scope of church life. My family will forever treasure the friendships and experiences gained there. The Trinity faculty and doctoral studies colleagues made my time at the Divinity School one of the most rewarding and stimulating times in my life. I am deeply grateful for their guidance in studies and their willingness to let me teach and find my calling in the classroom. The extensive constructive comments by Dr. Wayne Grudem and Dr. Robert Yarbrough made this book so much better than it would have been otherwise.

The last three years spent at Dallas Theological Seminary have fostered my personal and professional growth in ways I never would have imagined. I want to thank the Systematic Theology department, especially Lanier Burns and Bob Pyne, for taking a chance on hiring me, for freeing me to continue my work on my dissertation by protecting my schedule and teaching load, and all the while stretching and befriending me. I want to thank the administration, especially Mark Bailey and John Grassmick, for taking care of many thousands of dollars in fees and expenses as I continued my education, and I am profoundly grateful for this support. The library staff made this project so much easier by providing office space, handling voluminous inter-library loan requests, and sparing Jeff Webster for lengthy coffee breaks that broke up long days of study and inspired me to continue. Thanks also go to the several students who lightened my grading load and assisted in research, carving out many hours that I could spend concentrating on writing (thanks Rick, Ragan, Chris, Eric, Rachel, Paula, and so many others). Special thanks are due to my intern, Cory Kuhn, whose computer help and editing skills helped finish the job expeditiously.

Finally, thanks go to my family. Thank you, Mom and Dad, for teaching me to love the Lord and setting me on the course I continue to follow. My children, Jacob, Alan, and Jani—maybe someday you will understand what all of this business was about, and I hope you will learn to love the Lord with your heart, soul, and mind, too. As for my wife, Debbie, your encouragement means the world to me. "You are the wind beneath my wings." Thanks for being my best friend, and I love you.

Foreword

Nearly every book about the spiritual disciplines, and I can look through my personal shelves at more than two dozen of them, has a section on fasting. Each one of them exhorts us to fast more than we do – and most of us know we need to fast more – by trotting out a list of "benefits." In fact, benefit-itis, the inflammation of benefits coming to the person who fasts, has become fashionable. But, when a person turns to the Bible, one finds – unless I'm mistaken – not one instance of any biblical writer exhorting us to fast on the basis of the benefits we might receive.

Kent Berghuis' fine examination of fasting is a rare exception to the trend in literature about fasting. Instead of feasting on the benefits of fasting, Berghuis steers the conversation away from benefits toward the Lord of history and the vision toward which we are to orient our lives. And, Berghuis informs us, if we orient our lives toward that future, fasting will find its proper place in the Christian life.

Fasting isn't a trick. Nor is fasting a manipulative game we play with God as if we could eventually get God to give in to our wishes if we drum up sufficient courage to discipline our bodies rigorously enough to show God that we really do mean business about something.

Fasting, instead, is the natural physical manifestation of a Christian whose body is at one with her or his own spirit. In other words, the biblical saints fasted, not to bring the body into line with the spirit – as one finds among the monastics and (if the truth be told) anorexics who were also saints, but because the body was already in line with the spirit. It is the whole person – body, soul and spirit – coming to terms with God about something that matters deeply.

What were those matters? Not very interesting topics for many today: sin, repentance, atonement, pleading with God for something important, and mourning. Yet, there is one more topic that gave rise to biblical fasting, and it is a topic that is uniformly neglected in literature on fasting: eschatology. As Kent Berghuis avoided dabbling in benefits, so he also focused on this much-neglected theme. Jesus called his followers to fast until he came again.

One might, then, say that fasting is eschatological yearning – the Christian yearning with heart, soul and body for what God wills, the Christian yearning against what God is against, and the Christian turning his or her face toward God, looking up, awaiting that final redemption that God has promised. There is simply no book about fasting that is this biblical, and I'm grateful that it is now being offered to the public.

Scot McKnight
Karl A. Olsson Professor in Religious Studies
North Park University Chicago, Illinois

Introduction:
Contribution and Methodology

This book develops an integrative theology of fasting from an evangelical Christian perspective. This introduction will suggest the contribution the study makes to theological studies, briefly describe the methodology that has been followed, and succinctly present its thesis statement.

Contribution of the Study

As later chapters in this book will show, fasting has been largely overlooked as a topic for thorough theological study in the modern era. But in the latter part of the twentieth century, fasting practices began receiving more attention. The Roman Catholic Church reevaluated its stance toward fasting practices in and around the time of the Second Vatican Council, sponsoring renewed interest from that perspective.[1] Evangelical Protestants also began paying attention to fasting in the Bible and other church traditions, and this revitalized interest was seen in an increased number of popular books promoting fasting as a spiritual discipline.[2] A number of theses or minor dissertations have appeared, some of which are focused on various aspects of fasting.[3] Roman Catholic scholar Joseph Wimmer has written a significant work on fasting in the New Testament, and a handful of modern scholarly monographs have been devoted fasting in Christian history.[4] A few substantial articles on specific aspects of fasting have also appeared,[5] and there are several brief articles in standard reference works.[6] Yet no evangelical Christian has developed a comprehensive study of fasting that integrates biblical, historical and systematic theological insights into a cohesive framework.[7] This book is the most comprehensive attempt to date by an evangelical Protestant to synthetically work with the biblical texts in their cultural contexts, in conversation with the broader Christian tradition, in order to develop an integrated theology of fasting for Christians today.[8] It is hoped that fitting this work into that niche will make some modest contribution to academic studies and the church.

Additionally, this book has appended to it two sermons, *About Fasting*, Sermons 1 and 2, by St. Basil the Great, the fourth century Cappadocian church father.[9] These sermons are not readily available in English translation, and represent the most important, previously untranslated, extant patristic statements on fasting, ranking with works on fasting by

Tertullian, Augustine and Leo the Great in influence.[10] These sermons have been integrated into the conversation with patristic texts that takes place in this book, but it is hoped that including the complete translations also represents something of a contribution to readers of English that are interested in patristic literature, and Basil specifically.

Methodology

The basic methodology of this study is evangelical in character, and that perspective entails several convictions. These include the inspiration and authority of Scripture, an orthodox understanding of the Trinity (as expressed in the creeds of Nicea, Constantinople, and Chalcedon), and the Reformation understanding of salvation by grace through faith in Jesus Christ. These convictions will be assumed and not argued in the context of this book. This book is an attempt to develop a specifically Christian theology of fasting. As a result, it does not engage in discussions of fasting in non-Christian religions, or fasting for purposes of health, except where certain intersections might be used for background or application of ideas.

In holding scripture in high regard as the primary source for Christian theological reflection, the progress of revelation is seen as centering on the work of Jesus Christ in a canonical theology. Two chapters have been devoted to studying the references to fasting in scripture, one each on the Old and New Testaments. Various passages related to fasting are studied within their theological and textual contexts, raising attendant ideas that will relate to a theology of fasting.

This reflection is also done in conversation with the Christian community, both in its historical trajectories as well as contemporary forms. A chapter has been devoted to the extensive discussion of fasting in the patristic era, as well as another chapter that traces the history of fasting practices through monasticism, the Reformation, and into their decline in the modern era. In the final chapter of the body of the book, the contemporary reawakening to fasting in Catholic, Orthodox, and evangelical traditions is examined. The integrating eschatological motif of the nature of the age that is seen emerging from the larger study of fasting is then stated in a christocentric fashion within the context of the story of God's redemption. This synthetic theology is applied in the cultural context of evangelical Christianity in the beginning of the twenty-first century.

Christian fasting must ultimately be centered on Christ, reflect proper ways of engaging the human body in sanctification, and remember the corporate nature of the believer's community. Fasting has too easily been associated with a focus on human effort, a fixation on or deprecation of the body, or an individualism that disregards communitarian concerns. It is hoped that this thesis will set fasting in an appropriate, positive theological context, so that its biblical and Christian heritage might be embodied in renewed spiritual expressions.

§1
Fasting in the Old Testament and Ancient Judaism: Mourning, Repentance, and Prayer in Hope for God's Presence

By its very nature, fasting seems to suggest that something is wrong. Eating is a normal part of human existence, so abstaining from eating implies a disruption in the very rhythm of life. But it will be seen in this chapter that the OT uses fasting and abstinence from food to point to something even more necessary for life—communion with and dependence on God. Fasting behaviors were sometimes commanded, sometimes voluntary, and sometimes even ritualized, but the Hebrew Bible rather consistently portrays fasting in conjunction with themes of disruption and restoration. In the midst of disruption, fasting comes to symbolize hope. Through repentance and prayer, fasting can signify the centering of the self in humility, the renewal of the relationship to God's sustaining force. As such, fasting takes on a dual significance of mourning and hope. And the hope evidenced in the proper kinds of fasting in the OT is ultimately a hope in the fulfillment of the eschatological, messianic age. These themes that especially anticipate the NT theology of fasting as a symbol of eschatological, messianic fulfillment will be highlighted below, within the overall context of the nature and purposes of fasting in the OT and ancient Judaism.

It is reasonable to ask how theological applications might be derived from the biblical texts related to fasting. An attempt will be made to examine a wide number of biblical passages in order to arrive at what Gerald O'Collins and Daniel Kendall describe as "biblical convergence." They write that "the principle of convergence entails letting the broadest and most varied amount of biblical witness come to bear on the theological question at issue."[1] This will also entail acknowledging intersection with certain "metathemes and metanarratives" in key passages, as will be seen below in discussions of Adam and Eve in the Garden of Eden, Moses on Mt. Sinai, and the Day of Atonement, and how these kinds of themes find an answer in the NT literature (especially as discussed in the following chapter).[2]

In his discussion of moving from the text to application, Daniel Doriani lists seven biblical sources for application: (1) rules, (2) ideals, (3) doctrine, (4) redemptive acts in narrative, (5) exemplary acts in narrative,

(6) biblical images or symbols, and (7) songs and prayers.[3] Since most of the references to fasting occur in narrative literature, those points that relate to narrative will be most important. First and foremost, these narratives should be seen theologically as communicating the redemptive acts of God in the world. As Doriani suggests, "The central character in every Bible story is God, and some aspect of his redemptive purpose attaches to the main theme of every narrative. Therefore, while interpreters rightly draw moral lessons from biblical history, theological lessons should come first."[4] So as these passages related to fasting are discussed, a primary consideration will be given to the respective places of these narratives in the theological history of redemption that unites the larger biblical story. As one might expect, many of the instances of fasting in Scripture are presented as exemplary acts of biblical characters, and these will generally be seen to be reasonably straightforward in their presentation. There is almost no specific teaching about fasting in the OT, but as Doriani suggests, "where there is no direct teaching, narrative provides guidance," and "biblical narratives guide readers in their proper use."[5] But also of interest will be how fasting begins to be used as an image or symbol, and this will lay the foundation for how the NT uses fasting as an eschatological fulfillment motif.[6]

Backgrounds for Old Testament Fasting

As shown below, abstaining from food for essentially spiritual purposes was part of the fabric of ancient cultures. By the time such fasting appears in the biblical record, it was already a well-established feature of life in the Ancient Near Eastern context. When the Scriptures address fasting, it is often to criticize, modify, sanction, or appropriate behavior that is common to the human experience. But the Hebrew Bible also introduces particular theological emphases on dependence on God that manifest in messianic, corporate, and individual ascetic themes. The concept of fasting in the Bible should ultimately be subsumed under these larger, theological ideas. The following section briefly reflects on the place of religious fasting in ancient cultural backgrounds for studying the OT and introduces the main terminology that is used to describe fasting in the Hebrew Bible.

Ancient Cultural Backgrounds: Fasting as a Common Human Religious Activity

Fasting arose and was practiced as a human religious activity that transcended the cultures of the biblical narratives. H. A. Brongers writes:

> As a matter of fact fasting is by no means a [sic] Israelite monopoly. From earliest antiquity peoples scattered all over the

world have, for one reason or another, abstained themselves from food and drink for a shorter or longer time, as individuals or as a community. Instances collected from many books on ethnology and history of religion are abundant. They all demonstrate such a variety of forms and practices that it is almost impossible to classify them.... .

Now turning to our main subject it soon becomes clear that almost the whole range of fasting-rites we meet with in all parts of the world is present in Israel as well.[7]

The original motivations for ancient fasting are not entirely clear, although a few suggestions have been offered. Some have suggested a connection in mourning rituals to abstain from food so that the dead might make use of it, or in increasing susceptibility to visions and dreams, or in preparation for a sacred meal, or in humbling oneself before one's god.[8] But because of the variety of fasting practices, both religious and secular, it seems best to conclude with Brongers that there is likely no single origin to which all fasting could be traced.[9]

Fasting in the Bible can generally be viewed as an example of religious activity that would have been common in any number of cultures, and therefore subject to similar impulses. Certain Sumero-Akkadian documents describe instances of partial and absolute fasts, which R. Largement thinks may form a basis for (or at least a parallel to) the life of prayer required in the religion of YHWH, minus some of the magical components.[10] Stolz suggests that fasting survived as a remnant of the Canaanite cult of the dead because of the connection to weeping and mourning.[11] Proving direct historical connections like these seems tenuous, but they at least illustrate the commonality of fasting practices. It should not be surprising that occasionally the biblical record would view these religious impulses as misdirected, since the Bible frequently critiques the religious practices of both the believing community as well as outsider cultures. And it should also be understood that such practices could be beneficial if directed toward purposes consistent with the will of the God of the Bible.

Fasting Terms in the Hebrew Bible: Abstaining from Food to Humble Oneself Before God

The principal Hebrew term for fasting is the root צום. The verb occurs twenty-one times in the Hebrew Bible, all in the *qal* stem, and the noun צוֹם twenty-six times in scattered references.[12] The root form also appears in Arabic and Ethiopic "as a religious technical term."[13] Both the verb and noun forms refer exclusively to abstaining from food (and possibly drink), whether personal or corporate in nature, with the primary general occasions being mourning for the dead and worship.[14]

Verbs of interest associated with the noun include קָרָא, "to call" or "to proclaim" a fast (1 Kgs 21:9-12; Isa 58:5; Jer 36:9; Jon 3:5; Ezra 8:21; 2 Chr 20:3), קָדַשׁ, "to sanctify" a fast (Joel 1:14, 2:15), and the verb and noun together as וַיָּצָם צוֹם, "to keep a fast" (or literally, "to fast a fast," 2 Sam 12:16).[15] The term "belongs to the semantic field that also contains weep, mourn, wear sackcloth and ashes, deny oneself, and to do no work."[16]

The most important other term for this study in this semantic field is עִנָּה נֶפֶשׁ, to "afflict one's soul" (as in Lev 16:29, 31, KJV), to "humble one's soul" (NASB) or to "deny oneself" (NRSV, NIV). Forms of this phrase are found in apposition to צוֹם in Ps 35:13 and Isa 58:3 and Isa 58:5. While the derivative תַּעֲנִית (note the tractate of the Mishnah by that name) becomes a standard term for a fast in Judaism, Way is correct (in contrast to the NIV footnote on Lev 16:29) that the two terms should not be seen as complete synonyms.[17]

Rather, fasting would be a more specific means of accomplishing the self-denial enjoined by the public תַּעֲנִית. The relationship of these concepts will be discussed in more detail below, in reference to the Day of Atonement.

Besides these terms there are occasional references in narratives to persons who go without food or water (as in 1 Sam 28:20 and 30:12). The Hebrew term רָעֵב means "to hunger," and is used along with noun and adjective forms to describe the condition of hunger or famine. This descriptive term differs from fasting in that the condition typically is not intentionally self-imposed. צָמֵא, "to thirst," along with its noun and adjective forms, functions in a similarly descriptive manner, although it shares an assonance of sound with צוֹם.

Brongers lists the general occasions for fasting in the OT as related to: mourning a death, making war, preparing or introducing oneself to certain experiences, accompanying prayer, expiating sins, accompanying other activities, and ritualizing days of remembrance.[18] The collation of biblical purposes done for this study divides the bulk of the material from the OT prophets and writings into five positive categories: (1) fasting as a sign of grief or mourning, (2) as a sign of repentance and seeking forgiveness for sin, (3) as an aid in prayer, (4) as an experience of the presence of God that results in the endorsement of his messenger, and (5) as an act of ceremonial public worship.[19] For the purposes of this study, only those occasions in which food is purposely abstained from will be considered "fasting," and within that range most attention will be paid to those occasions that have a demonstrably spiritual purpose. But broader concepts, such as involuntary fasting (as in a siege or illness) or dietary restrictions could be considered in the degree to which they have direct bearing on the theological implications of fasting practices in general. They may help to color the contexts of the broader categories of self-denying behavior, which in turn help one to understand fasting more clearly.

Fasting in The Torah:
Returning to the Sustaining Presence of God

The Torah does not regulate or enjoin fasting *per se* on the people of the covenant.[20] But several key points emerge that contribute to and set the foundation for the rest of the biblical theology of fasting. Of the greatest significance are the nature of the food prohibition in the Garden of Eden, the supernatural fasting of Moses on Sinai, the injunction of personal affliction on the Day of Atonement, and the various dietary restrictions of the law. As seen in the following section, together these metathemes associate fasting with living in or returning to the sustaining presence of God.

The Prohibition in the Garden:
Abstinence as a Condition of Life with God

> Then the Lord God commanded the man, "You may freely eat fruit from every tree of the orchard, but you must not eat from the tree of the knowledge of good and evil, for when you eat from it you will surely die."
>
> Gen 2:16-17, NET

The first sin in the Bible was a violation of a dietary restriction. Even in the Garden of Eden, a restriction on dietary behavior was imposed. As Nahum Sarna comments, "Unrestricted freedom does not exist. Man is called upon by God to exercise restraint and self-discipline in the gratification of his appetite. This prohibition is the paradigm for the future Torah legislation relating to the dietary laws."[21]

After the wonders and methods of creation have been described, YHWH Elohim commands the man[22] in Gen 2:16, "Then the Lord God commanded the man, "You may freely eat fruit from every tree of the orchard, but you must not eat from the tree of the knowledge of good and evil, for when you eat from it you will surely die". Then the creation of the woman is juxtaposed, with the introduction that it was "not good for the man to be alone" (2:18), which stands in contrast to the repetition of the pronouncement after each day of creation in Genesis 1 that the works were "good," and "very good" in the conclusion of the sixth day which included man as male and female in Gen 1:31. Immediately after the creation of the woman the food prohibition is referred to again in Gen 3:1, creating a structure that interchanges the individual creation narratives with references to the food prohibition.[23] In Gen 3:1, the serpent questions the validity of the command to the woman.[24] In fact, the serpent contradicts the stated penalty of certain death, suggesting instead that they would become like Elohim, "knowing good and evil" (3:5).[25] The resulting reasoning process of the woman included three elements, "that the tree produced fruit that was good for food, was attractive to the eye, and was desirable for making one wise" (3:6, NASB). This led her to take it, eat it, and give it to her husband who also ate (3:7).

After the disobedient act, the couple knew they were naked and so they covered themselves and hid. When YHWH Elohim called to them, he immediately asked Adam if he had eaten from the tree (3:11).[26] The man responded that the woman whom God had given him gave him fruit from the tree and he ate, and the woman likewise defers to the deception of the serpent when she is interrogated. This launches the story into the curse format of Gen 3:14-19, in which God begins by pronouncing judgment on the serpent. Along with his penalty of going on his belly comes the statement that he will eat dust all the days of his life (3:14). As Sarna suggests, "The transgression involved eating, and so does the punishment. As the serpent slithers on its way, its flickering tongue appears to lick the dust."[27] There would be enmity between the serpent and the woman and her offspring, who would one day bruise the serpent on the head while being himself bruised in the heel.[28] The woman is assigned great pain in childbearing and a potentially dysfunctional relationship with her husband.[29] Because the man listened to his wife and ate what he was commanded not to eat, the ground is cursed, resulting in great toil to produce food to eat in the future (3:17-19). "Once again, the punishment is related to the offense. The sin of eating forbidden food results in complicating the production of goods."[30] Then the judgment of death is pronounced, with the foreboding words, "for you are dust, and to dust you will return" (3:19).

Of what significance is this account to fasting? At least three ideas present themselves that are picked up by the NT, referred to often in the Church Fathers, and prove foundational to a christocentric, biblical theology of fasting: (1) the notion that the created world, including food, may be regulated by God for his purposes, requiring disciplined obedience on the part of mankind; (2) the messianic idea that the offspring of the woman will reverse the effects of the fall, a theme which will later be symbolized by fasting passages; and (3) the unsettling reality that the body is somehow disconnected from the sustaining force of life. These aspects will be explored in further detail below.

- Food as a Tool of Divine Discipline

In the context of Genesis 2-3 we find that food is used as a tool of discipline by God both before and after the fall. As Thomas Brodie notes, "Among human needs and activities, eating is fundamental, thus making it a suitable representative for human conduct in general."[31] Before the fall, all manner of food was allowable (hardly a fast), with one exception. Was this a test by God to examine the loyalty of the man and woman? It would appear so, since a direct command was given and a penalty was prescribed for disobedience. Without speculating too much about the purposes of God (such as a "covenant of works" or the like, which are not readily discernible from the text), one may surmise a couple of relevant points. First, the creation should be viewed as fundamentally good, but even in the Garden of Eden potentially subversive elements lurked. The crafty serpent was ready to deceive, and the food that led to separation from God was readily available. Amidst all the glory and good of creation, God immediately called the woman and man to disciplined obedience, abstinence from something that might appear desirable. It is interesting to find that although the Mishnah and Talmud do not elaborate on the concept, "later Christian fathers and particularly Byzantine hymnographers, however, interpret the fall in terms of a failure to maintain a decreed fast."[32] Additionally, the intertestamental book of *The Life of Adam and Eve* 6:1 will add that Adam engaged in a forty-day fast in penitence for his fall (the Slavonic adds that Eve fasted forty-four days).[33] This would create an interesting correlation with the forty-day fasts of Moses, Elijah, and Jesus as discussed below, as well as the Christian idea of a forty-day Lenten fast.

In humanity's fallen condition, the disciplinary nature of food is heightened. The curse section repeatedly draws attention to the failure to obey the negative command not to eat by reinforcing penalties related to eating. The serpent will eat dust, mankind will wring their food from the sweat of their brow, eating from the painfully toilsome cultivation of the ground only to one day return to the very soil from which they derived their food. Perhaps this signifies their apparently ultimate defeat by the forces of nature, of which they are no longer clear masters (as in 1:26-30, 2:15). They are relegated to being participants in a hostile conflict they are doomed to lose. So food is used as a tool of discipline throughout the passage. Before the fall, it is part of a call to obedience, abstinence from one source in the midst of abundance, while afterward its difficult acquisition is part of the penalty. In the end, the ground becomes master of all life.

- Hope for Deliverance

It is difficult to assess the messianic role of Gen 3:15 in the immediate context. But there can be little doubt that the Bible picks up on the concept of a זֶרַע, "seed" or "offspring," bringing hope for God's people. Most notably this can be traced through the promise to Abraham of "descendants" (literally "seed," זֶרַע, Gen 12:7, 13:15-16, 15:3-18, 17:7-19) when he was as yet childless. After the birth of Isaac, he is pronounced to be the inheritor of the seed covenant of Abraham (21:12), though Ishmael receives blessing as still part of the seed without being the heir of promise (21:13). The seed promise is reiterated to Isaac (26:4, 24) and passed along to Jacob by Isaac (28:4) and God (28:13-14, 32:12, 35:12, 48:4). No doubt these passages nourished ancient Israel's concept of their nation as the chosen people, the promised seed of Abraham.[34] The literary connection of the prominence of the concept of זֶרַע, in Gen 3:15 and the rest of Genesis would in turn suggest that the chosen people, the seed of Abraham, were the potential fulfillment of the promise of victory over the serpent.

Besides the nation of Israel as the promised seed of Abraham, perhaps the most important narrowing of the concept is the specifying of David's royal line as a covenantally promised זֶרַע, whose throne would endure forever (2 Sam 7:12-17; Ps 89:4, 29, 36; Jer 33:26). It is this idea that allows the NT to connect Jesus Christ theologically back to the Garden of Eden. Christ, the heir of the royal seed promises to David (Matt 1:1; John 7:42; Rom 1:3), is the embodiment of the chosen people as the chosen seed (Gal 3:15-16), the second Adam (Rom 5:12-21), the ultimate seed of the woman (Gal 4:4-5).

Additionally, Jesus is presented in the NT through subtle literary food motifs as the restorer of paradise through his incarnation in at least two contexts (combining the synoptic accounts). First, he withstands the three-fold temptation by the devil in the wilderness during his forty days of fasting, showing himself as the new Adam who lives "not on bread alone, but on every word that proceeds out of the mouth of God" (Matt 4:4; this theme will be explored more fully below in the following chapter). This interpretation is commended by the points that the devil answers to the serpent, and the three temptations answer to the three qualities of the fruit of the tree in Gen 3:6. In the Garden, knowledge of good and evil was offered at the expense of death by eating; in the desert, Christ refuses to eat and so shows dependence on the true source of life, rejecting the devil's offer of dominion to acquire his own rightful title as seed of David, Abraham, and the woman.

Second, at his Last Supper, Jesus' actions recall Eve when she took the fruit of the tree, gave it to Adam, and ate it with him (Gen 3:6). Victor Hamilton comments on the "distinctive sonant structure in this verse" in the phrase וַתִּקַּח מִפִּרְיוֹ וַתֹּאכַל וַתִּתֵּן גַּם־לְאִישָׁהּ עִמָּהּ וַיֹּאכַל, "she took from its fruit and ate it; and she also gave some of it to her husband with her, and he ate it":

> The first four words—of which three are *waw*-consecutive imperfect—contain six instances of doubled consonants—"and she took," *wat-tiqqaḥ*; "of its fruit," *mippiryô*; "and she ate," *wattōʾkal*; "and she gave," *wattittēn*. Such "extremely difficult pronunciation … forces a merciless concentration on each word."[35]

It is interesting to consider how this language is similar to the solemn verbal formula of remembrance in the Lord's Supper. When Jesus "takes" the bread and cup, "giving" them to his disciples, instructing them to "take" and "eat" and drink, all of them together, the NT accounts of the Last Supper use the same verbs that the LXX used to translate Eve's taking of the fruit in Gen 3:6 (Matt 26:26-27; Mark 14:22-24; Luke 22:17-20; 1 Cor 11:23-26).[36] It seems reasonable, then, that in the NT accounts of the Last Supper Jesus is presented as offering his body and blood to his disciples as the remedy for original sin, which would also be consistent with the more immediate Passover imagery there of the substitutionary lamb. The "tree" of Christ's cross is also mentioned in 1 Peter 1:21-25, in a context that evokes Christ as the sinless substitute (second Adam imagery), connecting it with Isaiah 53 (Christ as the suffering servant of Israel, the ultimate "seed" upon whom God would look and be satisfied). Although Genesis itself does not elaborate much on the remedy for sin, in the Christian theological context, the fall of Adam and Eve is reversed in Christ. He is the second Adam and the ultimate seed of the woman, who himself dies on a tree to make himself the food that gives life to those who will take and eat.

Finally, Rev 22:1-3 presents a vision of the New Jerusalem in the New Heavens and Earth. Once again there is an answer to the fall in the Garden, but this time it is the once forbidden tree of life. Now it is presented as given for the "healing of the nations," and there will "no longer be any curse." This amplifies the eschatological banquet language that is common in the NT.[37] The ultimate hope of the believer is one of feasting and enjoying the life intended by God through the work of Christ, who kept the fast that humanity could not.

- ## The Body as Material

The account of the creation and fall of man raises questions about humanity's ambiguous relationship with the rest of the created order. On the one hand, it is obvious that man is very much a part of the material world in which he finds himself. Adam is created from the "dust of the ground" (Gen 2:7), a fact which God reminds him of in the curse narrative (3:19). The woman derives her life from the man when God fashions her from one of his ribs (2:21-23). The man and woman have material bodies that are organically connected to the ground on which they walk and from which they derive their life-sustaining food.

On the other hand, the couple is presented as more than just a part of nature. The creation of Adam involves the unique infusing of the "breath of life," which appears to be anthropomorphically transmitted directly to his nostrils from the nostrils of YHWH Elohim (2:7).[38] This act sets the man apart from the rest of creation as "a living soul," a נֶפֶשׁ חַיָה, who possessed the נְשָׁמָה, the breath of God himself. This animating aspect of humanity does not come from the ground, but instead the vibrant life force of his breath comes from God. This fact adds to the chill of the curse of Gen 3:19, because the penalty of death apparently means the cessation of the function of this infused life force. The נְשָׁמָה, the breath, cannot return to dust, since its source is not created material. Instead, the fall reorients man to his status as created, material being, deriving his life from the ground.

All of this sets up the tension inherent in theological anthropology. Von Rad writes:

> This man, however, formed from the earth, becomes a living creature only when inspired with the divine breath of life. [N^eshama] corresponds to our "breath." This divine vital power is personified, individualized, but only by its entry into the material body; and only this breath when united with the body makes man a "living creature." Thus v. 7 is a *locus classicus* of Old Testament anthropology. It distinguishes not body and "soul" but more realistically body and life. The divine breath of life which unites with the material body makes man a "living soul" both from the physical as well as from the psychical side. This life springs directly from God, as directly as the lifeless human body received breath from God's mouth when he bent over it! Nevertheless, the undertone of melancholy is unmistakable: a faint anticipation of the state of post-Adamic man! When God withdraws his breath (Ps. 104.29 f.; Job 34.14 f.), man reverts to dead corporeity.[39]

So humans are more than simply material beings that function like the rest of the created order, existing in a web of life in nature that includes but transcends them. The "living soul" still functions, pulling man toward his initial role as lord of creation in the image of God (1:26-30, 2:15). These concepts will affect one's view of the body and spiritual life, which will have implications for fasting in the traditions of both Judaism and Christianity.

Sometimes added to the biblical concepts will be the alien notion of a dualism between a pure spiritual world and a corrupt material world, which will complicate ascetic traditions through the ages. The biblical account of the creation and fall of mankind does not sanction a strict dualism between body and soul. Rather, humanity is viewed as both material and immaterial, created from the ground and infused with divine life. The curse of the fall clearly tells what happens to the material side of man at death—it returns to the ground from whence it came. But the ongoing, living, fallen status of the immaterial life force is left unaddressed, at least explicitly. But a clue that it continues (albeit in a fallen condition) is the fact that Adam and Eve did not physically die the day they ate from the fruit of the tree (after all, that was the stated consequence of the food prohibition in 2:17). So one is left wondering if they really died in some way when they ate (or was the serpent correct when he asserted, "You surely shall not die!"?). The material life did not cease, nor did the vivifying breath. Gen 5:1-5 says that Adam lived to be 930 years old before he died, and in the meantime the text explicitly states that he passed along the image and likeness of God to his offspring.

An implicit message of the account, then, would be that the nature of the punishment of Adam and Eve did indeed involve death, though they did not instantly die. The punishment of death was not merely a distant consequence. The very principle of death became operative in Adam and Eve as soon as they disobeyed God and ate the fruit. The account ties sin and death together in an organic, dissoluble union. Where sin exists, there death exists. Death is not only the punishment for sin (which it surely is on a basic level), but death actually is part and parcel of the concept of sin itself. The fingers of the grave reach out into the land of the living in every inclination toward evil.

Therefore the initial OT account presents man as a complex dichotomy. He exists in a fallen state, both materially and immaterially, and oriented by the curse more toward the material world. This will have implications for fasting in at least two other areas: the incarnation of Christ and the ongoing struggle for sanctification, addressed in more detail in later chapters.

Moses on Mount Sinai:
Fasting in the Sustaining Presence of God

> So he [Moses] was there with the Lord forty days and forty
> nights; he did not eat bread, and he did not drink water.
>
> Exod 34:28, NET

The first explicit reference to a case of total fasting one encounters in the biblical text is found in Exod 34:28. This second occasion of Moses on the mountain follows on the heels, however, of the first forty day period mentioned in Exod 24:18, and both incidents are acts of fasting, as Deut 9:9 and 10:10 make clear. In between the events, Deut 9:18 suggests that there was another intercessory period of forty days' fasting. So the story line as presented by Deuteronomy actually contains three incidents of Moses engaged in forty-day fasts from food and water on Sinai, although the Exodus account only explicitly mentions one fasting episode.[40]

While the intended chronology of the Sinai account is less than crystal clear, it appears that God spoke with Moses in the cloud, giving the instructions of Exodus 20-23. Then Moses came down and related the teachings to the people, writing them down and initiating a covenantal ceremony, before coming back up to receive the divinely inscribed tablets and further instructions (24:1-18). One interesting factor is that in Exod 24:11 the nobles of Israel (which must have included Moses, Aaron, Nadab, Abihu, and the seventy elders of 24:9) "beheld God, and they ate and drank." After this feasting in the presence of God, Moses is separated from them to go up on the mountain alone (with Joshua). After six days of the cloud of the glory of YHWH resting on the mountaintop, which appeared to the Israelites as a "consuming fire" (v. 17), God called to Moses, who entered the cloud for forty days (24:18). Presumably he received the instructions of Exodus 25-31 during this time, dealing primarily with tabernacle construction and worship regulations. The encounter ends with the story of the people's idolatry, Moses' repeated intercessions, his breaking of the tablets, and his destruction of the golden calf (32:1-35).

After these momentous happenings, the journey resumes on the ground, but the presence of God is reserved for Moses alone in the cloud in the tent, where they would speak face to face (33:11). Moses is granted a partial vision of YHWH in Exod 33:12-23, after which another invitation to go up Mt. Sinai is given, in order to replace the broken tablets (34:1). The teachings of the previous meeting are reiterated in Exod 34:10-26, apparently a summary of a much larger communication Moses received. Then the reader is informed that Moses was writing down these words, and "he was there with the Lord forty days and forty night; he did not eat bread or drink water" (34:18). When he descended, his face still shone with the glory of YHWH (34:29-35).

The retelling of the story in preparation to cross Jordan and enter Canaan in Deuteronomy 9-10 mainly contributes an emphasis on Moses' intercession for the people in the midst of their rebellion. Deut 9:4-6 mentions that the reason for Israel's possession of the land is not their own righteousness, but rather the combination of the wickedness of the inhabitants and the fulfillment of the patriarchal oath. Even the miraculous events of Sinai (called Horeb in 9:8), including the divine tablets of stone, Moses' supernatural sustenance, and the voice from the cloud and fire on the mountain had not kept the people from idolatry. Moses then again fasted from bread and water another forty days, "because of all your sin which you had committed in doing what was evil in the sight of the LORD to provoke Him to anger" (9:18). YHWH listened to Moses' intercession again (9:19). God called Moses back up on the mountain, and after a parenthetical account of the intervening journey (10:6-9), Moses says that he was again on the mountain "forty days and forty nights like the first time" (10:10), which, when correlated with Exod 34:18, meant another supernatural fast. Once again the emphasis is on intercession, because "the LORD listened to me that time also; the LORD was not willing to destroy you" (10:10b).

One main theological point of reflection about these fasts of Moses is the supernatural sustaining power of God for his servant. Under ordinary circumstances it would be difficult to fast from food for forty days, but not impossible. However, to go without water for more than just a few days would mean certain death from dehydration. Yet the text explicitly mentions Moses' abstinence from water on all three of these occasions. As Walter Kaiser comments, "That Moses was able to go for this length of time without food or water was a miracle requiring the Lord's supernatural care."[41] Similarly, Nahum Sarna elaborates on the reference to abstinence:

> In the presence of the ultimate Source of holiness and in communication with Him, Moses realizes a transformation of his self. He achieves a state that is beyond the ordinary range of human experience. In this extrasensuous world he transcends the constraints of time and is released from the demands of his physical being.

> This same phenomenon is included in the retrospective summary of the first theophany on Sinai found in Deuteronomy 9:9, 18, although it is omitted in the primary narrative in Exodus 24:18. Its emphasis here must be taken as

another indication that the thrust of this epilogue is to elevate the status of Moses. It serves as the background for the culminating and extraordinary experience recounted in the following verses.[42]

The apparent means of the sustaining of Moses' life is the near absorption of Moses into the glory of God. When he is in the presence of God on the mountain, he needs no food or drink, because God himself sustains him. Perhaps we should think then of God being pictured as the real source of life, in whose presence even earthly food and water might be unnecessary for a person, if God so chooses. Of significance is the fact that Moses was speaking with God. This comes on the heels of Deut 8:3, in which Moses recounted the story of the manna in the wilderness, asserting that the people were made to hunger, "that He might make you understand that man does not live by bread alone, but man lives by everything that proceeds out of the mouth of the LORD." Moses is being kept alive on the mountain, then, not by food and water, but by the mouth of YHWH. This recalls the creation of Adam from the breath of God, the life force being separate in source from the body itself, and ultimately divine in origin.

Another point of emphasis is on the contrast between Moses, the servant of God, and the nation for whom he was interceding. The people are pictured as in need of an intercessor, a mediator between them and God. Jeffrey Tigay comments:

> The phrase implies that Moses can, as it were, restrain God from destroying Israel. Midrashic commentaries understand it as a hint for Moses to do just that by praying on Israel's behalf. In other words, God is saying that by right Israel ought to be destroyed, but that He wants the prophet to make the case for sparing them. Prophets frequently play this intercessory role in the Bible in addition to their role as God's messengers to man. This is part of what God wants them to do.[43]

God's wrath is imminent, but it is averted when he is appeased through the prayers of his servant. The complete humility and dependence on God shown by Moses in his fasting plays a role in God's acceptance of his plea. Moses himself could have become the father of a new nation (Deut 9:14), but the covenantal, patriarchal promises are invoked and applied to the entire people (Deut 9:26-29).

The promise that God would raise up a prophet like Moses to whom the people would listen (Deut 18:15) is recalled in later biblical accounts through fasting motifs in two key instances. The first will be Elijah, who returns to Horeb on the strength of a food that enables a forty day fast (1

Kgs 19:8). The second, and most important for Christians, will be Jesus (as discussed more fully in the following chapter), who initiates his ministry with a forty day fast in the wilderness before presenting himself as the giver of the new law (Matt 4:2; Luke 4:2). As Eugene Merrill comments on the similarity in the gospels, "One cannot help but note the reference to bread and stones in light of the experience of Moses, who received the Word of God on stone tablets even while being denied physical food and drink."[44] The NT will pictures Jesus as a new Moses, the mediator of a new covenant. He is the One who is able to resist the temptation to make his own bread, and instead chooses to live on "every word that comes from the mouth of God" (Matt 4:4). This messianic function will be further reflected in the Davidic promise, and he is the "Son of God," and the people are commanded to "listen to Him!" (Mark 9:7). So these fasting passages contribute to the way the NT will coalesce several OT messianic images into Christ as the one central figure of biblical theology.

The Day of Atonement: Fasting as a Solemn Sign of Humility

> This is to be a perpetual statute for you. In the seventh month, on the tenth day of the month, you must humble yourselves and do no work, both the native citizen and the foreigner who resides in your midst, for on this day atonement is to be made for you to cleanse you from all your sins; you must be clean before the Lord. It is to be a Sabbath of complete restfulness for you, and you must humble yourselves. It is a perpetual statute.
>
> Lev 16:29-30

Secondary sources about fasting often mention that the only fast required by law in Judaism was the Day of Atonement as described in Lev 16:29-30, 23:27-32, and Num 29:7.[45] However, it is not specifically described as a "fast" in the Hebrew Bible, nor is fasting enjoined. That is, the words from the root צום are not employed, nor is there any explicit reference to abstaining from food. Instead, the Hebrew uses a broader term (תִּעֲנוּ אֶת־נִפְשֹׁתֵיכֶם, which may have included fasting as an understood application) and commands the people to "afflict," "deny," or "humble yourselves." Jewish tradition practiced fasting on that day, as also evidenced by the Targums (which actually used the Aramaic cognate of צום), the Qumran literature, and the NT.[46]

Since Jewish tradition universally has interpreted the instructions of these passages to include fasting as a sign of afflicting and humbling oneself, it is possible that other places in the Bible that mention humbling, affliction, and the like may have in fact tacitly included fasting. This connection is clear in Ps 35:13, "I humbled my soul with fasting" (עִנֵּיתִי בַצּוֹם נַפְשִׁי)(NASB). Here, fasting is explicitly the means of "humbling" oneself. Isa 58:3 similarly links these terms: "'Why don't you notice when we fast? Why don't you pay attention when we humble ourselves?'"[47] In this poetic text, צַמְנוּ stands in parallel relationship to עִנִּינוּ נַפְשֵׁנוּ in the next line. It is reasonable that a similar logical relationship exists with the Day of Atonement admonitions, even though the Hebrew text itself is not explicit. Fasting is a particular expression of the more general concept of humbling oneself.

The intended solemnity of such an occasion can be gauged by a review of the usage for the root ענה.[48] Of the approximately seventy-seven uses of this verb, about twenty-nine refer to suffering imposed by God, eighteen to suffering forcibly at the hands of others, and fifteen as a euphemism for rape or illicit carnal knowledge of a woman. Of the fifteen references to the possibility of self-imposed affliction, six fall in the Day of Atonement passages, and two are referenced above in connection with fasting. To afflict oneself, then, was a very serious concept, a way of identifying with suffering, often thought of in severe terms, usually imposed by God or through other means beyond one's control. This would result in a humble spirit as opposed to a proud or haughty one.[49] It would be a way of taking the part of the poor, suffering and afflicted in society. A survey of the related nouns עָנָו and עָנִי shows how this class often appears to have the special attention of God.[50] The NT will echo these themes, as Jesus himself identifies with the humble and afflicted in his life (Matt 11:28-29) and ultimately in his death (Phil 2:8), and in like manner, God's people are called to humble themselves in order to be exalted by God.[51]

Dietary Restrictions in the Law: God Setting Apart a People for Himself

While a full-scale examination of dietary regulations is outside the scope of this study, their similar relation to fasting would be difficult to avoid entirely. Their theological overlap eventually comes under the category of sanctification, although different purposes may be delineated.

• Kosher Restrictions: A National Community Set Apart

Food consumption is of course part of everyday life, and Judaism has been distinctive for its regulations of eating habits.[52] While both fasting and dietary restrictions at times have some kind of sanctification as their common end, kosher regulations can be seen to deal more with issues of ontological purity. The meat of certain animals is forbidden because they are "unclean." As is the case with fasting, the instructions and narratives are woven together in a complex web rather than dealt with systematically. Commenting on this, Neusner writes:

> What is new here is the equation of purity with holiness, a theme virtually absent in the narrative, prophetic, and sapiential materials we have just examined. But what we are not told is why these particular animals are unclean and lead to unholiness; the pre-history of the forbidden creatures is not recorded. All living creatures are simply divided into clean and unclean, without explanation.[53]

The primary lists of unclean animals may be found in Leviticus 11 and Deuteronomy 14.[54] The stated reason in Lev 11:44-45 for abstaining from such animals is simply YHWH's holiness and his desire for his people's holiness:

> I am the Lord your God and you are to sanctify yourselves and be holy because I am holy. You must not defile yourselves by any of the swarming things that creep on the ground, for I am the Lord who brought you up from the land of Egypt to be your God and you are to be holy because I am holy.

The main explanations offered for the rationale behind such regulations are cultic, hygienic and ethical considerations, although Bryan prefers some kind of an anthropological approach.[55] However, getting into the mind of the author (and contextually in this passage, that would include God!) is a difficult task (as Bryan admits). Perhaps the ethical approach that refuses to speculate into the rationale behind the commands provides a better framework for reflecting on the phenomenon of obedience to the commands themselves.

At any rate, these kosher regulations set the ancient people of Israel apart unto YHWH, and obedience to these laws protected ritual purity. Although this happens in the same general sphere of food intake regulation as fasting, one can see that their purposes ultimately diverge. These dietary restrictions were ways of normativizing a sanctified lifestyle, whereas fasting is generally an unusual behavior, an action taken that is conspicuously out of the ordinary. Yet there is a similarity in the kosher regulations for the people of Israel to the command in paradise to abstain from the fruit of the tree of the knowledge of good and evil. Both prohibitions require God's people to abstain from foods to demonstrate submission, obedience and loyalty to him. The command in the garden can be seen as anticipating these kosher regulations, or alternately, kosher regulations can be seen as reflecting the primeval ideal of obedient abstinence.

- The Nazirite Vow: A Special Class of Abstinence

Perhaps a slightly closer theological relative to later ascetic fasting behavior is the taking of a Nazirite vow, as discussed in Num 6:1-21. The only explicit food regulation was abstaining from any product of the grapevine, whether as food or wine (6:2). But the whole cluster of regulations suggests an ascetic lifestyle that was unusual, whether temporary or lifelong (as was intended in the case of Samson, Judg 13:5). In this example we see an intensification of the approach to sanctification, the idea that one must live a strictly disciplined lifestyle before God. This of course was not mandatory for the entire community (otherwise the very unusual characteristic of the lifestyle would lose its primary meaning), but rather reflected a specific calling. Christian monks and other ascetic characters in later ages can be seen as following in the train of these OT Nazirites who exemplified a special calling to a life of renunciation.

Fasting in the Prophets and Writings: Mourning that Converges on Eschatological Realization

The first use of צוֹם and the first narrative reference to fasting after Moses is Judg 20:26, when Israel fasted during the Benjamite civil war. Fasting accounts become more frequent in historical sections of Samuel and Kings, but none of these passages provides instruction on how fasting should be practiced or hint about the origins of the rite. As noted above, it would appear that this kind of fasting was a part of the normal cultural milieu in which the Bible exists, without Scripture dominating its early shaping.

In dealing with fasting beyond the Torah, it may be useful to categorize the instances by their occasions. These categories show fasting as (1) a sign of grief or mourning, (2) a sign of repentance and seeking forgiveness for sin, (3) an aid in prayer, (4) an experience of the presence of God that results in the endorsement of his messenger, and (5) an act of ceremonial public worship. Texts that specifically focus on fasting or raise the key theological themes that anticipate the Christian theology being explored in this book will be dealt with in more detail than those that mention fasting more incidentally. While fasting occurs for a variety of reasons in a variety of passages, the theological ideas attached to the practice seem to grow and converge in the prophetic anticipation of an eschatological fulfillment in an age when fasting and repentance will give way to the presence of gladness and justice.

- Fasting as a Sign of Grief or Mourning

When tragic events struck in ancient biblical communities, fasting was often an expected response. When the Israelites lost a battle to the Philistines, "all the people went up and came to Bethel and wept; thus they remained there before the LORD and fasted that day until evening" (Judg 20:26, NASB). When David and his men heard of the death of Saul and the loss of the battle, they tore their clothes, "They lamented and wept and fasted until evening because Saul, his son Jonathan, the Lord's people, and the house of Israel had fallen by the sword." (2 Sam 1:12).[56] When news of the king's death edict reached them, "there was considerable mourning among the Jews, along with fasting, weeping, and sorrow. Sackcloth and ashes were characteristic of many" (Esth 4:3, NASB). Community fasting was proclaimed for drought (Jer 14:1-12) and locust plagues (Joel 1:14, 2:12-15). Fasting also was often part of someone's personal sorrow or suffering, as we see in Hannah, Job, and David and other Psalmists (1 Sam 1:7-8, 20:34; Job 3:24; Pss 42:3, 102:4, 107:17-18).

This type of fasting is possibly its most basic expression. This shows fasting's role as part of the overall human experience, particularly in ancient cultural contexts. The disruption of the normal course of life caused by death or calamity is reflected in a behavior that disrupts the normal functions of life, as fasting does with eating. The act of fasting reflects the disrupted state of affairs in the circumstances around it, and also engages the person fasting in behavior that intensifies the experience of the sorrow and abnormality of the situation.

- Fasting as a Sign of Repentance and Seeking Forgiveness for Sin

In an expansion of the idea of fasting as grief or mourning as described immediately above, fasting in biblical contexts often was done as a sign of grief or mourning over sin as a show of repentance. This frequent occasion for fasting probably grows out of (or at the very least accompanies) the understanding of fasting as a means of humbling oneself. Several of the OT's specific references to fasting involve repentance from national or corporate sins. Several of the references dealt with under other headings also include elements of repentance, in addition to those highlighted here. Often leaders and prophets called for public fasting as a demonstration of humility and repentance:

> 1 Sam 7:5-6: "Then Samuel said, 'Gather all Israel to Mizpah, and I will pray to the LORD on your behalf.' After they had assembled at Mizpah, they drew water and poured it out before

the LORD. They fasted on that day, and they confessed there, 'We have sinned against the LORD.'"

Neh 9:1: "...the Israelites assembled; they were fasting and wearing sackcloth, their heads covered with dust."

Joel 1:14: "Announce a holy fast; proclaim a sacred assembly. Gather the elders and all the inhabitants of the land to the temple of the LORD your God, and cry out to the LORD."

Jonah 3:5: "The people of Nineveh believed in God, and they declared a fast and put on sackcloth, from the greatest to the least of them." [57]

We also see individuals such as David and Ahab fasting in repentance and prayer after their own sins. Righteous leaders mourned over and identified with the sins of their people as evidenced by Nehemiah and Daniel:

2 Sam 12:16: "David prayed to God for the child and fasted. He would even go and spend the night lying on the ground."

1 Kgs 21:27: "When Ahab heard these words, he tore his clothes, put on sackcloth, and fasted. He slept in sackcloth and walked around dejected."

Neh 1:4: "When I heard these things I slumped down, crying and mourning for several days. I continued fasting and praying before the God of heaven."

Dan 9:3: "So I turned my attention to the Lord God to implore him by prayer and supplications, with fasting, sackcloth, and ashes."

Ceremonial fast days seem to have been regarded as appropriate times for exposing the sins of people. The prophets Isaiah (Isa 58:1-5), Jeremiah (Jer 36:6-9), and Zechariah take advantage of these occasions to rebuke people who otherwise may have seemed hostile to their message. Even in the negative example of wicked Queen Jezebel, we see that she used a fast day to accuse Naboth under false pretenses (1 Kgs 21:9-12). While hardly exemplary, it shows that fasting was commonly viewed as appropriate behavior when dealing with matters of grave consequence.

- Fasting As an Aid in Prayer

Prayer and fasting are frequently connected in biblical texts. The examples already cited generally include prayer in their contexts, and there are several other situations in which prayer and fasting are connected in a general sense. Bible characters are often found fasting while in intercessory prayer for others (2 Sam 12:16-23; Neh 1:8-10; Ps

35:13; Dan 6:18, 9:15-19). Fasting is sometimes part of personal prayer (1 Sam 1:7-11; Neh 1:11; Ps 109:21-24; Dan 9:3, 10:1-3). Leaders pray and fast for success in battle (Judg 20:26; 1 Sam 7:6; 2 Chr 20:3), for relief from famine (Jer 14:1-12; Joel 1:14, 2:12-15), or for success in other endeavors, such as Ezra's return from the exile or Esther's success before the king (Ezra 8:21-23; Esth 4:16).

Fasting in such instances appears to be a kind of intensification of prayer. The humility associated with the act of fasting is demonstrated physically, perhaps as a sign of the special and serious nature of the petition being offered. This calls the believer into a physical enactment of the prayer, engaging the self more thoroughly into the religious action of prayer. Additionally, the petitioners may have hoped that God would see their seriousness and answer, as in the case of Daniel's intense conclusion to his prayer in Dan 9:19: "O Lord, hear! O Lord, forgive! O Lord, pay attention, and act! Don't delay, for your own sake, O my God! For you are identified with your city and with your people". We see also in the case of Daniel 9 and 10:1-3 prayer and fasting associated with receiving special revelations from God through angels.[58] Perhaps this suggests that biblical characters fasted in order to receive revelations, although that theme is certainly not very dominant.

- Fasting as an Experience of the Presence of God and Endorsement of His Messenger

As noted above, Moses is the prototype for this kind of fast. In an interesting parallel, Elijah visits Horeb (a variant name for Sinai) and is sustained by a supernatural meal for a similar forty-day period: "The Lord's angelic messenger came back again, touched him, and said, 'Get up and eat, for otherwise you won't be able to make the journey.' So he got up and ate and drank. That meal gave him the strength to travel forty days and forty nights until he reached the mountain of God in Horeb" (1 Kgs 19:7-8). This kind of fasting highlights the role of God as giver and sustainer of life, who can supply food at will, and sustain human life without food if necessary.

The fasting of Elijah also functions in a literary manner to further the redemptive-historical theology of the OT narrative. This recalls the promise of God raising up a prophet like Moses (Deut 18:15), with the implication that God will sustain his chosen servant, even by supernatural means.[59] Thomas Brodie notes the parallels between Moses and Elijah's trip to Horeb in "the thunderous meeting at the mountain, the supplying of food in the wilderness, the journey for forty years/days, and the appointment of a successor (Joshua/Elisha)."[60]

This fasting incident highlights the motif of the succession of the Mosaic prophet. R. P. Carroll has demonstrated convincingly that there is a theme of prophetic continuity in the OT, with Yahweh raising up prophets from time to time in succession and in the mold of Moses, as occasion demanded.[61] The NT interprets this Mosaic prophetic succession eschatologically as culminating in Christ, as can be seen in Acts 3:22 and 7:37. This helps us understand something of the way John the Baptist was referred to as "Elijah" by Christ (Matt 11:13-14). He was the last in a line of prophetic successors, initiated by Moses and epitomized by Elijah, and predicted to return in the eschatological day:

> Remember the law of my servant Moses, to whom at Horeb I gave rules and regulations for all Israel to obey. Look, I will send you Elijah the prophet before the great and terrible day of the Lord comes. He will encourage fathers and their children to return to me, so that I will not come and strike the earth with judgment (Mal 4:4-6).

All of God's true prophets were penultimately pointing toward Christ as the quintessential divine mediator. So when Christ fasts in the desert for forty days, he is demonstrating himself to be the fulfillment of the prophetic line from Moses through Elijah, who both also fasted forty days in the wilderness. The Elijah narrative picks up on the fasting aspect of Moses' experience, transforming it into a symbol of prophetic succession that the NT can apply to Christ in his messianic, prophetic role.

As in the cases of Moses and Elijah, fasting can be used to mark out God's messenger for ministry. This seems to highlight God's ability to sustain his prophet or servant by his own means, creating an aura of the supernatural around the messenger. This can also be seen in the rather obscure OT narrative of 1 Kgs 12:1-22, where an unnamed prophet was commanded to fast while on a specific mission. Perhaps this was associated with the need for purity when the prophet was speaking the words of the Lord, or of the solemnity of the message. This idea of God's leaders fasting in relation to specific ministries seems to find further expression in a few NT contexts as well. Jesus' forty-day fast came at the onset of his public ministry. Then in Acts we see the commissioning of Saul and Barnabas and the ordination of elders accompanied by fasting (Acts 13:2-3, 14:23). Paul said that he was in "fastings often" (2 Cor 6:5/11:27, NASB), which could refer to intentional fasting, or possibly the fact that he was forced to go hungry at times for the sake of the ministry (see discussion in the following chapter). In these instances, fasting associated with a specific ministry highlights God's endorsement of his messengers, as the messengers deny themselves food to deliver his words.

- Fasting as an Act of Ceremonial Public Worship

In addition to the Day of Atonement described above, several instances are recorded in the OT in which ceremonial fasts of Judaism are described. As these do not grow out of direct teachings of the law, the attitude of the people and not the ritual in itself was of greatest concern to God as speaking through his prophets. It is possible that the altogether human penchant for expanding on Scripture's admonitions gave rise to ritualistic fasting, which often was seen as problematic by the prophets. Isaiah 58 and Zech 7:3-14[62] provide powerful examples of Judaism's own prophets offering critiques of their religious fasting traditions, and will be dealt with in greater detail below. Even when the prophets offer their critiques of fasting, it is not the ceremony itself they attack, but merely the hypocritical spirit that accompanies it. The assumption is that the ceremony might have positive value if accompanied with righteousness. A couple of the most theologically important passages are worth dealing with in more detail as examples of the role of ceremonial fasting in the prophetic tradition. These passages look forward to an eschatological realization of the underlying purposes of fasting, a day when mourning gives way to gladness and justice.

Isaiah 58: True Fasting Must Include Justice. The prophet Isaiah gives an extended example of alternative fasting attitudes in OT Judaism.

> No, this is the kind of fast I want. I want you to remove the sinful chains, to tear away the ropes of the burdensome yoke, to set free the oppressed, and to break every burdensome yoke. I want you to share your food with the hungry and to provide shelter for homeless, oppressed people. When you see someone naked, clothe him! Don't turn your back on your own flesh and blood!
>
> Isa 58:6-7

The chapter begins with YHWH urging the prophet to expose the sins of his people (58:1) by raising his voice like a shofar (note the connection between the shofar and fasting in *Ta'anit*, below). Although the people appear to be acting in sincere desire (יֶחְפָּצוּן) for the Lord's favor (58:2), they feel that they have not been answered in their fasting, that God has not noticed (58:3).[63] The Lord responds that this is because they are actually seeking after their own desire (חֵפֶץ),[64] and exploiting workers (58:3). Such fasting does not merit God's attention. God has not chosen fasting to be a day for merely humbling oneself outwardly, as shown by the bending of the head and lying in sackcloth and ashes. Such displays seem to not even merit the title of fast, as the concluding question of Isa 58:5 suggests: "Is this really what you call a fast, a day that is pleasing to the LORD?" (NASB). Instead, God has chosen a fast in which one will make restitution for injustice, "to loosen the bonds of wickedness, to undo the bands of the yoke, and to let the oppressed go free, and break every yoke" (58:6). Additionally, it is a day for sharing food with the hungry and clothing the naked (58:7).

These social actions are actually considered to be a proper expression of the attitude of fasting and not a rejection of fasting altogether. As Barré observes, the passage uses "dialectic negation," which is characterized by "'exaggeration' ... in the negative member, which may often be characterized as a statement of contradiction," but this "contrasting-by-way-of-negating is intended for emphasis."[65]

> Isaiah 58 is not rejecting fasting but emphasizing that unless accompanied by actions of love of neighbor it is an empty ritual. As noted earlier, for the Israelites fasting was meant to be a "sign" of *repentance*, of turning back to God. A distinctive mark of Israelite (i.e., covenant) religion was that turning to God was inseparable from turning in love to one's neighbor. This is why Isaiah 58 uses "dialectic negation" to emphasize the fact that a sign of repentance means nothing if the neighbor is unaffected by it.[66]

When one makes oneself hungry by fasting, perhaps the plight of those who suffer hunger involuntarily will be more personalized, prompting sharing (58:7, 10). By humbling or afflicting one's own soul, one will enter vicariously into the suffering of those who are oppressed (וַתַּעֲנֶה וְנֶפֶשׁ), helping their needs to be satisfied (58:10). This will demonstrate a true righteousness, and result in God answering the people's cry. The reference to water on scorched land (58:11) may suggest that these fasts were linked to drought, perhaps being part of the tradition of fasting for rain preserved in the Mishnah tractate, *Ta'anit* (see below). The ones who bow themselves low will ultimately "ride on the heights of the earth" (58:13, NASB), and the one who has fasted and kept the sabbath for the Lord's delight will be fed "on the land I gave to your ancestor Jacob," apparently a reference to the covenanted blessings of Israel.[67]

> Fasting in Isaiah 58, then, is intended to be more than ritual. It is to be a true humbling of the heart that results not only in humility, but in actual identification with those who are lowly—the hungry and oppressed. This theme will later be appropriated by Christians who call for true forms of fasting as opposed to fasting for mere rituals.

Zechariah 7-8: Fasting Turned to Gladness. This passage forms a distinct literary unit, with sermonic material bracketed by references to fasting.[68]

> The sovereign Lord says, 'The fast of the fourth, fifth, seventh, and tenth months will become joyful and happy, pleasant feasts for the house of Judah, so love truth and peace.'
>
> Zech 8:19

The stated occasion for the Lord's reply is the question of an envoy from Bethel[69] to the priests and prophets in Jerusalem, asking if they should continue certain fasting days (7:2-3). Zechariah responds with a call to dedicate both fasting and feasts to God as opposed to themselves (7:4-7), and a call to social justice with themes reminiscent of Isaiah 58 (7:8-14). Then an eschatological vision of a restored Jerusalem ensues (8:1-23), which includes the turning of the people's fasts into feasts (8:19).

The fasts mentioned in the passage are specifically linked to the calendar. The first reference, in the question of the messengers from Bethel, is to a fast in the fifth month (7:3). The fifth month refers to the destruction of the temple by Nebuchadnezzar about seventy years earlier on the ninth of Ab (August 14, 586 BC).[70] The word employed here is הִנָּזֵר, a niphal infinitive absolute from נָזַר, "to devote" or "dedicate oneself unto."[71] The fact that this root is morphologically related to the Nazirite concept of consecration is significant. Since the context clearly includes fasting, it suggests that here fasting was seen as a communal act of consecration. In Zechariah's immediate response, he mentions fasts in the fifth and seventh months (7:5).[72] Then in Zech 8:19 four fasts are mentioned as being in the fourth (marking the breach of the wall of Jerusalem, the ninth of Tammuz), fifth, seventh and tenth (apparently commemorating the onset of the siege of Jerusalem on the tenth of Tebeth) months. So while the initial question mentions only one fasting occasion in the fifth month, it seems probable that the nature and legitimacy of a certain system of ritual fasts was being discussed.[73]

The eschatological nature of the question itself may be inferred from Zechariah's answer. Zerubbabel elsewhere has been presented as a potentially messianic figure (Zechariah 4). As Mason suggests, it would seem that the envoy is asking about the appropriateness of continued fasting, if indeed the exile is over, the temple is being rebuilt and a messianic figure is present:

> The force of the question seems to be, as Ackroyd has suggested, "Has the new age you have been predicting come or not?" It is universally agreed that the answer to the question

occurs in 8:18f., for only there is the question of whether to continue fasting, or stop it, dealt with. The section beginning in 7:4 is concerned more with the *motive* for fasting.[74]

While the prophet certainly desires to see the blessings he prophesies in Zechariah 8, the fulfillment appears to await an eschatological future when YHWH returns to dwell with the people in Jerusalem. Ackroyd thinks that Zech 8:19 "makes it clear that the new age has come."[75] Jewish sages took this to mean that when the temple was rebuilt, these ritual fasts were to be turned to times of rejoicing.[76] The post-exilic return to the land and the restored worship in Jerusalem were indeed an eschatological fulfillment, although that fulfillment may not yet have been exhausted. Willem VanGemeren places this discussion in this eschatological context, noting that "God's response is that the new era of restoration calls for rejoicing instead of fasting. Joy is more in accordance with the loving kindness of the Lord (8:19)."[77] But the social conditions suggested by the passage as prerequisite for such an age clearly were not being universally applied by the nation, and so it seems most reasonable that the new age was viewed as an ideal for which to strive. In a future, more realized age, Israel would be a spiritual leader among the nations, entreating the Lord even as the envoy from Bethel had done, and declaring their allegiance to Israel's God (8:20-23).[78] It would be brought about by the messianic figure and result in the kind of social justice the passage envisions, overturning the fasting and mourning into joyous feast days. The NT will pick up on these themes, identifying the appearance of Christ, the "bridegroom," as the beginning of that messianic age when mourning gives way to gladness (Matt 9:15; Mark 2:19; Luke 5:34).

Extrabiblical Literature: Fasting Established in Jewish Tradition

The fasting customs and theology of the Hebrew Bible are reflected and expanded in extrabiblical Jewish literature, establishing some identifiable fasting traditions. While these Jewish traditions find certain roots in biblical literature, it also becomes evident that various additions to that tradition form a backdrop that the NT can address in its own formation of a more specifically Christian theology of fasting. References to fasting in the apocrypha, pseudepigrapha and rabbinic literature will be examined briefly below.

- Fasting in the Apocrypha: Reflecting and Expanding Biblical Fasting Themes

There are several instances of fasting in the apocryphal books. 1 Esd 8:50 and 8:73 are similar to the stories in the canonical Ezra 8:21-23 and

10:6, with the first instance of fasting initiated for the journey of the exiles and the second in humiliation for the sins of the people.[79] When Baruch read the words of his book that recounted the destruction of Jerusalem to Judah's kings, nobles and people already in exile, "Then they wept, and fasted, and prayed before the Lord" (Bar 1:5, NRSV). In 2 Esd 5:13, Ezra is commanded by an angel to "pray again, and weep as you do now, and fast for seven days" in order to receive further apocalyptic revelations.[80] In 2 Esd 9:23 the seer is told not to fast this time. In this vision he sees a woman whose son died in his wedding chamber, and she says in 2 Esd 10:4 that she will "neither eat nor drink, but will mourn and fast continually until I die" (NRSV). This account turns out to be a metaphor for Jerusalem's desolation. Judith 4:13 describes a national fast as an act of repentance, and "The Lord heard their prayers and had regard for their distress; for the people fasted many days throughout Judea and in Jerusalem before the sanctuary of the Lord Almighty" (NRSV). In 1 Macc 3:47, the people fast in mourning over their devastated sanctuary and to seek counsel from God, and a similar fast is observed in 2 Macc 13:12. So in each of these passages, fasting is portrayed in mourning or repentance scenarios much as in the biblical literature already examined.

Other apocryphal references to fasting seem to parallel OT contexts. Sirach 34:26 (LXX, 34:31 NRSV) asks in a manner similar to the OT prophets, "So if one fasts for his sins, and goes again and does the same things, who will listen to his prayer? And what has he gained by humbling himself?" This suggests that fasting and prayer are of no use to the man who goes his way and continues in his sin, and his superficial humbling does not profit him unless accompanied by true life change. 1 Maccabees 3:17 tells of a victory in a guerilla-style battle accomplished while fasting. The question is raised whether they should engage in battle because of their faintness from fasting, but God provides the victory. This stands in interesting contrast to 1 Sam 14:24-46, in which Saul is viewed as foolish for forcing a fast on his army.

A couple of apocryphal texts use fasting in ways that appear to be echoed in the NT. An interesting passage in Tob 12:8-10 associates prayer, fasting and almsgiving with righteousness, themes elaborated by Jesus in Matthew 6. Except here we see almsgiving (and perhaps the other acts of righteousness by implication) as capable of purging sin and providing life:

> Prayer with fasting is good, but better than both is almsgiving with righteousness. A little with righteousness is better than wealth with wrongdoing. It is better to give alms than to lay up gold. For almsgiving saves from death and purges away every sin. Those who give alms will enjoy a full life, but those who

commit sin and do wrong are their own worst enemies. (Tob 12:8-10, NRSV).

It appears that here is an elaboration of the theme of Isaiah 58, that true fasting should be accompanied by sharing with those who have nothing to eat. However, the raising of this kind of righteousness to the status of purging sins seems to relocate the forgiveness in the action itself, something not stated explicitly in the biblical passages. In Jdt 8:6, Judith is described as a woman who "fasted all the days of her widowhood, except the day before the sabbath and the sabbath itself, the day before the new moon and the day of the new moon, and the festivals and days of rejoicing of the house of Israel" (NRSV). Presumably this was an extraordinary sign of mourning, and this long-term fasting as a sign of mourning for widowhood seems similar to the depiction of the NT Anna in Luke 2:37.[81] Additionally, the idea that Sabbaths and festival days were not to be days of fasting will be found in early Christian traditions that exempt Sabbaths, Sundays and certain feast days from fasting.

- Fasting in the Pseudepigrapha: Some Escalation of the Virtues of Fasting

The *Testaments of the Twelve Patriarchs* contains several references to fasting.[82] The *Testament of Simeon* 3:4 has Simeon say, "Two years therefore I afflicted my soul with fasting in the fear of the Lord," which he describes as fleeing to God in order to finally overcome the vice of envy.[83] Joseph says that he "fasted in those seven years" (*T. Jos.* 3:4) when he was tempted by the Egyptian woman, giving his bread to the poor. Afterward, he "appeared to the Egyptians as one living delicately, for they that fast for God's sake receive beauty of face" (*T. Jos.* 3:4).[84] Joseph even fasted in prison (9:2), and he attributes his accomplishments to prayer and fasting: "Ye see, therefore, my children, how great things patience worketh, and prayer with fasting" (10:2).[85] Rachel is said to have prayed and fasted while barren, with the result that Benjamin was born (*T. Ben.* 1:4). Fasting while continuing in sin is condemned as hypocrisy in *T. Ash.* 2:8, in a manner reminiscent of prophetic themes: "Another committeth adultery and fornication, and abstaineth from meats, and when he fasteth he doeth evil."[86] Reuben is said to have abstained from meat and wine in penance for seven years for his sin of fornication (*T. Reu.* 1:10), as did Judah until his old age (*T. Jud.* 15:4). These frequent references to fasting in the *Testaments of the Twelve Patriarchs* evidence an escalation in the attention being paid to the virtues of fasting, since the original biblical materials describing these figures never mention it.

1 Enoch 108:7-9 describes the humble as longing more for God than earthly food, which sounds ascetical in tone.[87] *Psalms of Solomon* 3:8 suggests that involuntary sins may be atoned through fasting, which may be an extension of the concept of fasting on the Day of Atonement: "[The righteous] maketh atonement for (sins of) ignorance by fasting and afflicting his soul, and the Lord counteth guiltless every pious man and his house."[88] As previously mentioned, in the *Life of Adam and Eve* 6:1, Adam fasted forty days, and the Slavonic version adds Eve fasting forty-four days, as penance.

Fasting was not always encouraged in pseudepigraphal literature, however. *Jubilees* 50:12 lists fasting as one of several things forbidden on the sabbath, on pain of death, and the *Fragments of a Zadokite Work* 13:13 makes a similar statement. But as Wimmer observes, "the command not to fast on the sabbath implies that some wanted to do just that."[89] So on the whole, when fasting is mentioned in the pseudepigraphal texts, there appears to be an escalation of its virtues.

- First-Century Jewish Literature: Fasting Evidence in Jewish Practices Contemporary with the NT

The Qumran literature and the authors Philo and Josephus offer glimpses into Jewish life in the first century, and they are briefly examined below. While the evidence from this material is not extensive, it does at least give some picture of Jewish fasting practices that were going on around the time of the events and writing of the NT.

Qumran Literature: Scanty Evidence from an Ascetic Community. Although the Qumran community practiced a life of discipline, in the Dead Sea Scrolls the only explicit mention of fasting is in reference to the dispute with the Jerusalem temple authorities over when to observe the Day of Atonement.[90] It is possible that the lifestyle of the community included ritual fasting, since asceticism was woven into the fabric of their lives.[91] But on the whole, the Qumran literature does not factor into this discussion of a theology of fasting in a very significant way.

Philo: Blending Jewish Religious Fasting with Greek Philosophies. Philo represents something of a blending of a Hebrew religious focus on fasting and some broader Greek ideas of bodily purity and receptivity. In rather Hebrew fashion, he describes the purpose of the Day of Atonement as humility before God and the putting away of boasting, which results in propitiation.[92] He contrasts the awe and reverence of the Jewish fast, which he says is kept more strictly and solemnly than the "holy month" of the Greeks, which he describes as gluttonous "fasts."[93] He contrasts drunkards with the sober and their clarity of the senses in a way that may reflect a more broadly Greek concept of purification:

> Though indeed, it is true that these sober ones are drunk in a sense, for all good things are united in the strong wine on which they feast, and they receive the loving-cup from perfect virtue; while those others who are drunk with the drunkenness of wine have lived fasting from prudence without ceasing, and no taste of it has come to their famine-stricken lips.[94]

In a similar vein, he says, "For understanding is starved when the senses feast, as on the other hand it makes merry when they are fasting."[95] In *De Vita Contemplativa*, Philo discusses approvingly the disciplined lifestyle, which included fasting and dietary regulations, of the "Therapeutae," a Jewish communal sect living on the shore of Lake Mareotis near Alexandria.[96] In all of these references, we see Philo's desire to honor the traditional practices of Jewish fasting and correlate them with an appeal to Greek notions of virtue.

Additionally, Philo connects gluttony with sexual indulgence:

> Gluttony is naturally followed by her attendant, sexual indulgence, bringing on extraordinary madness, fierce desire and most grievous frenzy. For when men have been loaded up with overeating and intoxication, they are no longer able to control themselves, but in haste to indulge their lusts they carry on their revels and beset doors until they have drained off the great vehemence of their passion and find it possible to be still. This is apparently why Nature placed the organs of sexual lust where she did, assuming that they do not like hunger, but are roused to their special activities when fulness of food leads the way.[97]

This connection between the belly and the genitals will be seen in the Church Fathers and become a point of a good deal of reflection in monasticism.[98]

Josephus: Fasting as Practiced in First-Century Judaism. Josephus does not add a great deal to the theology of fasting, but he "is an important witness to the Jewish institution of fasting and to its spirit of penance for sin and supplication for deliverance."[99] He frequently mentions fasting in his retelling of OT narratives, and refers to the Day of Atonement as "the Fast."[100] He also recounts an instance of wicked Ananias proposing a general fast day for the deceitful purpose of getting his enemies among the people, including Josephus, to lay down their weapons and catch them off guard.[101] He describes the prayer and fasting of King Izates when threatened by Parthian invaders.[102] He also "points out with pride that many nations have taken over Jewish beliefs and pious practices, including the fasts."[103] Like Philo, Josephus upholds Jewish fasting as a positive ideal, and reflects the general practice of Judaism in the first century.

- Fasting in the Mishnah and Talmud: Codifying and Qualifying Fasting in the Jewish Tradition

There are numerous references to fasting in rabbinic literature. Occasionally some of these discourage fasting, while others are more favorable. Of those that are favorable, they qualify fasting by considering whether or not the reasons are imperative, and whether those fasting go beyond mere mortification to true spiritual reappraisals of inner thoughts as well as actions.[104] Although the literature is diverse, evidence of some codification of fasting practices can clearly be seen. Some of the more important instances of fasting, especially the extended treatments, will be discussed below.

Ta'anit: *Regulating How to Fast for Rain*. Over time, Judaism grew keenly interested in ritual fasting, and a tractate of the Mishnah, *Ta'anit*, is devoted to certain fasting regulations.[105] The tractate is divided into four chapters, primarily dealing with drought in the rainy season. The first and longest chapter deals with the conditions of drought which would necessitate fasting and the prescribed days and regulations for doing so. The second details certain ceremonies to be performed on such days, as well as the potential calendar collision of fast days and festival days when fasting is prohibited. The third chapter discusses the appropriateness and methods of sounding the shofar for fast days at various times of calamity. The fourth discusses the relation of priestly orders and temple service to the fast days, and includes a recounting of the tragedies that befell the Jews on the seventeenth of Tammuz and the ninth of Ab.

According to *Ta'anit* chapter one, if rain had not begun to fall by the seventeenth of Marcheshvan, a series of fasts would be initiated. The first series was for individuals distinguished in the law. On the immediately following Monday, Thursday, and Monday they would fast during the day, but they were allowed to eat and drink after dark, and they were permitted to work, bathe, anoint themselves, wear shoes, and have marital relations (*m. Ta'an.* 1:4). If by the first of the next month, Kislev, rain had not arrived (about two weeks after the seventeenth of Marcheshvan), a series of three Monday-Thursday-Monday fasts was enjoined upon the entire community. They were allowed to eat and drink only during the day, and forbidden to work, bathe, anoint themselves, wear shoes or have marital relations. The bathhouses were to be locked (*m. Ta'an.* 1:6). If these passed without rain, seven more stringent fasts were enjoined, still following the Monday-Thursday pattern.

They were to sound the shofar and lock the stores. On Monday the store doors could be opened partially toward evening, and they could be open on Thursdays in preparation for the Sabbath. If these days passed, they were to "decrease" commerce, construction, planting, betrothals, marriages, and greeting one another. The distinguished individuals would resume the fasting until the end of Nissan, after which any rainfall would be symptomatic of a curse, since it would no longer be of benefit to the crops (*m. Ta'an.* 1:7).

As can be seen, there was an increased intensity in the nature of these fasts as time wore on: "Abstaining from food and drink on a public fast-day is not an end in itself, but the means by which the community is to arrive at a spiritual awakening and true repentance."[106] The rituals prescribed, however, are subject to a great deal of discussion about exceptions and exemptions, which leads to the observation that the acts could easily have been interpreted by the people as primarily symbolic. The fact that certain accompanying actions (work, bathing, laundering, anointing, sandals, and sex) are discussed tends to focus attention in their direction.[107] It is also interesting to observe the distinction between the fasting and prayers of those distinguished in the law and the community at large. The prayers of the leaders appear to be seen as more efficacious, as they begin the cycle (no point in bothering the entire community yet) and end it (there was little hope left, no point in disturbing the community further). In *Ta'anit*, then, fasting retains its role in repentance, but it also becomes more ritualized, codified, and elevated to a potentially elitist function. The Pharisee who fasted twice a week but was condemned by Jesus in a parable in Luke 18:12 seems to reflect such an elitist attitude toward his fasting.

Yoma: *Regulating Fasting on the Day of Atonement.* The tractate *Yoma* expands on the procedures of Leviticus 16 concerning the Day of Atonement. For the most part it discusses the preparation and function of the high priest and the service order for the day, including both the sacrifice and the scapegoat.

The eighth (and last) chapter deals some with the laws promoting repentance by regulating fasting and labor on the Day. Eating, drinking, washing, anointing, wearing shoes and cohabitation were all prohibited (*Yoma* 8:1).[108] One was not to eat more than the volume of a large date or drink more than both cheeks full (8:2). Sin offerings were prescribed for violating these limits (8:3). Children were not required to afflict themselves but were to be instructed in the procedures, and pregnant women and the sick were allowed exemptions from fasting (8:4-6). Similarly, work could be performed to clear a collapsed building if it threatened human life (8:7). Yom Kippur provided atonement for sins before God, provided repentance was genuine; but for sins against a fellow man reconciliation was first enjoined (8:8-9).

On the whole, *Yoma* does not add a great deal to the discussion of fasting, except to show the practical outworking of the practice on the Day of Atonement. The need for true repentance over against merely ritualistic conformity is stressed, although the ongoing discussion of related regulations may tend to obscure that basic point.

Fasting in Other Talmudic References: Diversity, with Some Extreme Tendencies. The Talmud contains a number of incidental references to fasting, and S. Lowy provides the best introduction.[109] The main purposes for voluntary fasting in the early talmudic period followed the biblical and apocryphal lead, and primarily focus on repentance, atonement, and the strengthening of prayer, while fasting as an expression of private mourning is discontinued.[110] Later, however, there are some examples of more extreme cases of fasting as examples of penitence, which are attributed to the Tannaim of the earlier period, even though tannaitic literature itself does not mention such things. There were attempts to curb or modify fasting, evidenced by Samuel's statement, "There are no public fasts in Babylonia except *Tish'ah be-'abh*" (*Pesah.* 54b), but Lowy says this qualification was not intended to be taken literally.[111] Some excessive examples include:

> R. Eleazar b. Azariah's teeth "were blackened from fasting" to atone for his sin of opposing a majority view (*y. Šabb.* 3.4, 7c.).

> R. Joshua used insulting words about an illogical opinion of the school of Shammai, and his "teeth were black from fasting" (*t. Ohol.* 5.11).

> R. Tarfon saved his own life by revealing his identity when accused of being a thief, and a later tradition says he fasted throughout his life for this sin (*y. Šeb.* 4.2, 35b, *b. Ned.* 62a).

> R. Simeon made a derogatory remark about R. 'Aqiba, and his "teeth were blackened from fasting" (*Naz.* 52b).

> R. Hiyya b. 'Ashi lived in sexual abstinence from his wife for years. His wife tested him by dressing as a harlot and seduced him. When he realized her identity, he was plagued by guilt, because he intended to sin, and he died from extensive fasting to expiate this sin (*Qidd.* 81b).

R. Hisda offended his teacher, R. Huna, with a comment, and both fasted forty fasts: R. Hisda because of the suffering caused his teacher, and R. Huna because he falsely suspected his pupil (*Bab. Mes.* 33a).

R. Papa fasted because of a slightly insulting expression about the sages (*Sanh.* 100a).

Mar b. Rabhina fasted the whole year except for some holidays (*Pesah.* 68b).

Rabbi Sadoq is described as having fasted forty years so that Jerusalem would not be destroyed. The context describes a famine, and a woman ate a date left by the Rabbi, who would allow himself to suck the juices of a fig to get well. When he ate something, it is said that the food could be seen in his throat (*b. Git.*56a).[112]

However, Lowy cautions us:

It would be wrong to assume that an ascetic tendency towards extensive fasting was prevalent. On the whole, Judaism was set against such extreme practices. From the very earliest times— even before the ascetic sects came into existence—down to the amoraic period such practices were generally discouraged. There were many limitations on fasting.[113]

Despite Lowy's cautions, we can see, however, that there were ample examples of rather excessive forms of fasting in certain rabbinic traditions. Additionally, the fasting practices reflected a division in society between great ascetic men, the middle class, and everyone else. It is easy to see how such a division associated with religious practices could lead to ritualization and potential abuse or neglect, as the case may be.

We should be careful not to stereotype traditional Jewish fasting as completely negative or hypocritical, which the Church Fathers occasionally did. [114] But we should take to heart both the OT prophets' admonitions as well as Jesus' later instruction in the Sermon on the Mount. Fasting can have its proper place in personal and corporate religious experience, but it can also degenerate into meaningless or even hypocritical ritual.

Conclusion

The various references to fasting in the Hebrew Bible and Jewish tradition begin to converge in several key theological themes. The most basic ancient purpose of fasting as a sign of mourning in times of death or disaster branches into two main theological ideas, namely fasting as repentance for sin and fasting to intensify prayer when seeking God's favor. Both of these ideas, however, presuppose an even more basic theological idea that the OT occasionally highlights through fasting references: that God is the ultimate source and sustainer of life, and human life depends on connection to his presence and obedience to his words. This theme that emerges already in the Garden of Eden is the basis for the fasting that highlights Moses as God's chosen leader, and sets in motion a messianic motif that God's chosen prophet will be like him. As the fasts of Israel turned routine, the prophets urged the people to true justice in anticipation of the eschatological day when their mourning would be turned to gladness, their fasting to feasting. Against the backdrop of Jewish fasting that occasionally obscured true humility, repentance and justice through hypocrisy and ritual, the eschatological realization of the ideal that fasting anticipated came in the person of Jesus Christ. To the theological discussion of fasting in the NT we now turn.

§2
Fasting in the New Testament:
Remembrance and Anticipation in the Messianic Age

A thoroughgoing Christian, evangelical, and canonical theology of fasting will seek to orient both testaments to the central figure of Christianity, Jesus. The OT will be seen as pointing forward toward him and the NT as pointing back to him. The NT presents Jesus as the pivotal, messianic figure who would usher in the kingdom of God. This chapter will seek to show that fasting plays a significant role in new covenant theology by symbolically contributing to this eschatological identity of Christ. Key fasting texts help Christians to understand the nature of the age, and fasting is described both didactically and by example.[1]

The most important theological ideas related to fasting texts in the NT will flow from this messianic center. In this chapter, Jesus himself is seen to be marked out by his fasting, as he identifies with Israel as its messianic prophet like Moses. He brings an end to the old covenant and the mourning for Israel's exile and would seem to be putting an end to the significance of the fasting motif. But then he ushers in a new age, one marked by his absence as well as his presence in the Spirit, and so fasting is reinvested with meaning. Fasting was never a sign of righteousness in itself, but humble, righteous people may indeed fast in any age. And so the early followers of Christ did fast, not out of a sense of obligation, but in a desire to seek the Lord's presence and out of necessity for the ministry of the gospel. Such discipline is encouraged as the Lord does his work through his people, but the act itself did not have the kind of formalized or ritualized meanings it occasionally had for contemporary Judaism, as seen in the last chapter.

In order to better understand the references to fasting in the NT, some further general background will first be presented below. Then a focus on the references to fasting in the gospels will establish the essentially messianic and eschatological character of fasting as a central aspect, as well as a recasting of fasting as an act of true humility before God. In the book of Acts and a couple of references in the epistles, fasting will be seen to function in a renewed form in the nascent new era. Finally, a few major text critical issues will show the bridge from NT fasting to the increasingly ascetic tendencies of the early Christian community.

Greek Background and Terminology
Fasting as Abstaining from Food,
Usually for Religious Reasons

Two of the most important pieces of academic work related to a biblical theology of fasting focus on the New Testament. One is a rather comprehensive dissertation by Marion Michael Fink, and the other a competent monograph by Joseph F. Wimmer, without reference to one another.[2] Fink presents fasting in the NT against the backdrop of Greco-Roman culture, generally following the lead of Rudolf Arbesmann.[3] He gives extensive citations of both primary and secondary sources in Graeco-Roman literature. But while the broader historical milieu of the NT era certainly plays a role in shaping contemporary attitudes toward fasting, one wonders if Fink has overstated the importance of non-Jewish sources on the NT. For instance, he convincingly argues that fasting did not play that great a role in the overall Graeco-Roman culture, yet he suggests that Christian fasting grew away from biblical descriptions: "Through the innocently applied examples of fasting in the New Testament, the early ascetics gained control of the import of the teachings in the New Testament; and fasting succumbed to the syncretistic influences."[4] This seems to result in a lack of balance in the work, with relatively little discussion of the OT precedents as compared to voluminous references to Greek and Latin literature. Such literature is more appropriately used to set a context for the later reception of Christianity in the broader Graeco-Roman world, especially when one considers the thoroughly Jewish character of Jesus, his Galilean disciples and the other protagonists of the NT.

Wimmer's work exemplifies some of the best of modern Catholic biblical scholarship. The writing is lucid and thorough, and the work is probably the best overall biblical study of fasting to date. While he engages in technical (and sometimes rather theoretical) reconstructive textual work, he keeps an eye on the hermeneutical, theological, and practical implications of his study for the life of the church. His conclusions, as seen below, place fasting in the context of a Catholic commitment to virtue theology (he says that fasting can "foster union with Christ," while Protestants might wish to emphasize that the gospel establishes that union). In summarizing the relevance of his study, he writes:

> We may conclude, then, that the eschatological acceptance of the kingdom, the kerygmatic union with Christ and the transcendental norms of faith, hope, and charity which flow from it are always valid, and that the perennial validity of

certain precepts of the New Testament's categorical morality is to be determined by the degree of their fidelity to the fundamental kerygma. The validity of fasting is judged ultimately by the same criteria, by the degree of its relationship to the fundamental aspects of Christian doctrine, by its ability to foster union with Christ in faith, hope, and love, and by its capacity to prepare us for eternal life.[5]

While these brief conclusions are appreciated, Wimmer leaves room for an expansion of key theological concepts, which he only touches on as he grounds his work textually. Both Fink and Wimmer provide commendable background studies for fasting in the NT. So it will only be necessary to briefly summarize some of the key features of this discussion here before moving on to the biblical and theological material.

The NT Greek terms relating directly to fasting are forms of the adjective νῆστις, the noun νηστεία, and the verb νηστεύω. Behm says that the basic word νῆστις "means generally 'one who has not eaten, who is empty,'" and when referring to abstention from food on religious grounds, it becomes the term for the one who fasts.[6] The noun form, νηστεία, can denote general hunger, but most often refers to fasting as a religious rite, whether public or private.[7] The verb νηστεύω "can also mean generally 'to be hungry, without food,' ... But it usually means 'to fast' in a religious and ritual sense."[8]

Louw and Nida discuss the basic terms under the domain of "physiological processes and states," and the subdomain of "eat, drink," with these comments:

> the state of being very hungry, presumably for a considerable period of time and as the result of necessity rather than choice (compare νηστεία[a] 'fasting,' 53.65)—'to be quite hungry, considerable hunger, lack of food.'[9]

Referring to the domain of "religious activities," "fasting" is given its own subdomain, and defined as "to go without food for a set time as a religious duty—'to fast, fasting.'"[10] The Day of Atonement is also recognized as a festival known simply as "the fast."[11]

Fink emphasizes the "tendency toward non-religious meanings" in the terms: "They were so fundamentally bound up in the physical state of not eating or of lacking food that they represented a spectrum of meanings from 'hungry' to 'hunger' to 'famished' to 'famine,' and they were even used to describe the state of unfed animals."[12] This supports his idea that Judaism and Christianity progressively influenced the Graeco-Roman culture to view fasting as being linked to religious observance, while that was not necessarily the case earlier.

According to Wimmer, "With the exception of oracular shrines, fasting played only a small part in the worship of ancient Greece."[13] The only common fast known was a fast on the second day of the three-day Thesmophoria festival, in honor of Demeter. Wimmer notes that fasting and food observance later became common through Oriental influence, as evidenced by initiation rites of mystery religions like Kybele and the Eleusinians. Those who gave oracles, as well as Pythagoreans, sometimes engaged in fasting or partial abstinence behaviors, perhaps having to do with symbolic or magical purification to allow for clarity in their mantic activities. It was "thought that the soul could reach its greatest power when it was independent of the digestive activity of the body and of the evil spirits that inhabit certain foods, so that it could then enter into free communion with the divine world and learn its mysteries through oracles and dreams."[14] The Cynics and Stoics practiced lives of self-control, which included dietary restrictions, to seek peace through simplicity.

As already seen, the Hebrew terms related to צוֹם certainly did have a specifically religious connotation. The LXX almost always employed νηστεύω for the Hebrew verb צוֹם and νηστεία for the noun צוֹם, with Behm calling them "the fixed equivalent."[15] With reference to the NT, then, the religious usage for νηστεύω words will be primary, but the broader, more general usage of the terms in Greek heritage may also occasionally be present.

Fasting in the Gospels: In Christ, Fulfillment Has Come

The synoptic gospels provide the basic material for a study of NT fasting, with several important contexts.[16] Two are treated in more than one gospel, the fasting of Jesus while he was tempted in the desert, dealt with in Matt 4:1-4 and Luke 4:1-4 (although Mark 1:12-13 refers to the incident without mentioning fasting), and his response to a question as to why his disciples did not fast, which is recorded in all three synoptics (Matt 9:14-17; Mark 2:18-22; Luke 5:33-39). Matthew records Jesus' teaching concerning fasting in the Sermon on the Mount (Matt 6:16-18), and Luke mentions the fasting of Anna in the temple (Luke 2:37) and a parable of a Pharisee who fasts (Luke 18:12). There is also a reference to the possibility of sending the crowd away "fasting," which raises the question of the less than distinct relationship between intentional fasting and hunger (Matt 15:32; Mark 8:3).

This chapter will suggest that the primary theological contribution of these texts is to highlight the pivotal, momentous eschatological change that has arrived in the person of Christ. The texts will be dealt with in a theologically prioritized order, to highlight the flow from the messianic, eschatological mission of Christ, to teachings about fasting, to less important examples that nonetheless contribute to the greater theology of fasting. First, Jesus' forty-day fast will be seen to mark him as the messianic figure, the promised prophet like Moses. The fasting query directed to Jesus will teach his followers about the eschatological nature of the age that follows his messianic appearance. The instructions in the Sermon on the Mount and the parable of the Pharisee will both highlight the nature of true righteousness as opposed to hypocrisy, suggesting the primacy of humility instead of hypocrisy in fasting. The fasting of Anna in the temple anticipates the eschatological fulfillment described above. And the feeding of the hungry crowd, whether it is to be considered fasting *per se* or not, only further highlights the messianic role of Christ as the giver and sustainer of life. Taken as a whole, it will become evident that fasting functions as an important, symbolic theological foil for the concept of promised fulfillment in Christ, and this theology provides a basis for renewed teaching for the practice of fasting in the life of his disciples.

Jesus' Fasting in the Desert: The Ultimate Messianic Figure Has Come (Matt 4:1-4; Luke 4:1-4)

> Then Jesus, full of the Holy Spirit, returned from the Jordan River and was led by the Spirit in the wilderness, where for forty days he endured temptations from the devil. He ate nothing during those days, and when they were completed, he was famished. The devil said to him, "If you are the Son of God, command this stone to become bread." Jesus answered him, "It is written, 'Man does not live by bread alone.'"
>
> Luke 4:1-4

The only narrative explicitly describing Jesus as fasting confronts the reader in context between his baptism and the beginning of his public ministry. The following discussion will show that in this strategic location, fasting contributes to the christological theme of identifying Jesus in his messianic mission. This will be seen primarily in his identification as the eschatological prophet like Moses, but also in his identity as the new Adam who faces temptation victoriously through the power of the Spirit.

It must be noted that Mark does not mention fasting in his brief account. Mark 1:12-13 reads: "The Spirit immediately drove him into the wilderness. He was in the wilderness forty days, enduring temptations from Satan. He was with wild animals, and angels were ministering to his needs.". Both Matt 4:1-11 and Luke 4:1-13 offer significantly expanded accounts, mentioning Jesus fasting for forty days as a segue into his dialogue with the devil. While Mark and Luke imply testing during the entire period, Hagner rightly notes that "Matthew's aorist participle νηστεύσας (and ὕστερον, "afterwards") puts the testing explicitly after the forty days and nights."[17]

A good deal of the scholarly discussion of this account has to do with the nature of the historical background. The expanded accounts in Matthew and Luke include private information, utilizing an omniscient narrator perspective literarily. The second and third specific temptations appear to transcend the simply literal, as it is difficult to imagine the devil transporting Jesus bodily to a pinnacle of the temple, or to the top of a mountain where he could view all the kingdoms of the world.[18] But this does not necessarily mean that the account should be considered purely a composition of the author. The following comments of Geerhardus Vos put it well:

> Much confusion of thought is created here by a failure to distinguish between the objectivity and corporealness of such a transaction. The second involves the first, but this cannot be reversed: an encounter between persons, especially in the supersensual world, can be perfectly objective without necessarily entering into the sphere of the corporeally perceptible.[19]

So one does not need to deny the objective fact of the temptation of Jesus by the devil, even though the exact physical nature of the temptations may not be entirely apparent. Perhaps Jesus in the desert experienced a kind of apocalyptic vision of the devil and these temptations, which might find some analogy in the OT prophet Ezekiel. In Ezek 8:3 and 11:1, Ezekiel was transported in vision to Jerusalem, though there is no reason to suppose he traveled there bodily. Rather, he would seem in these and other visions to be bringing a spiritual reality that intersects with earth at some other location into his present one. Similarly, Jesus' temptations had to do with his messianic calling, which would be centered in Jerusalem and have global implications, so that it is entirely understandable that these would be the subjects of his temptations. Perhaps we can think of the temptations as having truly happened, while also moving into a different dimension—a spiritual, or apocalyptic realm.

The primary purpose of the longer version in Matthew and Luke seems to be theologically oriented toward the identification of Jesus with Moses and Israel in the wilderness. Not only does the fact of Jesus' fasting for forty days recall Moses on Mt. Sinai going without food and drink (Exod 34:28; Deut 9:9, 18, 10:10), but it also recalls Elijah, who also went without food for forty days on his journey to Mt. Sinai in his role as a prophet like Moses (1 Kgs 19:8). Additionally, the texts Jesus will cite in his rebuke of the devil all come from the context of Deuteronomy 6-8, in which the narrative of Israel in the wilderness is retold by Moses, with Moses' forty-day fasting explicitly mentioned in the context in Deut 9:9: "When I ascended the mountain to receive the stone tablets, the tablets of the covenant that the LORD made with you, I remained there forty days and nights, eating and drinking nothing". The story of Jesus' fasting, therefore, highlights Jesus' role as the new Moses, leading his people into the promised New Covenant.

Such a role is inherently messianic. All three synoptics place the wilderness temptation just after Jesus' baptism by John, each concluding the baptism event with the pronouncement from heaven that Jesus is God's beloved Son, in whom he is well pleased (Matt 3:17; Mark 1:11; Luke 3:22). This identification highlights Jesus' messianic role as Son of God, derived from imagery surrounding the Davidic dynasty (2 Sam 7:14; Ps 2:7). Vos comments that "the Spirit leading Him into the temptation was the Holy Spirit in His Messianic aspect. The close sequence between the accounts of the baptism and that of the temptation puts this beyond all doubt."[20]

Interestingly, Luke inserts the genealogy of Jesus immediately after the heavenly pronouncement and before the temptation account. Luke's genealogy ends with the phrases, "son of Adam, the son of God" (Luke 3:38). With this juxtaposition, Luke suggests a three-fold meaning for the identification of Jesus in the temptation narrative: He is the eschatological prophet like Moses, the messianic Son of God as son of David, as well as the Son of God as the son of Adam, the head of a new, redeemed humanity.[21] Matthew continues the theme of Jesus as the new Moses in the next chapter in the Sermon on the Mount, where Jesus authoritatively recalls the ancient laws written on stone, but now pushes them further, suggesting that he is the one who will write the law on the hearts of his people. This creates a "context of messianic and eschatological fulfillment," as D. A. Carson says.[22]

As Hendriksen points out, the temptation of Jesus by Satan is an attempt to cause Christ as the last Adam "to fail even as the first Adam had failed, in both cases in connection with food consumption."[23] However, Christ found himself at great disadvantage, humanly speaking, when compared to the situation of Adam and Even when confronted by the tempter. Adam and Eve were in paradise, enjoying the fullness of God's created provision, with the freedom to eat from every tree of the garden. In contrast, Christ was in the wilderness, experiencing his humanity in its weakest condition, eating nothing.[24] Jesus' successful resistance of the devil while in his weakest physical state reinforces the truth of his quotation, "Man does not live by bread alone." His true life is sustained by his Father, "on every word that proceeds out of the mouth of God" (Matt 4:4).

The literary connection of the themes relating Jesus to Moses and Israel, and the identification of Jesus as Son of God, are really quite overwhelming. In commenting on the devil's opening words to Jesus in questioning his identity as Son of God, Wimmer writes:

> This suggests those passages from the Old Testament which connect the ideas of desert, forty, temptation, Spirit, and Son of God. Those most applicable refer to Israel. If we substitute "Lord your God" for "Spirit," then *all* of these themes are present in Dt 8:2-5: "And you shall remember all the ways in which the *Lord your God* has *led* you these *forty* years in the *desert*, that he might humble you, *testing* you... . As a man disciplines his *son*, the Lord your God disciplines you." Ex 4:22f also contains the fundamental idea of Israel as son, going into the desert: "You shall say to Pharaoh, Thus says the Lord, Israel is my first-born *son*, and I say to you, let my *son* go that he may serve me." The themes of Spirit and desert with the Israelites are found also in Nm 11: 16-30; Is 63:8-14; and Neh 9:19-21. A consideration of the individual images leads to the same conclusion.[25]

So as Israel was tested in the desert, Jesus as the new Moses and representative of his people Israel was tempted in the desert; but unlike Israel, so frequently rebelling in the wilderness in the midst of testing, Jesus emerged victorious. As the new Adam, Christ endures temptations in the inverse of the ideal conditions of paradise, bringing humanity at its weakest into complete submission to the will of God, resisting the devil and showing that indeed humanity can be united to divinity. So fasting is used both as a means to prepare Jesus for his messianic ministry, and to identify him in that role. Jesus, through fasting, shows himself to be able to withstand the temptation to disobey God in satisfying his human appetites, unlike Adam and Eve, Israel in the desert, and by implication the rest of humanity. And that very act of fasting reminds his followers of the messianic promise of the raising up of the prophet like Moses, whose words would be heeded by the people of the covenant.

The Fasting Query: The Messiah Has Come, But an Age of Anticipation Will Go On (Matt 9:14-17; Mark 2:18-22; Luke 5:33-39)

> Then they said to him, "John's disciples frequently fast and pray, and so do the disciples of the Pharisees, but yours continue to eat and drink."
>
> So Jesus said to them, "You cannot make the wedding guests fast while the bridegroom is with them, can you? But those days are coming, and when the bridegroom is taken from them, at that time they will fast."
>
> He also told them a parable: "No one tears a patch from a new garment and sews it on an old garment. If he does, he will have torn the new, and the piece from the new will not match the old. And no one pours new wine into old wineskins. If he does, the new wine will burst the skins and will be spilled, and the skins will be destroyed. Instead new wine must be poured into new wineskins. And no one after drinking old wine wants the new, for he says, 'The old is good enough.'"
>
> Luke 5:33-39

Just what is the nature of this age?[26] How did the advent of Christ change history and how God's people should perceive their time? These eschatological questions are christocentrically located. The fasting dialogue quoted above tackles the issue of the nature of the age in a moment when Jesus and his disciples are portrayed on the hinge of history. The disciples of John and the Pharisees are part of the old order, and a new order has come—but days will come when elements of the past age are once again present.

How can this be so? After the advent of Christ do we not possess the realization of the ancient hopes? Christ's ascension and outpouring of his Spirit on the Day of Pentecost demonstrate his lordship over the age. But there are constant reminders that although the victory has been won, the battle is still being fought—both in the world, with its spiritual warfare for the souls of men, and in the flesh, with its ongoing struggle between residual sin and the indwelling Spirit. So this age must be understood in terms of the "already but not yet."

The following discussion will show that the teaching of this fasting question can play a key role in a balanced understanding of the nature of the age. Not only do we have explicit teaching that should guide our understanding of our time, but we have a tangible practice that links us to both ancient and contemporary communities of faith that wait for God's redemption. There is continuity with the past in that both fasting and feasting mark our experience. But since Christ has come, their significance has been reversed. Where once the faithful feasted in hope, we may feast in realization of hope fulfilled. Where once the community fasted in mourning, we may fast because of Christ's absence and in anticipation of the return of our beloved.

Here is the central contribution of this fasting question and answer: this age is appropriately one of fasting, even though the messiah has come. It could also be regarded as an age of feasting since he has come. The "already but not yet" character of the age calls for both expressions in the rhythm of our spiritual seasons, which can move from dry to satisfied, to dry to satisfied again. This will be demonstrated by examining this central passage in greater detail, reviewing the movement from Jewish to Christian fasting, and reflecting on the implications in our eschatology.

- Synoptic Issues: A Central Eschatological Episode

This pericope appears in all three synoptics (Luke 5:33-39; Mark 2:18-22; Matt 9:14-17), which suggests something about the theological centrality of its teaching. Bock (based on Fitzmyer and Marshall) mentions nine synoptic differences, listed here with a couple of expansions and an additional tenth point:

1. Luke includes or at least suggests that the Pharisees participated in the questioning. Matthew has the question on the lips of John's disciples, while Mark is more ambiguous, perhaps suggesting that it comes from the crowd.
2. Luke alone ties prayer to the fasting issue.
3. Like Matt. 9:15, Luke 5:34 relates a shortened form of the wedding image reply, phrased as a question. Mark has Jesus both asking and answering the question.
4. Luke alone calls the final verses parabolic.
5. Like Matthew, Luke has no allusion to the fasting practice of others before the event, in contrast to Mark 2:18.
6. Luke 5:35 speaks of *days* when fasting will occur, while Mark 2:20 speaks of a *day* of fasting, a remark that is clearly intended nonetheless to refer to a period of time, as the plural at the beginning of Mark 2:20 makes clear.
7. Luke 5:33 alone speaks of eating and drinking as the issue, a remark that alludes back to 5:30.
8. Luke 5:36b refers to "a patch cut out of a new garment," a variation of Mark 2:21 ("a piece of unshrunk cloth").
9. Luke 5:39 is a proverb unique to Luke's version.

10. Matthew 9:17 includes the phrase, "and both are preserved," which Mark omits, as apparently Luke does as well, although it shows up in textual variants in the Byzantine family.[27]

On the whole, the synoptic differences are relatively minor, but they do demonstrate the difficulty of strict historical/chronological harmonization. Additionally, the agreement of Luke and Matthew against Mark on a couple of points shows the difficulty of maintaining a simplistic two-source hypothesis. But the fact that all three keep the fasting query with the wineskin and garment metaphors suggests that the theological force of all three is the same: the old age is passing away, and it is time for a new age in the person of Christ. The metaphors are of such a nature that they look like they could stand alone, and perhaps in the teaching ministry of Christ they may have been together or separate at times. But in Scripture they stand together because of their similar eschatological teaching. In fact, there is a fascinating correlation of the concepts of eating, drinking, and the wearing of clothes in several NT contexts.[28]

- The Fasting Question and Its Answer: Fasting Ends with Christ, but Days for Fasting Will Return

The fasting query asserts that both John the Baptist and the Pharisees were characteristic of the old era. Fasting in Judaism was often associated with the destruction of the temple. As demonstrated in the previous chapter's discussion of Zechariah 7-8, the fasts of the fourth, fifth, seventh and tenth months mentioned in Zech 8:19 were all "linked to events connected with the destruction of Jerusalem by the Babylonians; keeping them was a reminder that Israel was still waiting for her real redemption from exile."[29] With Jesus a new "temple" was being erected. This new temple was his body, which metaphorically becomes the church in the epistles (Mark 14:58/Matt 26:61; John 2:19-22; 2 Cor 6:16; Eph 2:22, 4:15-16). The Jews also fasted ceremonially on the Day of Atonement, but in Christ atonement was being made. But the metaphor Jesus chooses is that of the bridegroom and his friends (literally, "the sons of the bridechamber"). The bridegroom's presence is a cause for rejoicing and feasting—it would be a sad wedding indeed if fasting was called for! But then that is just what Jesus announces: "when the bridegroom is taken away from them, then they will fast in those days" (Luke 5:35, NASB). The feast will be aborted, and fasting will take its place. Clearly Christ implies here that he will leave his disciples, and their fasting would be an expression of their sadness at his absence.

In fact, this metaphor of the bridegroom and his wedding feast is found throughout the NT in "already but not yet" contexts.[30] In Isa 25:6 the great eschatological day was pictured as lavish, joyous banquet with wine flowing in abundance, and it would seem that Jesus is picking up on this apocalyptic theme.[31] Luke 12:35-37 describes the need for disciples of Christ to await the return of the bridegroom from his wedding feast, and be ready when he comes knocking. Matthew 22:1-14 describes the master's wedding feast and the invitations that must be heeded to attend. Matthew 25:1-13 tells the story of the ten virgins awaiting the bridegroom's arrival at the feast. Ephesians 5:22-33 describes the church as the bride of Christ, already married but awaiting presentation to the bridegroom. Revelation 19:7-10 again links the bridegroom to feasting, and the bride's clothing is explicitly noted, as the New Jerusalem of Rev 21:2 is also described. The time of Christ's earthly ministry is a critical moment in history. The bridegroom is present, but the consummation is in the indefinite future. In the scope of God's plan it is already begun in the presence of Christ, but from our human perspective it may be distant.

But it certainly sounds very negative to say that the time of the bridegroom's absence will be a time that is marked by fasting. It is so negative that scholars have had a tendency to relegate this time of fasting to the period immediately following the crucifixion and prior to the resurrection. I. Howard Marshall argues for this,[32] citing 4 Esd 10:1-4 as a significant parallel, where a woman (representing Zion) fasted in mourning after her son died in his wedding-chamber. He also ties the thought to John 16:16-24, in which Jesus tells his disciples that they will mourn after he is taken away, but that they will rejoice when they see him again. But it is difficult to imagine the first century church receiving this story off the pens of the evangelists and recognizing in it a historical fulfillment only. In fact, the early church practiced fasting (Acts 13:2-3, 14:23), and these words from Jesus could easily have been seen as validation of the practice. There is at least evidence that some of the Church Fathers understood the passage to be encouraging fasting in this age.[33]

Marshall deals with the possibility by saying that the fasting of the early church was an accompaniment of prayer for guidance rather than an expression of mourning for Christ's absence. However, the need for guidance actually begs the fact of Christ's absence! In his presence, guidance is embodied, and there is a walk of sight, not just faith. When believers are in the presence of Christ, the faith becomes sight—so in this age of faith, Christ's absence, while vicariously filled by the Spirit, is still a true absence that creates longing in the heart. John Piper's penetrating devotional questions from his reflection on this passage illustrate a relevant application of this point:

Fasting poses the question: do we miss him? How hungry are we for him to come? The almost universal absence of regular fasting for the Lord's return is a witness to our satisfaction with the presence of the world and the absence of the Lord. This is not the way it should be.[34]

- ### The Garments and the Wineskins: The Better Nature of the New Age That Comes

In Luke 5:36-37 Jesus tells brief parables about garments and wineskins. Old garments are not patched with new cloth, and new wine is not put in old wineskins, because in either case, the old would be destroyed. Rather, "new wine must be put into fresh wineskins" (Luke 5:38, NASB). The comparison of the New Covenant age to the new garment and the new wineskins gives a much more positive impression of the new era. As Carson says, "they go beyond the question of fasting only to lay the groundwork for the coherence of Jesus' answer about fasting."[35]

Luke 5:39 is a fascinating commentary on the nature of the reception of the new age in Christ: "And no one, after drinking old wine wishes for new; for he says, 'The old is good enough'" (NASB). On an initial reading, one might think that this is making a positive statement about old wine, since fine wine is generally aged. But there is a danger in loving old wine too much. The new wine may be better, but because of satisfaction with the old, the pseudo-aficionado might not bother. "The old is good enough," he says.

With reflection on Jesus' use of irony here, one is forced to ask: "Is the old good enough?" Is it better than the new outpouring offered by Christ? After all, there is a mark of fasting in both eras. But indeed, the new is much better. The old is not bad, but it must be drunk in its own context (the old wineskins). The new wine of Christ's teaching and Spirit ministry will burst the categories of the old contexts of the law and the all too limited expectation of the messiah. The new righteousness of the garments of Christ cannot be a suitable patch for the old era; it must be a new garment all of its own. The new cloth will cause the old to tear—far better to rend one's own garments in repentance and accept the new era's new garment intact, without patching a piece of the new to the old, thereby destroying both.

- ### The Lord's Supper and This Eschatology: Fasting and Communing with Him

In light of the immediately preceding discussion of the theology of the fasting query (Luke 5:33-39 and parallels), the institution of the Lord's Supper or Eucharist can be seen as epitomizing this essentially christological eschatology. The Last Supper of Jesus' passion week of course took place during the Jewish feast of Passover. His words that night showed that he anticipated sharing with his disciples in the eschatological banquet of the kingdom of God (Luke 22:16-18; Matt 26:29; Mark 14:25). Further, he says that he will be abstaining from eating and drinking "until it is fulfilled in the kingdom of God" (Luke 22:16, 18, NASB). Perhaps at that moment in the Last Supper the disciples thought of the coming kingdom as imminent, since Jesus would not eat or drink until it came. Yet as time passed in the intervening years, the church had to come to terms with the nature of a new era, one that was better than, though perhaps unlike, that which the disciples had originally anticipated.

And yet the early church met together after Pentecost for the breaking of bread (Acts 2:42). They believed that the Lord Jesus was with them always, just as he had promised (Matt 28:20), and this was a promise until the end of the age—apparently not only the old covenant age that was passing away, but until his ultimate return as well. Paul described the Lord's Supper as a remembering and proclaiming of the Lord's death until he comes (1 Cor 11:23-26).

So when the church gathers and partakes of the Lord's Supper in remembrance, it also does so in anticipation. And, by faith and by his Holy Spirit, believers affirm that Jesus is there, communing with them, partaking of that Passover feast fulfilled in the kingdom of God. This is the realization of biblical eschatology, but cast in an age in which we still await its realization yet again. It looks back to promises fulfilled, and forward in hope to promises yet to be manifested. The eternal kingdom of God forever returns believers to their hope for paradise, for citizenship in the New Jerusalem, where access to eating the fruit of the primeval tree of life is continually open (Rev 22:2). Jenks summarizes the meaning of the images of eating as a communal, eschatological banquet:

> These scenes of eschatological dining complete the symbolic journeys whose trajectories began in Israel's most ancient scriptures. In the end time, in a perfect way never quite experienced in this world, food and drink represent fellowship with other men and women, communion with God through covenant and cult, and the gifts of God to Israel and to all mankind through history and through nature. In the time of God's final victory, the texts affirm, the life force itself will be eternally nourished as the plenty and joy of Eden are restored. The way to the Tree of Life, lost through a primal meal in the Garden, will no longer be barred to a hungering human race.[36]

Through Christ, these scenes have been fulfilled, and will yet be fulfilled. In one sense, Christ and his followers commune together in the bread and the cup, enjoying the fulfillment of his kingdom age. Yet in another sense, Christ and his believers continue their fast, awaiting a time when the Bridegroom is finally present with his friends once again.

- N. T. Wright's Very Realized Eschatology and His Use of the Fasting Query

N. T. Wright has offered an important theology of the realized eschatology of the NT.[37] His christological thesis is that Jesus came to announce the return of God's people from their spiritual exile, and to find the fulfillment of their hopes in him. So the fasting practices of Judaism find their feasting end in Jesus, the fulfillment of Israel's hopes. Wright notes that the feasts of Israel, while agrarian in nature, also looked back for Israel on the great acts of God in her history in the barley harvest of Passover, wheat harvest and the giving of the Torah at Pentecost, and grape harvest and the wilderness wanderings in the feast of tabernacles. Jesus presented himself as the embodiment of all of these feasts—he is the lamb that was slain (answering to Passover), the completion of the law (answering to Pentecost), and the new Moses who leads his people (answering to the feast of tabernacles).[38]

Wright's use of this fasting pericope provides some telling insights into his commitment to a very realized eschatology in the NT. Commenting on the fasting query (Mark 2:19-21/Matt 9:15-16/Luke 5:34-36) Wright notes well the thrust of the incident:

> Fasting in this period was not, for Jews, simply an ascetic discipline, part of the general practice of piety. It had to do with Israel's present condition: she was still in exile. More specifically, it had to do with commemorating the destruction of the Temple. Zechariah's promise that the fasts would turn into feasts could come true only when YHWH restored the fortunes of his people. That, of course, was precisely what Jesus' cryptic comments implied.
>
> ... In other words, the party is in full swing, and nobody wants glum faces at a wedding. This is not a piece of 'teaching' about 'religion' or 'morality'; nor is it the dissemination of a timeless truth. It is a claim about eschatology. The time is fulfilled; the exile is over; the bridegroom is at hand.[39]

There is reason for full agreement so far. But this is the end of Wright's discussion of the passage. Why does he not discuss the rather glaring part about the bridegroom being taken away, which will once again usher in a time of fasting? Does he think this is a later interpolation, as Joseph Wimmer concludes?[40] As Keith Main suggests, that would be an unlikely supposition, because the community would be advocating a practice their Lord had apparently thrust off.[41] But Wright chooses not to even address this issue, and the reason may be that it would complicate his thesis. The drumbeat of realized eschatology so prevalent in Wright's work is interrupted by this little text on fasting. In the words of Jesus that Wright fails to mention, "But the days will come; and when the bridegroom is taken away from them, then they will fast in those days" (Luke 5:35, NASB). Another period of waiting, after the earthly life of Christ is over, is introduced. This is a period that will again be marked by fasting.

Wright could easily enough incorporate this into his eschatology, but it would call for a finer nuancing of his thesis.[42] Although he opts for a preterist reading of the majority of eschatological passages in the NT, he does leave room for a shifting of focus and a redrawing of the fulfillment of them for later Christianity. In his discussion of the Christian hope and its movement past the destruction of the temple, he discusses the fact that Christians have always been waiting for Christ's second appearing.[43] Yes, Christ does fulfill Jewish hope—but the NT church is also called to live in hope for an even fuller realization of our Christology and eschatology. It is best to conclude that this teaching actually goes right back to Jesus himself, as evidenced by this fasting text, in which case there is a more complex and earlier version of the "already but not yet" eschatology than Wright seems to allow.

A Fasting Instruction in the Sermon on the Mount: The Messiah Teaches True Humility (Matt 6:16-18)

> And whenever you fast, do not put on a gloomy face as the hypocrites do, for they neglect their appearance in order to be seen fasting by men. Truly I say to you, they have their reward in full. But you, when you fast, anoint your head, and wash your face so that you may not be seen fasting by men, but by your Father who is in secret; and your Father who sees in secret will repay you.
>
> Matthew 6:16-18 (NASB)

This saying of Jesus in the Sermon on the Mount is probably the passage that most readily comes to mind when Christians think of fasting. As already noted, the Sermon on the Mount follows contextually in Matthew relatively near to the account of Jesus fasting in the wilderness, and the theological connection between the two strongly suggests the identification of Jesus as the new Moses. As the messianic Moses, Jesus transcends the older Mosaic categories here as he gives his "Messianic Torah." W. D. Davies has summarized this aspect of the Sermon's identification of Jesus:

> The case would seem to be that, while the category of a New Moses and a New Sinai is present in v-vii, as elsewhere in Matthew, the strictly Mosaic traits in the figure of the Matthaean Christ, both there and in other parts of the Gospel, have been taken up into a deeper and higher context. He is not Moses come as Messiah, if we may so put it, so much as Messiah, Son of Man, Emmanuel, who has absorbed the Mosaic function. The Sermon on the Mount is therefore ambiguous: suggestive of the Law of a New Moses, it is also the authoritative word of the Lord, the Messiah: it is the Messianic Torah.[44]

This fasting instruction falls in the literary unit of Matt 6:1-18, in which almsgiving, prayer and fasting are treated in parallel sections (although considerably more space is given over to prayer, with the inclusion of the Lord's prayer occupying the prominent position). In this context, Jesus treats fasting on par with almsgiving and prayer as an "act of righteousness,"[45] and following Jesus' lead, later Christian tradition will frequently link these three elements together.[46] Betz classifies the genre of the section as a "cultic *didache*," referring to its reforming approach to religious behavior, the phrase of Matt 7:28 which calls the Sermon a *didache* (διδαχή, or "teaching"), and the similarities in structure with sections of the early Christian document of that name.[47] Carson suggests that these three "acts of righteousness" are chosen to represent all other similar acts, and that the section as a whole is a denunciation of religious hypocrisy in general, and ostentatious piety in particular.[48]

Jesus does not attack the institution of fasting in Matt 6:16-18. Instead, he warns against hypocritical or ostentatious fasting, which includes putting on a gloomy face and neglecting personal appearance in order to appear to be fasting. It has already been noted in the previous chapter that in Jewish practice, outward rituals such as abstaining from anointing, sexual activity and even the wearing of sandals, as well as the putting on of sackcloth and smearing the body or face with ashes, often accompanied fasting.[49] Betz suggests that this characterization of the gloomy-faced worshipper "points to a stock figure in Greco-Roman literature, in particular in texts having to do with the critique of religion and philosophy."[50] Such practices led the Romans to view the God of the

Jews as a sad god.[51] Betz also calls attention to a parallel from Greek literature in Pseudo-Plato's *Alcibiades Minor* in the dialogue "On Prayer:"

> In this text Alcibiades is on the way to offer a prayer to the gods when Socrates stops him because of the sullen look on his face. The dialogue on the whole has its purpose in changing Alcibiades' sullen look into cheerfulness, so that at the end he is ready to crown Socrates with a wreath. Alcibiades' gloomy look is, as we learn, the result of his wrong ideas about prayer and what to expect from it.[52]

Such parallels in the broader literature could suggest that the hypocrisy evident in certain ostentatious displays of Judaism was already under the critique of the pagans. There seems to be something of a hierarchy of practical righteousness being set up here, with the lowest rung being hypocrisy, which the best of pagans rise above, to the highest level of true, heart worship of the all-seeing God, that is demanded of Jesus' disciples.

Jesus assumes that his disciples will fast, and instructs them that whenever they fast[53] they should anoint their heads, wash their faces, and fast in order to be seen by God in secret. This passage then contrasts proper and improper motives and methods for fasting—fast sincerely for God alone, and not publicly for the purpose of being seen by others. Jesus urged his disciples to fast in a manner that was different from the hypocrites. As will be discussed in the following chapter, this is echoed in the *Didache* 8.1, but unfortunately it sees the difference in terms of which days of the week fasting should be done: "But do not let your fasts coincide with those of the hypocrites. They fast on Monday and Thursday, so you must fast on Wednesday and Friday."[54] This hardly seems consistent with the Lord's warnings, which have to do with appearing before others as fasting instead of before God, the true audience of our righteous behaviors.

When the disciples do fast to be seen by God, Jesus promises that they will be rewarded. As Carson notes, "Jesus does not discuss the locale and nature of the reward; but we will not be far from the NT evidence if we understand it to be 'both in time and in eternity, both in character and in felicity.'"[55] Here, then, is a clear teaching that Jesus' disciples can expect spiritual blessings if they fast in a manner that God views as righteous.

In summary then, the theological ethic of fasting in the Sermon on the Mount requires and assumes the theological perspective of the two fasting accounts previously examined in this chapter.[56] In the Sermon on the Mount, the messianic Moses is giving his new law, written on the hearts of his followers. He assumes that they will be acting out their righteousness in a period of time in which fasting is appropriate, because of the nature of the age. But this is a superior kind of righteousness, based not on one's own actions but proceeding from and reflecting a faith in and right standing before the unseen God. Jesus promises that such acts of righteousness will be rewarded, and therefore fasting based on confidence in the unseen God's reward reflects faith in and obedience to the Messiah in the inaugurated but unfinished messianic age.

A Pharisee's Fasting in a Parable: God Justifies the Repentant and Humble, but Rejects the Hypocrite (Luke 18:9-14)

> And He also told this parable to certain ones who trusted in themselves that they were righteous, and viewed others with contempt: "Two men went up into the temple to pray, one a Pharisee, and the other a tax-gatherer. The Pharisee stood and was praying thus to himself, 'God, I thank Thee that I am not like other people: swindlers, unjust, adulterers, or even like this tax-gatherer. I fast twice a week; I pay tithes of all that I get.' But the tax-gatherer, standing some distance away, was even unwilling to lift up his eyes to heaven, but was beating his breast, saying, 'God, be merciful to me, the sinner!' I tell you, this man went down to his house justified rather than the other; for everyone who exalts himself shall be humbled, but he who humbles himself shall be exalted."
>
> Luke 18:9-14 (NASB)

Jesus frequently found himself in conflict with the Pharisees, and no doubt this parable did little to ease the tension with this group. Luke 18:1-8 begins with a parable on prayer, the parable about a widow who wore out a judge with her constant petitioning. Jesus uses her as an example of continual prayer. Then Luke 18:9-14 contains the second parable of the chapter, this parable about the Pharisee and a tax-gatherer, which also is about prayer; but it goes further, to the issue of heart righteousness.

C. F. Evans suggested that the central section of Luke's gospel (Luke 9:51-18:14) intentionally corresponds to Deuteronomy 1-26.[57] Craig A. Evans has sought to demonstrate the relationship of this pericope, the last in Luke's central section, with Deuteronomy 26, which describes the requirements of tithes and obedience for the feast of the firstfruits in Judaism.[58] Craig Evans explores four areas of parallelism: verbal coherence, thematic coherence, exegetical coherence in Jewish sources, and the parable's meaning in the context of Luke's central section. Verbally, there are parallels with the concept of tithing all (Luke 18:12;

Deut 26:12), humbling and exaltation (Luke 18: 14; Deut 26:6-8), righteousness (Luke 18:9, 14; Deut 26:16-17), and looking to or from heaven (Luke 18:13; Deut 26:15). Josephus paraphrases Deuteronomy 26 to include words that correspond even more strongly, adding phrases about standing before God, giving thanks to God, and God being merciful.[59] Thematically, the Pharisee is one who would consider himself to be a keeper of the Sinai covenant, whereas the tax-gatherer has been disobedient and cannot consider himself righteous by means of the covenant. The parallel between the prayer of the Pharisee here and the farmer's speech at the feast of firstfruits (Deut 26:13-14) is very interesting:

> When you have finished paying all the tithe of your increase in the third year, the year of tithing, then you shall give it to the Levite, to the stranger, to the orphan and to the widow, that they may eat in your towns, and be satisfied. And you shall say before the LORD your God, 'I have removed the sacred portion from my house, and also have given it to the Levite and the alien, the orphan and the widow, according to all Thy commandments which Thou hast commanded me; I have not transgressed or forgotten any of Thy commandments. 'I have not eaten of it while mourning, nor have I removed any of it while I was unclean, nor offered any of it to the dead. I have listened to the voice of the LORD my God; I have done according to all that Thou hast commanded me.' (NASB)

Exegetically, the reference in Deuteronomy 26 to the place where Israel would worship is now the temple in Luke, and numerous Jewish sources exclude tax-gatherers from the covenant, associating them with robbers and thieves. Contextually, Evans believes that the story forms a fitting conclusion to Luke's central section, as each part deals with election in some way:

> The parable of the Pharisee and the publican brings the Central Section to a fitting end by summing up what is for Luke the essence of the gospel message, as it pertains to the question of election: anyone, no matter how far estranged from the covenant of Moses, can repent and be brought back to God. If there is genuine repentance, genuine faith, acts of charity and expressions of thanksgiving, then restoration is possible. This can happen, Luke believes, through the message of the 'prophet like Moses' (Deut 18:15-19; cf. Acts 3:22-23; 7:37). Just as obedience to Moses' teaching would assure possession of the promised land and prosperity within it, so obedience to Jesus'

teaching will assure entry into the kingdom of God and great reward.[60]

While Evans admits that the results of his study are suggestive and not conclusive, the parallelism is indeed striking. When one considers the general theology of fasting flowing from the messianic Christ as fulfillment of the covenant and the one who ushers in the eschatological age, the hypothesis linking Deuteronomy 26 with Luke 18:9-14 appears entirely reasonable.[61] Fredrick Holmgren offers a nice summary of the possible use of the two texts:

> Deuteronomy 26:1-15 could well be read as a companion text to the parable of the Pharisee and the Tax Collector when the latter is the focus of the sermon. The Deuteronomic text provides a needed critique to the prideful attitude that has ensnared the Pharisee, but it also serves as a rebuke to the self-deprecatory stance that often tempts tax collector types. The *Pharisee* is to remember, first of all, that *he is the recipient of the full grace of God* (Deut. 26:5-11), who has accepted him as a covenant partner.[62] The *tax collector*, on the other hand, should listen attentively to Deuteronomy 26:12-15, in which the farmer is *charged to witness to what he has done and not done*.[63]

Luke introduces the unit by saying that Jesus told the parable "to certain ones who trusted in themselves that they were righteous, and viewed others with contempt" (v. 9, NASB). With this theme of righteousness, already one can see the theological parallel with Jesus' discussion of fasting in the Sermon on the Mount in Matthew 6. Although each of these accounts is unique to its respective writer, it is interesting that both use essentially the same theological base for dealing with fasting in the context of righteousness. The Pharisee in this parable considers himself to be righteous, and fasting is listed alongside of tithing as a positive example of his acts of righteousness, contrasted with the negative examples he lists in Luke 18:11 and assumes for the tax-gatherer next to him.[64] But Jesus declares that the tax-gatherer, who humbly begged for God's mercy and declared himself to be a sinner, actually went away justified rather than the Pharisee.[65] The unit ends with the proverbial expression, "for every one who exalts himself shall be humbled, but he who humbles himself shall be exalted" (18:14, NASB). So in this passage fasting is linked to an act of righteousness, but in this instance it is done by one who is a negative example, like the hypocrites Jesus described in Matthew 6. Instead, the truly humble one is the tax-gatherer who confesses his sinfulness and goes away justified. His attitude was actually more consistent with the proper purposes of fasting and repentance in the tradition of the OT prophets. He has genuinely humbled himself with all his heart, as Joel 2:12-13 called for, and he found the gracious and merciful God he was seeking.

As for the reference to fasting, the Pharisee says he fasts twice per week. This would apparently have been a voluntary act, as Jews were traditionally required to fast universally only on the Day of Atonement. As previously discussed, some religiously oriented individuals might have fasted in various mourning ceremonies over the fall of Jerusalem or for the need for rain. Beyond even that, some pious individuals apparently developed those traditional occasions for fasting into a disciplined, regular routine.[66] The Pharasaic tradition of twice a week fasting mentioned here was done on Monday and Thursday, and may have meant taking only bread and water during daylight hours. In Jewish society, Mondays and Thursdays were market days and court days, when public assemblies and Torah readings were common.[67] The tradition was apparently grounded in the days Moses ascended and descended from Mount Sinai. This traditional reason is preserved in *Midrash Tanhuma*:

> Let our master instruct us: When a court has ordained a fast for the community so that rains may come down, and they do come down on that day, is it correct for them to finish it? Thus have our masters taught (in *Ta'an.* 25b [bar.]): IF THEY WERE FASTING, AND THE RAINS CAME DOWN BEFORE THE RISING OF THE SUN, THEY SHALL NOT FINISH IT. AFTER THE RISING OF THE SUN THEY SHALL FINISH IT. <THESE ARE> THE WORDS OF R. ME'IR, BUT R. JUDAH SAYS: BEFORE NOON THEY DO NOT COMPLETE IT; AFTER NOON THEY COMPLETE IT. And where did the generations (i.e., the sages) find support that they should fast on Monday and Thursday? <It is> simply <that>, when Israel committed that act (i.e., of the golden calf), Moses went up <onto the mountain> on a Thursday and came down on a Monday. How is it shown? R. Levi said: He went up on a Thursday. Now from Thursday through <the following> Thursday to the Thursday <after that> there are fifteen <days>. And from Sabbath eve through <the following> Sabbath eve to the Sabbath eve <after that> there are fifteen <days>, for a total of thirty. Also from Sabbath to Sabbath there are eight <days>, for a total of thirty-eight. Then a Sunday and a Monday make forty <days>. Therefore, the sages have ruled that one should fast on Monday and on Thursday, on <the day of> Moses' ascent and on <that of> his

descent. Now at the end of forty days they fasted and wept before Moses, so that the Holy One was filled with mercy for them and appointed that day for them as a day of atoning for their sins. And this was the Day of Atonement, as stated (in Lev. 16:30): FOR ON THIS DAY ATONEMENT SHALL BE MADE FOR YOU TO CLEANSE YOU. See how lovely repentance (rt.: *ShVB*) is![68]

In this important passage, the connection can be seen between the fasting of Moses for forty days on Sinai, the Day of Atonement fasting practice, the tradition of fasting for rain as outlined in Mishnah tractate *Ta'anit*, and the Pharasaic practice of fasting mentioned in Jesus' parable. While the connection may at first seem less than obvious, fasting forms the key thread, and the final exclamation cited above shows that the theological link for the rabbis was *repentance*. Fascinatingly, in Luke 18 the Pharisee is carrying out deeds designed to show repentance with an unrepentant heart, while the tax-gatherer exemplifies repentance.

In summary, then, the Pharisee of Luke 18 provides a negative illustration of the kind of fasting Jesus warned against in Matthew 6. While the tax-gatherer of Luke 18 is not described specifically as fasting, he does indeed provide a positive illustration of the repentant heart attitude that is acceptable righteousness before God. Clearly, then, when Jesus' disciples fast, they must fast with hearts that are truly repentant. They should not assume that fasting itself will somehow garner merit with God, but rather they must take the part of the sinner and trust a gracious, merciful God to justify and bless them.

The Fasting of Anna the Prophetess: The Promised Redemption Has Come (Luke 2:36-38)

And there was a prophetess, Anna the daughter of Phanuel, of the tribe of Asher. She was advanced in years, having lived with a husband seven years after her marriage, and then as a widow to the age of eighty-four. And she never left the temple, serving night and day with fastings and prayers. And at that very moment she came up and *began* giving thanks to God, and continued to speak of Him to all those who were looking for the redemption of Jerusalem.

Luke 2:36-38 (NASB)

This incidental reference to fasting occurs in an explicitly eschatological context.[69] She is literally coupled with a male counterpart, Simeon, whose similar but longer account is written in the immediately preceding context of Luke 2:25-35. Both Simeon and Anna were vessels of prophetic, revelatory gifts. Specifically, Simeon had earlier received a divine promise that he would not see death before he would see the Messiah (2:26). Anna spoke of seeing the Messiah to "all those who were looking for the redemption of Jerusalem" (2:38), implying that there were a sizeable number of people with eschatological, messianic hopes at that time. The account of the Christ-child appearing in the temple to these two saints of the old covenant clearly speaks of Jesus' messianic identity and the fulfillment of the covenantal promises of restoration for Israel.

Anna's name also recalls her OT namesake of Hannah (1 Samuel 1), who fasted and prayed in the temple (or tabernacle) before Eli the priest so that she might have a son. In that story, a barren woman was given the gift of a child as the answer to her prayers. In this story, an old widow saw the Christ-child as the answer to her prayers. Bart J. Koet has pointed out the similarities between Luke 2:22-39 and another document whose origins probably go back to first century Judaism, Pseudo-Philo's *Liber Antiquitatum Biblicarum* (LAB).[70] LAB 49-51 is a retelling of the story of Samuel's birth narrative, and chapter 51 paraphrases 1 Sam 1:20-2:11, Hannah's dedication of Samuel and her song of thanksgiving. There are several commonalities between Luke 2:22-39 and LAB 50-51, including the use of the phrase "light of the Gentiles/nations," the sanctuary, prominent women both named H/Anna/h, and the prophetic utterances of songs in praise of young boys of promise.[71] Koet's thesis is that "the author of Luke-Acts uses themes of the Hanna-traditions such as those in LAB as a background to Luke 2:22-39."[72] This idea appears sustainable and coincides well with the nuance of Luke's use of OT characters offered by Raymond Brown. Brown points out that Mary's "Magnificat" of Luke 1:46-55 also bears striking resemblance to Hannah's song from 1 Samuel 2. These similarities associate the NT characters with OT ones, while allowing room for differences in development that can accommodate both the historical situation and the new covenant theology. Brown makes this insightful comment: "Luke's method is not one of identifying figures in the infancy narrative with OT characters; rather he uses pigments taken from OT narratives to color in the infancy narrative."[73]

Even Anna's lineage from the tribe of Asher, which may appear incidental, in fact highlights new covenant expectation.[74] Jeremiah 31:31 stated that a new covenant would be made with both the house of Judah and the house of Israel, meaning the northern tribes. Although the northern tribes had been largely assimilated into the surrounding nations following their Assyrian captivity, some maintained their Jewish identity. Anna's tribe of Asher would have been one of those northern tribes. She is linked contextually with Simeon, whose lineage is not mentioned, but whose name at least literarily recalls another tribe. This also follows the story of John the Baptist's birth, which highlights the priestly tribe of Levi, and Jesus' own lineage from Judah.

Max Wilcox has suggested that Anna is linked to another character from Jewish tradition, Serah daughter of Asher, whose name is mentioned as going down into Egypt with Jacob in Gen 46:17, and in the family rolls of Num 26:46 (from which later Jewish works inferred that she survived until the Exodus).[75] She appears in later Jewish works as a heroine on a couple of occasions. Parallels can be seen between the reference to Asher, the great age of the characters, their exceptional piety, as well as the redemptive expectations of their respective traditions. In a Jewish midrashic work, *Pirqe de Rabbi Eliezer* 48:82-84, Serah identifies Moses as the liberator of Israel in a similar way to how Anna identifies Jesus.[76] She also is said to have brought Jacob the news that Joseph was still alive, which resulted in angels carrying her to paradise (literally, the Garden of Eden) while still alive (*Tg. Ps.-J.* Gen 46:17, Num 26:46). She is regarded as a woman of great wisdom in some other references (*Qoh.R.* 9; *Yalkut Sam* 152; *Gen.R.* 94, 8-9), and possibly as a prophetess (*b. Meg.* 14a).[77] These writings are later than the gospel of Luke and no literary dependence can be affirmed. But perhaps Wilcox is right that some of the Jewish community of the first century would have been aware of the Serah daughter of Asher motif. Whether or not this is so, it does at least show that there were similar characters in Jewish culture that transmitted redemptive eschatological motifs through their portrayal in their stories.

What is really carried on this OT pigmentation, then, is the theology of expectation and fulfillment. The fasting of Anna may play a role in highlighting this eschatological anticipation. In her fasting she shows herself to be part of a righteous remnant anticipating the messianic New Covenant. As an exemplary character, she fasts in humility, righteousness of heart, and in identification with her people's mourning and need for repentance.[78] This godly woman epitomizes the theme of righteous fasting in anticipation of restoration in the messianic age. And she is rewarded with seeing the Christ child, in whom the promised redemption had come.

Feeding a Crowd that Had Nothing to Eat: The Source and Sustainer of Life Has Come (Matt 15:32; Mark 8:2-3)

> And Jesus called His disciples to Him, and said, "I feel compassion for the multitude, because they have remained with Me now three days and have nothing to eat; and I do not wish to send them away hungry, lest they faint on the way."

Matthew 15:32 (NASB)

This passage (and the parallel in Mark 8:2-3), in the story of the feeding of the four thousand, is of relatively minor relevance to this study, though it does use the term νῆστεις to describe the crowd. This seems to be a general description of the condition they were in after three days of being with Jesus in a deserted area. They were lacking food (perhaps they had actually brought some along, but had run out). It does not appear to be an intentional, religiously oriented fast, but Jesus does take the occasion to feed them miraculously, which points to the presence of the eschatological Messiah. He was able to satisfy the hungry crowd, which is a picture of his new covenant ministry.

Fasting in Acts and the Epistles: The New Era Moves Forward

The following section deals with references to fasting in the NT outside of the synoptic gospels, and these are found in Acts and 2 Corinthians. There are several contexts that include fasting in the book of Acts. The first explicit reference is related to Saul's conversion, and may function theologically to illustrate the move from the old to new covenant in an individual Israelite. Two corporate prayer and fasting references would seem to answer positively the question of whether fasting is to be viewed as an ongoing practice in the Christian era. They occur after the outpouring of the Spirit at Pentecost, which marked the ushering in of the new covenant. Some passing references of relatively minor significance also occur, which will receive only a brief mention. Then in two passages in 2 Corinthians, Paul lists fasting with his hardships he suffered for the sake of the gospel, suggesting that in this age believers might willingly subject themselves to disciplined behaviors, and even disruption of normal lifestyles, for the sake of ministry. While none of these passages alone contributes a great deal to a theology of fasting individually, taken together, they will show that fasting did indeed play a role in the earliest Christian community, as the new era of messianic fulfillment and anticipation took shape.

Saul Fasts Three Days Waiting for Sight and the Holy Spirit: A Blinded Israelite Enters the New Covenant (Acts 9:9)

And he was three days without sight, and neither ate nor drank.

Acts 9:9 (NASB)

The story of Saul's conversion includes this account of him fasting. Although Bruce says this was "probably from shock," Saul's meeting with Christ was a religious experience of the first order, and his abstinence from food should not be seen as merely incidental.[79] When he encountered the risen Jesus on the road to Damascus, the accompanying flash of light blinded Saul, and although his eyes were open he could not see (9:3, 8, 22:11). His companions heard the voice but saw no one (9:7), and Acts 22:9 adds that they also saw the light though they did not understand the voice. Saul remained in this condition for three days, during which time he did not eat or drink (9:9). Then Ananias came and laid hands on him, commanding him to be filled with the Holy Spirit, and something like scales fell from his eyes so that he could regain his sight (9:18). After this, Saul was baptized and he took food (9:18-19).

In this fascinating story Saul may be viewed theologically as representing a prototypical conversion of an Israelite. Before his conversion, he thought he was the greatest keeper of the law, like the Pharisee in Jesus' parable in Luke 18:9-14.[80] In this state, he thought he could "see," but he was blinded to the spiritual reality of Jesus as messiah. When he met the risen Christ, the light shone on him, which ironically blinded him. His true spiritual state was exposed, one of inability to "see" the truth right before his eyes. When he received the Holy Spirit with the laying on of hands by Ananias, the scales fell off his eyes, and he could truly see. The Holy Spirit in the new covenant enabled him to see what his previously blinded eyes missed, though the truth was right in front of him. Acts 26:18 provides an expanded statement of Paul's mission, in which Jesus tells him that he will be sent to the Gentiles "to open their eyes so that they may turn from darkness to light and from the dominion of Satan to God, in order that they may receive forgiveness of sins and an inheritance among those who have been sanctified by faith in Me" (NASB). Perhaps this vivid personal experience informs Paul's use of OT blindness imagery as applied to Israel in passages like Rom 11:8, "Eyes to see not and ears to hear not."

Perhaps Saul's fasting in recorded in Acts 9:9 contributes to this theme in his conversion experience. He identifies with Israel as a self-righteous covenant keeper who blindly persecuted Christ. Now in his fasting, he has the appearance of a man truly humbled, even stupefied, by his new awareness of messianic realities. The fast ends with his receiving of the Holy Spirit and the ritual of baptism, as he fully enters into the blessings and ministry of the new covenant.

Fasting and Prayer in the New Community:
The Church Seeks and Finds Guidance and Leadership
(Acts 13:1-3, 14:23)

> Now there were at Antioch, in the church that was there, prophets and teachers: Barnabas, and Simeon who was called Niger, and Lucius of Cyrene, and Manaen who had been brought up with Herod the tetrarch, and Saul. And while they were ministering to the Lord and fasting, the Holy Spirit said, "Set apart for Me Barnabas and Saul for the work to which I have called them." Then, when they had fasted and prayed and laid their hands on them, they sent them away.
>
> Acts 13:1-3 (NASB)

> And when they [Paul and Barnabas] had appointed elders for them in every church, having prayed with fasting, they commended them to the Lord in whom they had believed.
>
> Acts 14:23 (NASB)

These two passages suggest that fasting was indeed part of the practice of the earliest Christian communities. In these verses it is clear that it was done as an accompaniment of corporate prayer. Both contexts have to do with the choice of leaders for the new community. While some commentators think it is important to note that these are not formal ordination services, Fitzmyer is right that such a distinction is basically "meaningless. It is not a question of a transfer of power, but of a Spirit-guided commission."[81] The first incident commissions Barnabas and Saul for their first missionary journey, and the second passage refers to the selection of local church leaders in the new communities that formed as a result of that missionary journey. As Johnson says, the prayer and fasting in the second incident "makes the ordination echo the appointment of Paul and Barnabas themselves as they began the mission."[82]

These passages illustrate a proper kind of application of the eschatological pronouncement of Jesus in the synoptic fasting query (Matt 9:14-15; Mark 2:18-20; Luke 5:33-35). The new covenant indeed had come—and yet this proved to be a time for fasting. But what these passages show is that such fasting is not necessarily like old covenant fasting, such as in mourning over exile. Rather, in the absence of the Messiah, these disciples prayed and fasted, with the result that the Holy Spirit of that very same Messiah ministered among them, and their Lord's presence was felt and his will was made known. It is a present era application of the reality of living between the realized and unrealized eschaton. The fasting of the earliest Christians bears witness to their inward, spiritual hunger, their longing for Jesus to be among them. They were rewarded with guidance from the Spirit of Christ as a token of his actual presence. So in this age, the Christian community expects the Spirit to minister in the absence of the Messiah himself, and fasting can demonstrate our desire for that presence in our lives.[83]

A Wicked Fast as an Oath
(Acts 23:12-14)

> And when it was day, the Jews formed a conspiracy and bound themselves under an oath, saying that they would neither eat nor drink until they had killed Paul. And there were more than forty who formed this plot. And they came to the chief priests and the elders, and said, "We have bound ourselves under a solemn oath to taste nothing until we have killed Paul."
>
> Acts 23:12-14 (NASB)

This plot by the forty Jews to kill Paul involved a total fast, apparently as a sign of their seriousness. This wicked, hypocritical use of fasting, normally a religious act of piety, may recall the OT king Saul's foolish oath imposed on his army (1 Sam 14:24-46), or Queen Jezebel's hypocritical fasting assembly to condemn innocent Naboth (1 Kgs 21:9-12). While hardly advancing the theology of fasting in any positive direction, it does show that religious actions that can be used for good may also be appropriated by evil, which only heightens the hypocrisy. As Fitzmyer says, "one may wonder about the binding character of such an oath."[84] Since the plot failed, one can only surmise that these conspirators proved themselves to be oath breakers as well, as it seems unlikely that they really kept their oath not to eat or drink until Paul was killed. Witherington notes that "Jewish law, however, specified that if one was unable to fulfill an oath due to circumstances beyond one's control, one could be let off the hook."[85] Such a use of the law, however, only further contrasts these men with Jesus' words in the Sermon on the Mount (Matt 5:20), "unless your righteousness surpasses that of the scribes and Pharisees, you shall not enter the kingdom of heaven."

A Passing Reference to the Day of Atonement
(Acts 27:9)

> ... the voyage was now dangerous, since even the fast was already over.
>
> Acts 27:9 (NASB)

This reference to "the fast" serves basically as a calendar notation.[86] The point of the passage is that in October the winter storms were making a sea voyage dangerous. The text contributes little to the theology of fasting, and serves only as a witness to the universal understanding of the Day of Atonement as a fast. The term had become basically synonymous for the Jewish holiday.

A Ship's Crew Eats Nothing for Fourteen Days (Acts 27:33)

> And until the day was about to dawn, Paul was encouraging them all to take some food, saying, "Today is the fourteenth day that you have been constantly watching and going without eating, having taken nothing."
>
> Acts 27:33 (NASB)

It is highly unlikely that this was an intentional or religious fast. Rather, because the storm caused extreme conditions on the ship, the crew likely could not find a good time to eat, and with the likelihood of seasickness, may not have wanted to do so. The Greek word used is ἄσιτοι, which tends to be more descriptive of the physical condition of hunger. Witherington says, "This may perhaps mean that there had been no formally prepared meals during the storm," and "Paul is probably speaking somewhat hyperbolically here to get his point across."[87]

Paul's Fasts Evidence the Hardship He Endured for the Gospel (2 Cor 6:4-7, 11:27)

> But in everything commending ourselves as servants of God, in much endurance, in afflictions, in hardships, in distresses, in beatings, in imprisonments, in tumults, in labors, in sleeplessness, in hunger, in purity, in knowledge, in patience, in kindness, in the Holy Spirit, in genuine love, in the word of truth, in the power of God; by the weapons of righteousness for the right hand and the left, ...
>
> 2 Cor 6:4-7 (NASB)

> I have been in labor and hardship, through many sleepless nights, in hunger and thirst, often without food, in cold and exposure.
>
> 2 Cor 11:27 (NASB)

The NASB used "hunger" to translate νηστείαις in 2 Cor 6:5, but this could be a reference to intentional fasting by the apostle Paul.[88] Several reasons have been proposed for Paul's mention of "fastings" here. If the word is more closely associated with the preceding terms, it might appear to be an affliction imposed from without, suggesting that circumstances forced him to go hungry. However, if it is read in connection with the context of the following terms in 2 Cor 6:6-7, it could be understood as a cultivation of virtue. Additionally, "sleeplessness" (here the plural of ἀγρυπνία) could refer to lack of sleep due to circumstances, or the kind of intentional vigil that would forego sleep for ministerial purposes. Since it is coupled with the "labors" (plural of κόπος) in the context, some have suggested that Paul performed secular work in order to support himself while in the ministry so as not to burden the churches, and as a result he may have had to work through the night, forego eating, or perhaps not even be able to afford food.[89] If this is the case, it would appear that this kind of fasting is of a sort of intentional but unintentional nature, not specifically religious but a willing suffering of hardship for the sake of the ministry.

Similarly, 2 Cor 11:27 is a bit ambiguous, where the reference to being "often without food" in the NASB translates ἐν νηστείαις πολλάκις. This follows an explicit reference to being in hunger and thirst (ἐν λιμῷ καὶ δίψει), so perhaps the context here is more clearly in line with hardships suffered rather than self-imposed disciplines.[90] Since it is coupled again with sleeplessness (ἀγρυπνία), it seems reasonable that one's conclusion would be the same for both passages, and that the reason for sleeplessness and fasting would also likely be the same. Though it is difficult to be sure, it seems best to conclude that both references to fasting in 2 Corinthians refer to hardships, the entering into circumstances in which eating had to be foregone. However, it should not be forgotten that the apostle entered into this state of affairs willingly. Perhaps Paul could refer to a variety of kinds of experiences of going without food, whether intentional or not, as "fasting." But in sum, his approach to ministry was indeed one of intentional discipline, though such circumstances as going without food (as referred to here) were in themselves not considered desirable.

The Lack of Fasting in the Epistles and Related Ideas

Apart from the two references in 2 Corinthians, the rest of the epistles and Revelation do not explicitly mention fasting. This might lead to the idea that the practice was not important to the early church, or perhaps even viewed negatively. Fink goes so far as to say that even the interest in fasting shown in Luke-Acts departs from the teachings of Jesus.[91] Keith Main stresses the Pauline doctrine of justification by faith so much that for him fasting seems to imperil Christian doctrine.[92] On the other hand, if the references to fasting in the NT already discussed (especially those mentioned in Acts) are understood as indicating that fasting was an accepted part of the life of the early church, then perhaps the absence of explicit references means very little. Perhaps the practice was assumed, and the examples in the synoptics and Acts serve as a kind of narrative teaching, so that the lack of didactic teaching on fasting should not be overvalued.[93]

Within the backdrop of the theology of the changing of the ages in Christ is the apparent abolition of dietary regulations. This is most clearly seen in the account of Peter's vision in Acts 10:9-23. The discourse begins with the intriguing statement that Peter "became hungry, and was desiring to eat" (10:10). Peter was commanded by the divine voice to "kill and eat!" While the account is first to be understood as about the acceptance of the Gentiles, it should also be noted that the Jewish concern about Peter was not that he preached to them, but that he "ate with them" (11:3). Whether or not this means he ate food that was not kosher is not explicit, but it is clear that Jew and Gentile were to enjoy table fellowship, and the revocation of food regulations is clearly implied (it was Peter, the Jew, who was commanded to eat the unclean food). This should also be read in conjunction with Mark 7:19. Here during a discourse of Jesus on internal versus external forms of righteousness, the writer inserts the parenthetical comment, "Thus he declared all foods clean." Clearly the early church was coming to a position that the old covenant food regulations had been done away in the new era. This raised sensitive cultural issues for Jews, especially when added to the thorny association of eating foods sacrificed to idols. The apostolic council of Acts 15 specifically concluded against those arguing that the Gentiles needed to "observe the Law of Moses" (Acts 15:5). But in a kind of position of deference, they wrote that they should still abstain from food sacrificed to idols, from blood and things strangled, as well as fornication (Acts 15:20, 28-29). Paul addressed these concerns by also taking a middle road, clearly affirming that food regulations were not a part of Christian practice, but readily deferring to others' sensitivities (Romans 14; 1 Corinthians 8). Yet the writer of Revelation could condemn a "Jezebel" who encouraged Christians to eat things sacrificed to idols (Rev 2:20). So this theme of the abolition of dietary regulations implies that fasting could not be made mandatory in the New Covenant community. Yet at times, some forms of abstinence would be desirable to maintain personal purity and harmony within the community. The application to fasting would be that Christians should not presume to mandate such practices, but fasting could at least be a live option. Hopefully such fasting would promote purity and harmony.

A decent case study might be made of Paul's discussion of bodily disciplines. In Col 2:16-23 he appears to take a dim view of regulating food, drink, and holiday observances. He refers to such things as acts of "self-abasement" (2:18, 23, NASB, translating ταπεινοφροσύνη) that are "of no value against fleshly indulgence." The word ταπεινοφροσύνη and related terms are sometimes used to refer to fasting in the LXX.[94] Some commentators, like Markus Barth and Helmut Blanke, do not think this text has anything to do with fasting.[95] On the other hand, John Muddiman says this is "probably a Semiticism for fasting, since the practice is coupled with 'angel worship,' i.e., it was intended to induce visions of angels."[96] Perhaps a middle ground is best. As argued previously in relation to the Day of Atonement passages, the "self-abasement" in view may include fasting as an understood application, but is larger in scope. As Francis says, the term is "bound up with regulations of much broader effect than fasting."[97] So Paul is strongly opposed to the kind of regulatory actions (which would likely include certain kinds of fasting) in certain instances, such as that described in this passage. Yet he is not entirely opposed to voluntarily abstaining from foods, as his discussion of questionable eating practices in Romans 14 and 1 Corinthians 8 proves. He describes "bodily discipline" as of some value in 1 Tim 4:8.[98] He also condemns those who live by their appetites, which might tacitly condone fasting (Phil 3:19; Rom 16:18; Titus 1:12). Additionally, the other NT appearances of the word ταπεινοφροσύνη from Col 2:18 and Col 2:23 are all used positively (including a use in the very next chapter), as a virtue Christians are to cultivate (Acts 20:19; Eph 4:2; Phil 2:3; Col 3:12; 1 Pet 5:5). Louw and Nida offer this comment on the term in context:

> The rendering of ταπεινοφροσύνη in Col 2.18 as 'false humility' is justified in terms of the context, but there is nothing in the word ταπεινοφροσύνη itself which means 'false.' It would be possible to render ταπεινοφροσύνη in Col 2.18 as 'subjection to,' and one might render the entire expression as 'in abject worship of angels.' In other languages 'false humility' may be rendered as 'just pretending to be humble' or 'appearing to be humble but really being proud.'[99]

It would seem reasonable that Paul would not outright reject a practice that he himself practiced, as evidenced in other texts. Rather, it would be consistent to see a passage like Col 2:16-23 functioning similarly to Jesus' strong criticisms of certain kinds of fasting behaviors in Matthew 6 or Luke 18. It is not fasting itself, or bodily discipline in general, that are condemned, but rather the hypocrisy and poor theology that so often accompany them. In fact, it is reasonable to believe that the apostles and early Christians thought that fasting would be an appropriate means of bodily discipline if it were encouraging genuine humility.

Textual Variants That Add Fasting to Biblical Texts

A handful of passages of Scripture have had phrases related to fasting added into their textual traditions in the early centuries of the church. In each case, fasting is added as a sort of tag on to a reference to prayer. In *The Text of the New Testament*, Bruce Metzger treats these passages under the heading of "Alterations Made Because of Doctrinal Considerations," and he writes:

> In view of the increasing emphasis on asceticism in the early Church and the corresponding insistence upon fasting as an obligation laid on all Christians, it is not surprising that monks, in their work of transcribing manuscripts, should have introduced several references to fasting, particularly in connexion with prayer. This has happened in numerous manuscripts at Mark ix. 29, Acts x. 30, and 1 Cor. vii. 5. In Rom. xiv. 17, where the kingdom of God is said to be not eating and drinking, 'but righteousness and peace and joy in the Holy Spirit', codex 4 inserts after 'righteousness' the words 'and asceticism' (καὶ ἄσκησις). Such interpolations abound in chapter vii of 1 Corinthians.[100]

Metzger's decision to treat these texts basically as a unit has been highly influential, as will be seen in the following discussion. Assuming that Metzger's line of reasoning is correct, the tendency to add fasting to the text of Scripture raises a couple of interesting questions about the role of tradition and Scripture. Should these additions be regarded as intrusive, reflecting a later and perhaps contradictory theology of fasting? Or are they merely clarifications, so that their addition accurately reflects the earliest church's theology and practice, making explicit what was previously merely implicit? Both of these (or something else) may be going on, and so a case-by-case analysis may be in order.

Mark 9:29 and Matt 17:21:
Balancing Spiritual Warfare Against Magical Powers

καὶ εἶπεν αὐτοῖς· τοῦτο τὸ γένος ἐν οὐδενὶ δύναται ἐξελθεῖν εἰ μὴ ἐν προσευχῇ (καὶ νηστείᾳ).

And He said to them, "This kind cannot come out by anything but prayer [and fasting]."

Mark 9:29 (NASB)

This verse occurs in a context in which the disciples were unable to cast a demon out of a boy. After Jesus performed the exorcism, they asked him why they could not do it, and this was his response. The fact that τοῦτο τὸ γένος is neuter would suggest that Jesus was referring to the unclean spirit, and that perhaps a special power was required for casting it out. This special power would come through prayer—and perhaps also fasting?

Mark 9:29 ends with "prayer" (προσευχῇ) in Vaticanus, the original hand of Sinaiticus, and several minor witnesses. But a corrector of Sinaiticus, 𝔓45vid, and a large number of later uncials and minuscules add "and fasting" (καὶ νηστείᾳ), and a few minor versions add "fasting and" before prayer. While it is possible that the manuscripts that omitted the reference to fasting did so in an attempt to harmonize the passage with Mark 2:18 that presents Jesus as speaking against fasting, this would posit an unlikely tendency in early monks to minimize the role of fasting because they found it inconsistent with the words of Jesus. Instead, recognizing the opposite scribal tendencies, the United Bible Societies' fourth edition of *The Greek New Testament* (UBS[4]) assigned the omission an {A} rating, and the reader is referred to 1 Cor 7:5. Metzger comments,

> In light of the increasing emphasis in the early church on the necessity of fasting, it is understandable that καὶ νηστείᾳ is a gloss that found its way into most witnesses. Among the witnesses that resisted such an accretion are important representatives of the Alexandrian and the Western types of text.[101]

All of the modern English translations based on the critical text of the NT omit the reference to fasting in the text of Mark 9:29. Similarly, contemporary commentators almost unanimously agree with Metzger's reasoning.[102]

The entire verse of Matt 17:21 (which reads with the long ending of Mark 9:29 as above) is well attested in the Byzantine witnesses, but omitted from Vaticanus, the original hand of Sinaiticus, and a number of other manuscripts. For this reason, and because it was likely assimilated to the parallel in Mark, the omission was assigned an {A} rating in UBS[4] (upgraded from a {B} rating in UBS[3]). According to Kurt Aland and Barbara Aland, "The relative lack of support here for the lectio brevior is not surprising in view of the significance of fasting and the respect for it characteristic not only of the early Church but also of monasticism throughout the medieval period."[103] Again, modern English translations based on the critical text of the NT follow this reasoning and so omit the verse, and contemporary commentators agree. Carson writes:

"But this kind does not go out except by prayer and fasting" is omitted by a powerful combination of witnesses. It is obviously an assimilation to the synoptic parallel in Mark 9:29. There is no obvious reason why, if original, it should have been omitted; and textual harmonization is quite demonstrably a secondary process.[104]

Similarly, Craig Keener writes:

17:21 is missing from some of the best manuscripts. Although its wide geographical distribution could favor its inclusion, it is easily explained as a harmonization with the wording of Mk 9:29, scribes being dissatisfied with Matthew's twofold use of Mk 11:23.... . Matthew omits some Markan material here; e.g., probably due to the danger of false prophets to his community (7:15; 24:24) he omits Mark's account of the exorcist outside their circle... . Despite the syncretic character of most exorcisms in the magical papyri, many early Christians continued to expel demons immediately by a command (Minucius Felix *Octavius* 24-27) and found fasting an important weapon against more powerful demons (Tert. *On Fasting* 8.8; Jerome *Against Jovinianus* 2.15; the variant reading in Mk 9:29).[105]

There appears to be nearly a consensus among scholars as to how to deal with the textual evidence in these cases. However, questions remain as to how certainly such conclusions can be asserted. The omission of fasting in Mark 9:29 is based on only a handful of manuscripts, and only two that might be considered major.[106] Elsewhere Jesus gave express directions about fasting (Matt 6:16-18), and the early church practiced fasting (Acts 13:2-3, 14:23), so there is no inherent reason why a reference to fasting could not be original. There is also the idea that adding fasting would create a harder reading, given Jesus' earlier statements in Mark 2:18. Additionally, the consensus regarding Matt 17:21 relies on the assumption that Matthew is literarily dependent on Mark, which could possibly be subject to future nuances. In total, it seems reasonable to follow Metzger's reasoning that scribes tended to add references to fasting to these texts that mention prayer, but one should be cautious not to oversimplify these textual issues.

Now, theologically, one must ask whether adding fasting is theologically intrusive, or if it could be understood as complementary to the original context. On the negative side, one needs to avoid the idea that prayer and fasting could intrinsically impart a magical sense of power over demons. On the other hand, if fasting is seen as an appropriate intensifier and accompaniment to prayer, then fasting might merely complement the original saying of Jesus. Seeing fasting as having an intrinsic, magical power should be rejected by Christians, and this passage as originally recorded (assuming the reference to fasting is not original) gives no warrant for pursuing fasting to increase abilities in exorcism. However, it is possible that humble, intense prayer may bring one into a state of dependence on God and close relationship to him. This could allow a person to accomplish his will more completely, and fasting may play a role in such prayer. There is clearly biblical precedent for connecting prayer and fasting, as already discussed.[107] Perhaps balancing these two ideas will help one to avoid the danger of fasting as a magical practice on the one hand, and the tendency to ignore spiritual warfare altogether on the other. In any case, fasting can be coupled by Christians with prayer as a means of intensifying the experience, but whether or not this would give specific spiritual powers would be up to God.

Acts 10:30: Describing Piety

καὶ ὁ Κορνήλιος ἔφη· ἀπὸ τετάρτης ἡμέρας μέχρι ταύτης τῆς ὥρας ἤμην τὴν ἐνάτην προσευχόμενος ἐν τῷ οἴκῳ μου, καὶ ἰδοὺ ἀνὴρ ἔστη ἐνώπιον μου ἐν ἐσθῆτι λαμπρᾷ

And Cornelius said, "Four days ago to this hour, I was praying in my house during the ninth hour; and behold, a man stood before me in shining garments."

Acts 10:30, NASB

Metzger describes this interesting text critical problem in some detail:

The Textus Receptus, supported by a diversified and respectable array of witnesses, appears to be clear and straightforward: Ἀπὸ τετάρτης ἡμέρας μέχρι ταύτης τῆς ὥρας ἤμην νηστεύων, καὶ τὴν ἐνάτην προσευχόμενος ἐν τῷ οἴκῳ μου, which ought to mean, "From the fourth day until this hour I was fasting, and while keeping the ninth hour of prayer in my house" ... The superficial impression, however, that Cornelius had been fasting for the immediately preceding four days is clearly erroneous, for the terminus of the fasting was the sudden appearance of a man in bright clothing who told him to send to Joppa, etc.[108]

The reference to fasting is omitted in Sinaiticus, the original hand of Alexandrinus, Vaticanus, 𝔓74, and several other witnesses, while being found in most of the Byzantine and a number of Western manuscripts.

Previous editions of the UBS Greek NT gave the reading that lacked the reference to fasting a {D} rating; the {B} rating in the UBS[4] seems to be a little optimistic.[109] Perhaps this growing confidence is due to the idea of treating all the textual variants related to fasting together as a kind of commonly themed unit. Metzger writes: "Although the words νηστεύων καί may have been deleted in some copies because nothing is said in the previous account of Cornelius's fasting, it is more probable that they were added to the text by those who thought that fasting should precede baptism (compare 9.9 and Didache 7.4 κελεύσεις δὲ νηστεῦσαι τὸν βαπτιζόμενον πρὸ μιᾶς ἢ δύο)."[110]

If the reference to fasting here is not original, then evidence of fasting in the early church drawn from the statement of Cornelius could only be coming from scribal additions. Cornelius's piety could have included fasting with his prayers, even though he likely was not originally presented as explicitly fasting. It is possible that in the original context his prayers could have included fasting, but there is no real way to confirm or deny such a thing. Perhaps early scribes sought to validate Christian fasting practices related to baptism, as noted above, by adding it to positive biblical texts like this one. There does not seem to be any real theological intrusion by the addition, and the problem seems to be one that is basically incidental.

1 Cor 7:5: Linking Fasting to Sexual Abstinence

μὴ ἀποστερεῖτε ἀλλήλους, εἰ μήτι ἂν ἐκ συμφώνου πρὸς καιρόν, ἵνα σχολάσητε τῇ (νηστείᾳ καὶ τῇ) προσευχῇ καὶ πάλιν ἐπὶ τὸ αὐτὸ ἦτε, ἵνα μὴ πειράζῃ ὑμᾶς ὁ σατανᾶς διὰ τὴν ἀκρασίαν ὑμῶν.

Stop depriving one another, except by agreement for a time that you may devote yourselves to [fasting and to] prayer, and come together again lest Satan tempt you because of your lack of self-control.

1 Cor 7:5, NASB

The reference to "fasting" in this verse is omitted by almost all of the Alexandrian and Western witnesses, with the Byzantine including it. The UBS[4] assigns the omission a certainty of {A}, apparently seeing this textual addition as informing Mark 9:29 and Matt 17:21 as well. Metzger describes the additions of fasting as "interpolations, introduced in the interest of asceticism. The shorter text is decisively supported by all the early and best witnesses."[111]

This text is of particular interest for fasting, in that the addition of fasting to the act of prayer here also associates the concept with sexual abstinence. This ascetic association of fasting and sexual abstinence cannot be found clearly in either the OT or NT, but it did appear in both Jewish and early Christian literature. Therefore it is not surprising to see fasting making its way into this context, much like the Aramaic Targums added fasting and sexual abstinence to the Day of Atonement passages already discussed. So here we see a very similar tendency toward textual addition by Christian scribes. Just as Jewish tradition sought to apply humiliation passages with the inclusion of fasting, it appears that Christians were attempting to associate fasting not only with prayer, but also as an accompaniment of sexual abstinence.

Summary of the Nature of Textual Fasting Additions: Increased Awareness, Without Subversion

What do these textual variants suggest about the relationship of fasting to the theology of the NT? A balanced approach seems best, one that is in line with what O'Collins and Kendall cite as "The principle of exegetical consensus: Where available, the consensus of centrist exegetes guides systematic theology."[112] On the one hand, it should be candidly acknowledged that these references to fasting are most likely not part of the original text of the NT, and so do not bear the kind of authority that inclusion in the NT would imply. However, that does not necessarily mean that the simple addition of "fasting" to references to prayer should be seen as subversive. The given theology of any of the above passages is not really changed by the references to fasting, since in each case the reference to prayer alone would have basically the same function. Fasting merely serves to intensify the references to prayer. This suggests that the early Christians who added fasting to these texts saw fasting as an appropriate way of applying the passages before them, and perhaps they saw this reflected in their own communities of faith. If fasting is seen as connected to prayer, it is difficult to see how adding a more intense action as part of prayer subverts the meaning of Scripture.[113] There may be evidence in the cumulative effect of these additions of an increase in ascetic behaviors in the early Christians over time, but that alone is not necessarily subversive, either. More appropriately, one would need to evaluate the forms that asceticism took, rather than merely dismiss it altogether. Such a discussion will be engaged in the following chapters.

Conclusion: Fasting as Remembrance and Anticipation in the Messianic Age

The NT uses fasting as a way of symbolizing the anticipation of the messianic age. Jesus fasted in the wilderness, and this helps to identify him as the messianic prophet like Moses, and as the second Adam who could withstand temptation and teach us not to live by bread alone (Matt 4:1-4; Luke 4:1-4). The godly Anna fasted in anticipation of his messianic appearance, and was rewarded with seeing him (Luke 2:37). His disciples could not fast in his presence, because the messianic bridegroom was with them. But, the nature of the age would turn, the bridegroom would be taken away, and this age is seen to be an age when fasting is once again appropriate (Matt 9:14-17; Mark 2:18-22; Luke 5:33-39). In this age, the teaching of Jesus in the Sermon on the Mount governs the way his disciples should fast—not hypocritically (like the Pharisee in Luke 18:12) or ostentatiously, but humbly before God, who will reward them (Matt 6:16-18). In the New Covenant community, the early Christians fast and pray, seeking the presence and guiding of their Lord, and his Holy Spirit leads them to build up his church (Acts 13:1-3, 14:23).

Now, in the messianic age since Christ has returned to his Father in heaven, fasting can become a way of both remembering him and anticipating his presence. As the texts that have been examined show, the NT certainly qualifies the religious practice of fasting, and Christians should not assume that fasting has any particular merit in and of itself. Additionally, the texts examined do not explicitly command fasting as an obligation for believers, either. But on the positive side, as Christians grapple with the nature of the age in which they find themselves, fasting appropriately could help center the believer and believing community in its life between the times. We now turn to a study of Christian history, to see how Christ's followers have sought to use fasting in the practice of their faith.

§3
Fasting Through the Patristic Era

The Development Of A Christian Religious Practice

The early Christian community practiced fasting, as already evidenced by the references in the NT. As the Christians reflected on their newly emerging eschatological identity, their fasting practices took on distinctly Christian theological explanations. This chapter will explore a number of fasting passages in important early Christian literature, then focus on writings that specifically address fasting by leading theologians of the patristic era, and finally trace the development of official church practices regarding fasting.

Joan Brueggemann Rufe offers a rather comprehensive examination of fasting in the early church, focusing on Christian references to fasting through A.D. 230. She notes that both Jews and Gentiles in the early church had backgrounds that included fasting, and the early community incorporated the practice for similar, but often reinterpreted, reasons. She summarizes the occasions and theological motivations:

> These early Christian texts show Christians fasting to prepare for baptism, to mourn and commemorate Jesus' death (for many their only routine practice of fasting as a ritual act of lamentation), to better resist temptation, to obtain revelation, as part of their observance of stations, in response to persecution, and to care for the poor and address community needs and support community goals. This fasting practice, in addition to being separate and distinctive, reflected two strongly-held convictions: (1) because Christians were living in an age of joy inaugurated by their risen Lord, fasting routinely practiced as a ritual act of lamentation was no longer appropriate behavior; and (2) because God's demands that justice and righteousness be done were primary, fasting was acceptable to God only when or as those demands were also met.[1]

This early emphasis would be consistent with the underlying perception of the church as the eschatological new community. As Rufe herself notes, there was fasting in commemoration of Jesus' death that became embedded in the Christian calendar. This reflects an awareness of something like the already/not yet understanding of the nature of the age. As time went on, it seems reasonable to think that the newness of the Christian situation would gradually be replaced by a more settled sense of awareness of the Christian experience as a pilgrimage, in a still fallen world, but awaiting consummation. Perhaps that theology at least partly explains the growing tendency toward asceticism in the church from the early centuries through the medieval period.

Herbert Musurillo produced an important survey of fasting in Greek patristic literature, taking a phenomenological, inductive approach. The variety of fasting practices and themes associated with them, he says, "defeats any attempt in the direction of precise categorization or unification."[2] He does offer, however, nine sections in which he examines major emphases, some of which live in tension with one another. These are:

> 1. 'Exempla' of Fasting and the 'Laudes Monachorum' (5-11), which show how Church Fathers listed positive and negative examples from sacred history;
>
> 2. Philosophic Motifs (11-16), which traces how Pythagorean, Neoplatonic and Stoic ideas on the relationship of the body and soul influenced fasting;
>
> 3. Hygienic Fasting (17-19), which shows the patristic awareness of medical ideas of the time, and fasting's presumed positive role in health;
>
> 4. Daemonic Motif (19-23), which reflects their belief in fasting having a role in spiritual warfare;
>
> 5. Christian Fasting as a Mourning-Fast (23-25), which suggests that the early church used fasting to acknowledge grief for Adam's sin as well as Christ, the bridegroom, being absent;
>
> 6. Abnormality in the Practice of Fasting (25-35), which surveys competitive or eccentric fasting approaches among monks, such as the stylites;
>
> 7. Spiritual Fasting (35-42), which highlights the emphasis patristic writers had on true, internal elements (like humility, justice, service) in fasting taking precedence over the form;
>
> 8. Fasting as a Means of Self-Conquest (42-55), which shows the desire for self-control and discipline;
>
> 9. The Martyrdom of Asceticism (55-62), which suggests that after the persecutions waned and the empire became Christian, asceticism was a way of identifying with the call to suffering and martyrdom as was required in former days.

Musurillo concludes that these varied strands work together in a conglomeration of themes that affect fasting practice and teachings about them in the patristic era. He highlights three main internal tensions here: (1) the polarity between spiritual and bodily emphases; (2) the conflict between rigorous asceticism and the exhortation to moderation; and (3) the contrast between the ascetical approach and the more mystical elements often associated with it.[3] When all is said and done, Musurillo offers this observation about fasting practices in the patristic era:

> [A]usterity of all kinds (and especially fasting) would appear to be nothing more than the vital reaction of the Christian, in the concrete circumstances and psychological presuppositions of his milieu, to the call of Jesus in the Gospels. And the words, 'Take up your cross and follow me' have been transposed from the messianic message of Christ to the precarious position of the Christian community placed between the Resurrection and the Parousia.[4]

So while there is a good deal of diversity in references to fasting in the history of the church, Musurillo is fundamentally right that this discussion is about appropriating human religious actions in the context of a theological understanding of the nature of the age in which Christians find themselves. This eschatological motif is a significant component underlying Christian fasting, however haltingly the theology may be understood at any given time, or however loosely Christians practicing fasting may see the connections.

References to Fasting in Early Christian Literature: The Growth and Idealization of Fasting

Since Rufe and Musurillo have provided such a thorough analysis of early Christian fasting, it will not be necessary here to go into the background and detail that they have already done. Instead, various authors and texts will be treated on their own terms, in order to paint something of a portrait of how fasting factored into their understanding of their place in the new Christian era. Hopefully, then, a synthetic picture will emerge that can help summarize the main contributions fasting practices offer in the emerging theological context of early Christianity. The two categories of literature that will be addressed in this section are the writings known as the Apostolic Fathers and the New Testament Apocrypha. In this literature, it will be seen that the emerging Christian community had a growing awareness of the role of fasting, and fasting became part of an idealized description of the disciplined Christian life.

Fasting in the Apostolic Fathers:
Its Growth in the Emerging Christian Community

One can observe from the following discussion that fasting played an important role in the self-understanding of the early Christian community. Fasting is mentioned and discussed more frequently in the early decades after the first apostles than in the NT itself. During this time or soon after, the several fasting variants discussed in the previous chapter found their way into the NT manuscript tradition, which also gives some indication of the growing importance of fasting. Key passages in the following documents find their way into church tradition as well, becoming authoritative for later patristic writers as they will mold fasting practices into what they hope will be meaningful, ritualized behaviors. The following survey examines all of the references to fasting in the documents that are commonly collected as the "Apostolic Fathers," with special attention paid to the emerging sense of Christians as an eschatological community.

- Clement of Rome: Fasting Identifies with God's People, Reflects Righteousness, and Intensifies Prayer

First Clement 53.2 (from around the end of the first century) gives a passing reference to the fasting of Moses forty days on the mountain in a passage that holds him up as a positive example of a leader identifying with his people in prayer and seeking forgiveness. *First Clement* 55.6 also mentions the fasting of Esther in context as a positive example of self-sacrifice. *Second Clement* 16.4 (from near the middle of the second century) says,

> Almsgiving is therefore good even as penitence for sin; fasting is better than prayer, but the giving of alms is better than both; and love "covers a multitude of sins," but prayer from a good conscience rescues from death. Blessed is every man who is found full of these things; for almsgiving lightens sin.[5]

Here we see the connection with the deeds of righteousness Jesus spoke of in Matthew 6, with a prioritization of the practices being given, apparently, relative to their intensity (fasting as better than prayer) and efficacy (almsgiving better than both, in accord with the law of love). All three fall under the category here of blessed things. The scriptural allusion to love covering a multitude of sins (1 Pet 4:8; Jas 5:20) is expanded to say that almsgiving actually "lightens" sin, and linked here to penitence, suggests a gradualistic approach to forgiveness and judgment.

- Polycarp: Fasting Aids Against Temptation

Polycarp's *Letter to the Philippians* 7 (ca. 150) warns against the temptation of false teachers and heresy, and believers are urged in 7.2:

> ... let us turn back to the word which was delivered to us in the beginning, "watching unto prayer" and persevering in fasting, beseeching the all-seeing God in our supplications "to lead us not into temptation," even as the Lord said, "The spirit is willing, but the flesh is weak."[6]

Here fasting is connected to the disciplining of the flesh to obey the spirit in avoiding temptation.

- Barnabas and Diognetus: Fasting Requires Justice and Must Differ from Judaism

The Epistle of Barnabas (probably early second century) includes two passages that refer to fasting. *Barn.* 3.1-5 quotes Isa 58:4-10, referring to God's rejection of the fasting that is not accompanied by humility, justice and generosity to the poor. The text is used to show that even in the OT God desired "guilelessness," and that the people of God in the new Christian community should not be "shipwrecked by conversion to their law," that is, to revert to Judaism.[7] *Barn.* 7 uses typological interpretation to show Christ as the scapegoat for sin on the day Atonement in his crucifixion. While the people fasted on that day, Christ broke his fast when he was given vinegar and gall to drink. By this action, he both identified with the people who could not avoid sin under the law, and became a curse for them. So here fasting is used as a foil to teach substitutionary atonement (even though the correspondence of Passover to the specifics of the Day of Atonement appears strained, as the people were not actually fasting during the crucifixion). Both of the passages in *Barnabas* highlight the early community's need to distinguish itself from Judaism through a christological interpretation of the OT.

Similarly, *The Epistle to Diognetus* (from the late second to early third century) contrasts the Christian community with the Jews. *Diogn.* 4.1 mentions the Jewish "hypocrisy about fasting" in context with the Sabbath, circumcision and new moons, as "ridiculous and not worth discussing."[8]

- *The Didache*: Fasting as a Part of Christian Self-Identity

The Didache contains three explicit references to fasting: 1.3, 7.4, and 8.1.[9] Clearly fasting was an accepted part of life for the early Christian community being addressed, and the practice is given certain practical associations and distinctions. The main themes that emerge are that fasting and prayer should be done for the sake of one's enemies, fasting is part of the preparation for baptism, and fasting should be practiced on different days from the Jews.

Fasting and Praying for Enemies. Did. 1.3 is an interesting reference to fasting comes in the midst of a chapter that presents a remolding of ethical teaching, largely drawn from the Sermon on the Mount tradition, and headed by an introduction of a "Two Ways" theme that reflects Jewish wisdom literature.

> Now, the teaching of these words is this: "Bless those that curse you, and pray for your enemies, and fast for those that persecute you. For what credit is it to you if you love those that love you? Do not even the heathen do the same?" But, for your part, "love those that hate you," and you will have no enemy.[10]

The explicit fasting reference here reworks the phrases from Matt 5:44, ἀγαπᾶτε τοὺς ἐχθροὺς ὑμῶν καὶ προσεύχεσθε ὑπὲρ τῶν διωκόντων ὑμᾶς.[11] The phrase in the *Didache* in Greek is προσεύχεσθε ὑπὲρ τῶν ἐχθρῶν, νηστεύετε δὲ ὑπὲρ τῶν διωκόντων ὑμᾶς. What results is a form of parallelism between prayer and fasting in the phrases. The text presupposes persecution in the early Christian community, and like the gospels, enjoins prayer for their enemies.[12] In the midst of persecution, fasting would be an appropriate sign of the manifestation of suffering and seeking the Lord's presence. But it is significant to note that the Christians do this *on behalf of* their enemies. Their fasting, like their prayer, is seen as a benevolent act of mercy that engenders love. This clearly evidences a radically new kind of commandment in the tradition of Jesus, and so this kind of fasting demonstrates an outward, rather than an inward, focus.

Fasting Before Baptism. Didache 7 discusses the Christian rite of baptism, invoking the Triune name (7.1), prioritizing mode (7.2-3), and associating fasting with baptism (7.4). Specifically, 7.4 reads:

> And before the baptism let the baptiser and him who is to be baptised fast, and any others who are able. And thou shalt bid him who is to be baptised to fast one or two days before.[13]

A couple of observations are of interest. First, the verb used for fasting here, προνηστευσάτω (a third person singular imperative), is unusual.[14] The addition of the prefix may reflect the discussion at hand of fasting "before" the baptism, and this kind of prefixing appears in 7.1, προειπόντες. Another observation is the fact that not only the candidate was commanded to fast, but also the baptizer, as well as others from the community who were able (καὶ εἴ τινες ἄλλοι δύνανται). This association of fasting with baptism has seeds in the NT, with Jesus' baptism preceding his fast in the wilderness, and Saul fasting following his conversion experience and prior to his baptism (Acts 9:9). Baptism in the NT was generally seen as an act of repentance, and repentance often had fasting associations implied in Jewish practice.[15] Additionally, as baptism was a preparation for partaking in the Eucharist, the community of those already baptized may have practiced fasting with the baptismal candidate as an act of solidarity for the special occasion.[16] This description of fasting prior to baptism in the *Didache* may be a link in a chain that gave rise to the more full-blown Easter preparations in the church year. Willy Rordorf cites J. Schümmer and comments:

> A remark of J. Schümmer seems particularly pertinent to me: "The custom of fasting with the person to be baptized is possibly even older than the general Easter fast (cf. Didache) and it could in its turn, after the transfer of the time of baptism to the Easter celebration, have contributed to first making the Easter fast into a general practice." The trajectory then passed from the *Didache* to Justin (*1 Apol* 61), to Tertullian (*Bapt* 19f) and to Hippolytus (*ApTrad* 21).[17]

Linking baptism with fasting, then, showed the connection of both with the idea of repentance. But further, baptism became the singular mark of the new community, and so linking fasting to that act also associates it with new rituals that commenced and were invested with new meaning with the coming of the Gospel.

Fasting on Different Days Than Jews. The final reference to fasting in *Did.* 8.1 follows immediately the reference in 7.4, and so fasting becomes the transitional hinge to a further brief discussion of prayer. The text reads: "Let not your fasts be with the hypocrites, for they fast on Mondays and Thursdays, but do you fast on Wednesdays and Fridays."[18] This is clearly similar to Matt 6:16, with the next verse following suit echoing Matt 6:5, "And do not pray as the hypocrites," and finishing up with the Lord's prayer that is similar in wording to Matt 6:9-13.[19] Included in this passage is the not-so-subtle implication that the term "hypocrites" referred to by Jesus in the Sermon on the Mount is being applied to practitioners of Jewish fasting generally. As already seen, certain members of the Jewish community fasted twice a week (like the Pharisee in Luke 18:12), on Mondays and Thursdays. Here the Christians are instructed to change their fasting days to Wednesdays and Fridays, and the imperative mood (ὑμεῖς δὲ νηστεύσατε) suggests to some that this fasting may have been compulsory, though that is not certain.[20] The references to the days of the week the hypocrites fast (δευτέρα σαββάτων καὶ πέμπτῃ) are in the dative, while the days enjoined here are in the accusative (τετράδα καὶ παρασκευήν). The shift in case is best explained as reflecting a difference between the dative referring to point in time (i.e., fasting on those particular days) and the accusative referring to extent of time (i.e., throughout those particular days),[21] which would actually mean an intensification of the fasting practice.

The only clear differentiation being made between Jewish and Christian fasting here is the days on which it is to be done. While this could imply that there was relatively little difference between their fasting practices, it could also be the case that fasting on the same days was the only common denominator left between the two practices, and now this link was also being severed.[22] Fasting on Wednesdays and Fridays could commemorate Jesus' betrayal and crucifixion, as well as distinguishing Christian practice from Judaism. Since Jews prepared meals for the Sabbath on Fridays, it was a day of extra food preparation, and Christian fasting on Friday would imply breaking with Jewish Sabbath observance as well. By marking out different days for fasting, the Christians represented by the writing of the *Didache* appear to be using fasting as a means of self-identity.[23] This at least shows an awareness that they believed they were a new community, while still being linked through Christ, the promised fulfillment, to the old.

- *The Shepherd of Hermas*: Fasting for Visions and Righteous Conduct

Another important early witness to Christian fasting practices is *The Shepherd of Hermas*, a text originating in central Italy and probably addressed to Rome, written sometime between the last years of the first century and the first half of the second century.[24] The several references to fasting in *The Shepherd of Hermas* can readily be dealt with in two categories. First, the author associates fasting with the obtaining of visions in four places. Second, an extended discussion of fasting broadens the scope of fasting to greater acts of righteous conduct and minimizes fasting as ritual, all in a manner reminiscent of biblical discussions of fasting.

Fasting for Visions. The first reference to fasting occurs in *Vis.* 2.2.1. In the previous chapter, the author had received a book with instructions to copy it, although he could not understand it. Now, after fifteen days of fasting and much prayer, the writing was revealed to him. The content of the vision is primarily a call to repentance for the author and his family, which includes treating his wife as a "sister" (2.2.3, which probably means sexual abstinence) from that time forward.[25] *Vision* 3.1.2 functions similarly, with the author receiving an explanatory vision from an ancient lady, symbolic of the church, after fasting for a long time (νηστεύσας πολλάκις). Again Hermas is viewed as in the midst of confession of sins, and the vision he receives pertains to the building up of the church in righteousness. These fasts remind the reader of the fasting and visions of Daniel (Dan 9:3, 10:2-3).

In *Vis.* 3.10.6-7 he requests understanding of the three forms in which he has seen the lady appear to him, and she replies,

> "Every request needs humility: fast therefore and you shall receive what you ask from the Lord." So I fasted one day and in the same night a young man appeared to me and said to me, "Why do you ask constantly for revelations in your prayer? Take care lest by your many requests you injure your flesh."[26]

While Hermas receives the answer to his question, this passage has an intriguing turn to it. Fasting is here associated with humility, and will result in receiving an answer to the request. Yet, when the answer comes, there is a kind of castigating of the importunity of the questioner (reminiscent perhaps of Jesus' parable of the woman and the unjust judge). While fasting is an ingredient in receiving his request, he is cautioned that he may indeed injure his flesh (perhaps by too much fasting), and it seems to imply a possible danger in progressing too far down this road—but it is a road Hermas insists on traveling, and his wish is granted.

Similitude 9.11.6-8 could similarly be classed as fasting relating to the receiving of visions, though it does not refer to fasting explicitly. Rather, Hermas spends a night with some maidens in prayer and sleeping. When the shepherd appears in the morning, he asks if they supped, and Hermas replies that he supped "on the words of the Lord the whole night." This motif might be considered fasting, in line with Jesus' words during his fast about man not living by bread alone, but by every word that proceeds from the mouth of God. In response to Hermas' words, he receives further vision and explanation. Like Daniel in the OT (Dan 9:3, 20, 10:1-5), Hermas has linked fasting with revelations and angelic visitations from God.

Fasting for Righteous Conduct. The most important discussion of fasting in *The Shepherd of Hermas* is found in three chapters in *Sim.* 5.1-3. Hermas was fasting and sitting on a certain mountain when he saw the shepherd sitting by him. When the shepherd asked what he was doing, he replied that he had a "station" (στατίωνα). The station suggests the Christian fasting during part of the day as a sort of spiritual watch, like a soldier on guard duty, who spends the time in spiritual meditation and prayer.[27] Pressed further, he explained that he was fasting as he had been accustomed (Ὡς εἰώθειν, ... οὕτω νηστεύω). The shepherd replies that this fast is useless, and is not really a fast to the Lord (5.1.3). Rather, God is looking for a fast from evil, a keeping of the heart pure and obedience to his commandments (5.1.5). He proceeds to tell a parable (5.2) that he says concerns fasting (though later chapters reveal that there is a great deal more meaning in the symbolism than strictly about fasting). This parable of a vineyard describes a faithful servant who weeds and cares for what his master gave him.[28] After some time, the master is pleased with the servant, and makes him a joint-heir with his son. When he sent a feast to the servant to celebrate the announcement, the servant kept a small portion for himself, and shared the rest with fellow servants. This pleased the master even further. The next chapter (5.3) begins to explain the parable. Hermas is told that there is a fast that is very good for him to keep. First, he should keep himself from evil words and desires. Then, on the day of his fast, he is to eat only bread and water, and take the price of the food he would have eaten otherwise, and give it to a widow or orphan or someone else who is destitute (5.3.7).[29] This would demonstrate true humility and "fill his soul" (ἵν᾽ ἐκ τῆς ταπεινοφροσύνης σου ὁ εἰληφὼς ἐμπλήσῃ τὴν ἑαυτοῦ ψυχὴν, 5.3.7), and be credited as acceptable before God. This passage reminds the reader of Isaiah 58 and other OT prophets on fasting. What is acceptable to God is righteousness and care for the poor, more than ritual.

This OT theme of justice superceding fasting finds frequent use in Christian writings. And, as noted above, the "station" fast mentioned in the *Didache* and *Hermas* was apparently being practiced by the early Christians with some regularity. The admonitions about justice and the like never really seem to have deterred them from practicing fasting, but rather served to qualify the relative merit of the practice. So we see again how the early Christians drew from the common practice of fasting, which was virtuous in the Old Covenant, and brought it into the new age with what they hoped would be appropriate reinterpretations.

Fasting in Early Christian Apocryphal Writings: Part of an Idealized, Ascetic Life

The early Christian apocryphal writings bear testimony to the importance of fasting in the early Christian community. Although orthodox Christians do not look at these writings as authoritative in doctrinal matters, it is fairly clear that they at least represent a link in the chain of historical traditions concerning fasting. These texts present an idealized portrait of early Christians as disciplined, ascetic people who fast.

- Apocryphal Gospels: Fasting Remembers Christ, Imitates Him, and Associates Heroic Figures with Him

The apocryphal gospels mention fasting in several contexts, and as might be expected, these are generally associated with the central figure of Jesus. However, the focus of these texts is often not on Jesus himself, but on the heroic figures around him that are being addressed, or the disciples of Jesus and how they are to respond to him. The following examination of these texts shows that fasting was used as a motif for associating Christ's followers with him, and sometimes by more or less orthodox means.

The Gospels of Hebrews *and* Peter: *Disciples Fasting for Jesus' Crucifixion.* The Gospel According to the Hebrews was written at the beginning of the second century and is not extant, but Jerome mentions that he translated it. He quotes from it in *De vir. Ill.* 2, saying that "James had taken an oath that he would not eat bread from that hour on which he had drunk the cup of the Lord till he saw him risen from the dead." When the risen Jesus appeared to James, he gave him bread to eat in celebration of his resurrection.[30] *The Gospel of Peter* (probably from the second half of the second century) 7.27 similarly says that after the crucifixion of Jesus, the disciples were in hiding because the Jewish leaders were seeking them, and they "were fasting and sat mourning and weeping night and day until the Sabbath."[31] Whether or not the stories reflect historical fasting accounts of the disciples, these references do at least show that early Christians viewed the crucifixion as a time of mourning, a time appropriate for fasting. Perhaps these kinds of texts show a bridge to later, more developed Lenten fasting practices that commemorated Christ's death.

The Gospel of Thomas: *Fasting as a Step of Repentance, Unnecessary for Those Who Have Attained.* The Gospel of Thomas contains four specific references to fasting. First these references will be presented, and then an attempt will be made to interpret them in light of the unorthodox theology of the community that produced them. It appears that these references see fasting as part of repentance, but that prayer and fasting could be rendered unnecessary by the spiritual disciple who has achieved a perfect state of righteousness.

Gospel of Thomas 6 has the disciples asking Jesus, "Do you want us to fast? How shall we pray, and shall we give alms, and what diet shall we keep?" (paralleling the deeds of righteousness of Matthew 6, with the addition of diet). Jesus' response is only "Do not lie and do not do what you hate, because all things are revealed in the sight of Heaven."[32] Again, *Gos. Thom.* 14 links fasting, prayer, and almsgiving, with Jesus saying, "If you fast, you will bring sin upon yourselves and, if you pray, you will condemn yourselves, and, if you give alms, you will do evil to your spirits."[33] *Gospel of Thomas* 27 has Jesus saying, "If you do not fast with respect to the kingdom of the world, you will not find the Kingdom; if you do not keep the Sabbath as Sabbath, you will not see the Father."[34] *Gospel of Thomas* 104 parallels the synoptic fasting question, with the disciples here saying that they would pray and fast on a certain day. Jesus responds, "Why? What sin have I committed or how have I been conquered? But after the bridegroom has left the bridechamber then let people fast and pray."[35] In this reference, it is clear that fasting would be associated with repentance or mourning, and this would not be appropriate in Jesus' presence, but afterward it would be.

These references to fasting are difficult to harmonize theologically, leaving the impression that they do not represent a consistent approach, even for the community that is responsible for the writing or collecting of the sayings.[36] The first two appear to view fasting very negatively, the third encourages it, and the fourth distinguishes between the presence and absence of Christ. It is possible that there is no coherent theology in these diverse logia, and that they are a conflicted collection. However, Antti Marjanen suggests that these statements can be interpreted in light of what is communicated by the imagery of the bridal chamber, which represents a kind of pinnacle of existence for the Thomasine theology, one in which the believer becomes his own master:

> Therefore, it seems best to understand Jesus' response to the disciples as a paradoxical statement according to which 'masterless' Christians need never practice fasting and prayer because after having entered the bridal chamber they should not leave it at all. But whenever some do and thus commit sin and become defeated in the midst of worldly allurements, they are in need of fasting and prayer.[37]

It is likely, then, that at least in the majority of examples, the *Gospel of Thomas* views practices like fasting, prayer and almsgiving as evidence, and perhaps even further causes of, the infection of sin. The one who is purified of sin would not need to practice them, and Jesus is presented in the book as an example and teacher of this theology. This presupposes an appropriate ground for fasting as an act of repentance, while adding a grossly unorthodox theology of spiritual perfectionism that, if attained, would do away with the need for things like prayer and fasting. Jesus' disciples would not have to do what they hate doing, because that would make them liars.

So by this theology, fasting (along with its classic partners, prayer and almsgiving) is made an intermediate step in mastering righteousness. By doing so, this takes a truth from the nature of the age—that Jesus is absent and it is a time for fasting—and combines it with a heretical notion, that in this life the followers of Jesus can attain a level of godhood that separates them from the need for penitent attitudes and behaviors.

The Protoevangelium of James: *Fasting Associates Mary's Parents with Messianic Expectation*. The *Protoevangelium of James* (from the second half of the second century) 1.4 presents Mary's father, Joachim, as going down to the wilderness where he "fasted forty days and forty nights, saying to himself, 'I shall not go down either for food or for drink until the Lord my God visits me; my prayer shall be food and drink.'"[38] Joachim and his wife, Anna, were childless. Anna received an angelic vision and Mary was conceived. Along with the association of mourning for childlessness and the seeing of heavenly visions, this text adds Mary's father to the forty-day fasting motif of Jesus from the Gospels in the line of Moses and Elijah. By doing so, it elevates the status of the conception of Mary to something messianic, "and it may be said with some confidence that the developed doctrines of Mariology can be traced to this book."[39] This apocryphal story shows that the forty-day fast was enough of a stock image in early Christian theology that a writer would use it to associate his heroic characters with Christ.

- Apocryphal Acts: Idealized Apostles
  Live Wondrously and Perform Great Deeds by Fasting

There are several apocryphal *Acts* that present the apostles as idealized Christian leaders. Fasting plays an integral part in the portrait these books paint of the first Christians, and so we can see that fasting played a significant role in the life of these early church communities. The apostles are presented as characters that fast and pray, and are enabled by God to receive supernatural revelations, do mighty miracles, and confound their enemies. They are held up as examples for the early church, and so one can surely infer that the apostles' fasting was also being imitated.

The Acts of John and Paul: *Idealized Apostles Make the Unusual Act of Fasting the Norm for Miraculous Living*. The *Acts of John* (late second century) 84 lists fastings in a long list of the righteous activities of the saints (of which Fortunatus, an unbeliever raised from the dead by Christians and remaining in opposition, would never partake).[40] *The Acts of Paul* (from the end of the second century) contains several references to fasting, some of which are surmised from fragments. Paul finds the Christian community in Damascus fasting when he arrives after his conversion (*Acts Paul* 1).[41] Paul "was fasting with Onesiphorus and his wife and his children in a new tomb" for the sake of Thecla, who was miraculously spared execution (*Acts Paul* 3.23).[42] When Paul was captured and had to face a lion, Artemilla and Eubula "mourned not a little, fasting," and of course, Paul was spared (*Acts Paul* 7).[43] Similarly, in a fragmentary account about another woman condemned, Paul "laboured and fasted in great cheerfulness for two days with the prisoners" (*Acts Paul* 8).[44] The people of the church in Corinth "were distressed and fasted" for Paul when he announced that he would go to Rome, because they believed he would be killed there. But when the Spirit spoke through a certain woman, Myrta, that it was for the greater glory of God, "each one partook of the bread and feasted according to custom" (*Acts Paul* 9).[45] On the ship to Rome, Paul was "fatigued by the fastings and the night watches with the brethren" (*Acts Paul* 10).[46]

These references to fasting present an idealized picture of the apostles, one in which they fast and pray and perform miracles. Fasting functions to present them as ideal examples to the Christian community, but it also appears to set them apart as especially holy, powerful Christians. These two ideas held together show something of the paradoxical nature of fasting for Christian spirituality: an inherently unusual activity is promoted as exemplary (hence normal), but results in unusual characters being the most likely to live out the ideal.

The Acts of Peter: *Fasting for Guidance and Visions in the New Community. The Acts of Peter* (from around the end of the second century) contains several references to fasting.[47] In 2.1.1 Paul "fasted for three days and asked of the Lord what was right for him," and he received a vision instructing him to go to Spain.[48] Paul is described as contending with the Jewish teachers, teaching that Christ had "abolished their sabbath and fasts and festivals and circumcision and he abolished the doctrines of men and the other traditions."[49] After an apostasy, some faithful members of the church in Rome fasted and mourned awaiting the arrival of Peter, while Peter himself fasted aboard the ship on his voyage there (*Acts Pet.* 2.2.5). Peter "fasted for three days and prayed" in response to a crime of a wicked Simon, and was rewarded with a vision of the true nature of the crime, whereupon he urged the people to fast and pray yet again (*Acts Pet.* 2.6.17-18).[50] In preparation before Peter was forced to face Simon in the forum, he "continued (in prayer) tasting nothing, but fasting, that he may overcome the wicked enemy and persecutor of the Lord's truth," and his companions received encouraging visions of success (*Acts Pet.* 2.7.22).[51]

In a manner similar to the *Acts of John* and *Acts of Paul* above, the *Acts of Peter* presents fasting as a powerful tool in the hands of early Christians faced with a hostile world. The apostles see themselves as members of a new community that has differentiated itself from the Jewish fasting practices, but they still fast and pray for guidance and visions. The Christians who produced these writings apparently saw fasting as a sacrificial action that accompanied the fervent prayer of the apostles and their companions, prompting God to respond with appropriate blessings and interventions on their behalf.

The Acts of Thomas: *The Ascetic, Idealized Apostle Fasts Serenely for the Sake of the Gospel.* The *Acts of Thomas* dates from the beginning of the third century, and was incorporated into the Manichean canon in place of the orthodox, canonical book of Acts.[52] The book stresses the ascetic life of its hero, Thomas, taking a somewhat hostile attitude toward worldly things. It portrays the apostle as "a wanderer and traveller [*sic*] who rescues souls for the army of the Great General and Athlete."[53] Thomas travels to India with a merchant, and on the way comes to a king's feast, but Thomas fasts, saying, "For something greater than food or drink am I come hither" (*Acts Thom.* 1.5).[54] When he settled in a city, his reputation was of one who traveled house to house preaching the gospel; "continually he fasts and prays, and eats only bread and salt, and his drink is water, and he wears one garment" (*Acts Thom.* 2.20).[55] Thomas fasted all night before the Lord's day and the celebration of the Eucharist. While he received gifts of food from well-wishers, "he himself continued in his fasting, for the Lord's day was about to dawn," and the passage goes on to say how he received a vision (*Acts Thom.* 2.29).[56] In speaking on meekness, temperance and holiness as the three heads that portray Christ; "for forty days and forty nights he fasted, tasting nothing. And he who observes it (temperance) shall dwell in it as a mountain" (*Acts Thom.* 9.86).[57]

The *Acts of Thomas* presents the hero as an idealized, ascetic apostle. He fasts regularly, living a life of austerity with a serene attitude for the sake of evangelism. This noble, if idealized, portrait of Thomas captures at least something of how many in the early church viewed fasting. Its heroes were champions of humility, and fasting was a component in showing how far they could go in renouncing worldliness for the sake of the Kingdom of God.

- Pseudo-Clementine Literature: Fasting Associated with Rituals of Baptism, Lent, and Stations

The Pseudo-Clementine literature consists of texts attributed to Clement of Rome, but that probably came into existence around the beginning of the 4th century or up to a few decades before.[58] In the *Ps.-Cl. Homilies* 35 there is an instruction that those who are going to be baptized should fast three days, but this section is possibly an Ebionite insertion because of its later references to James.[59] *Ps.-Clem. Hom.* 13.9-12 has instructions that purport to go back to Peter. The children of Simon the magician beg for their mother to be baptized, and Peter commands her to fast the day before. She already had been fasting for joy for two days anyway. But Peter still required another day, and he and the others joined in this fast.[60]

The *Apostolical Constitutions* require the one being baptized to first fast,

> for even the Lord, when He was first baptized by John, and abode in the wilderness, did afterward fast forty days and forty nights. But he was baptized, and then fasted, not having Himself any need of cleansing, or of fasting, or of purgation, who was by nature pure and holy; but that He might testify the truth to John, and afford an example to us (*Apos. Con.* 7.22).[61]

Similarly, the Pseudo-Clementine *Recognitions* that mention fasting are also in contexts having to do with baptismal instruction.[62]

The next chapter of the *Apostolical Constitutions* goes on to teach concerning what days to fast. Similarly to *Did.* 8.1, *Apos. Con.* 7.23 says to fast either:

> ... the entire five days, or on the fourth day of the week, and on the day of the preparation, because on the fourth day the condemnation went out against the Lord, Judas then promising to betray Him for money; and you must fast on the day of the preparation, because on that day the Lord suffered the death of the cross under Pontius Pilate.[63]

The only Sabbath to be observed by Christians in the year is the one before Easter, and that Christians Sabbath remembers Christ's burial with a fast. The Lenten fast of eating only bread, salt, herbs and water (though all who are able are asked to fast entirely on the day of preparation and the Sabbath) is commanded in *Apos. Con.* 5.13, 15, and 18-19, to be observed beginning on the second day of the week before Passover, broken after the day of preparation, then resumed for the Passover (for the sake of weeping for the Jews).[64] These fasts recall the words of Jesus, "When the bridegroom shall be taken away from them, in those days shall they fast" (Matt 9:15; Mark 2:20; Luke 5:35).

These texts further demonstrate the association of fasting with baptism, stations, and early Lenten practices, as well as the further distinction from Judaism. Although not genuinely going back to Clement, they do reflect practices that were generally a part of the practice of mainstream Christianity in the early centuries of the church. From this evidence it is clear that fasting was becoming thoroughly normalized into Christian rituals.

Fasting Texts in Select Church Fathers: Promoting and Defining Fasting

Fasting references in patristic literature become more numerous as time goes by. The significant contributions of selected authors will be examined, with the hope that a general picture of fasting and its theological associations in the mainstream Christian community will emerge.

First, references to fasting in Justin Martyr and Clement of Alexandria will be examined, to get a general sense of how early orthodox church leaders viewed fasting. Then four Church Fathers who wrote significant homilies about fasting will be examined, beginning with the earliest, Tertullian, who critiques orthodox fasting from his own more rigorous Montanist perspective. Basil the Great wrote important homilies that were influential in Eastern Orthodoxy, and Augustine likewise wrote on fasting and was so influential in Western Christianity. Finally, Leo the Great will be examined as a link to medieval, papal Roman Catholicism's approach to fasting. Fasting in the monastic tradition, which certainly overlaps the patristic era some, will be treated in its own category in the next chapter.

Through these fathers who developed fasting themes directly, it is hoped that a fair representation of patristic fasting can be seen from early to late periods, in both the East and West.[65] It is clear that these fathers promoted fasting, while defining and qualifying it for the faithful.

Justin Martyr: Fasting as Genuine Repentance, and Jewish Fasts Prefigured Christ

Justin Martyr (ca. 100-165) was an important early Christian apologist, and as his name suggests, martyr. In works dating from between A.D. 150-160, Justin mentions fasting in several places. In his *First Apology* 37 he defends the prophets, and quotes Isa 58:6-7 to argue that God prefers justice over rituals (including fasts).[66] In describing preparation for baptism, he says that Christians "pray and ask God with fasting for the remission of their past sins, while we pray and fast with them" (*First Apol.* 61.2.3).[67] He again cites Isaiah 58 in an extended quotation to urge Jews to humble their hearts before God, repent and become Christians: "In order to please God you must, therefore, learn to observe God's true fast" (*Dialogue with Trypho* 15).[68] He describes the Jewish Day of Atonement as a fast[69] that had to take place in Jerusalem, making a typology between the two goats offered and Christ. The goats refer to Christ's two advents, because at the first advent Christ suffered for the people's sins, but at the second advent the people will repent "and comply with that fast which Isaias prescribed" (*Dial. Tr.* 40.4-5).[70] He mentions the fasting of the Ninevites at the preaching of Jonah as a sign of the repentance that is needed by the Jews to accept Christ (*Dial. Tr.* 107.2.12).

Justin's statements on fasting, repentance, humility, and justice sound a familiar chord from the OT prophets. Justin uses these motifs in a direct challenge to Jews to turn to Christ, advancing themes present since the apostolic fathers. So for Justin, Christ fulfilled the OT promises typologically embedded in the fasting rituals of Judaism, and fasting ought to be a mark of the true humility that is required to come to Christ.

Clement of Alexandria: Fasting as a Christian Practice of Humility that Leads to Blessing

Writing around the beginning of the third century, Clement of Alexandria (ca. 155-ca. 220) mentions fasting on a few occasions.[71] He mentions the fasting of Esther when listing women who had attained high levels of spiritual perfection (*Strom.* 4.19). He cites Tob. 12:8, "Fasting with prayer is a good thing" (*Strom.* 6.12). He says that station fasts of the fourth and preparation days are practiced in order to help repel the temptations of covetousness and voluptuousness, because one must learn to abstain from pleasure to attain true spiritual knowledge (*Strom.* 7.12). He tells a story of a disciple of the Apostle John who had turned to a life of crime, but repented with serious prayers and fasting, and was restored (*Quis dives salv.* 42).[72] He lists numerous good works that may be performed by Christians, and recalls Isaiah 58 when discussing fasting to insure that truly good deeds must be prioritized above ritual (*Paed.*, or *The Instructor*, 3.12). Fasting is described as being done as preparation for baptism in *Exc. ex. Theod.* 83-85. This is because it is a time of fear and vulnerability, "since unclean spirits often go down into the water with some, and these spirits following and gaining the seal together with the candidate become impossible to cure for the future."[73] Therefore fasting is part of the purification ritual before baptism, which is thought to parallel

Christ's fasting in the desert following his baptism, in preparation to meet temptation. Since food is a source of earthly life and absence of food symbolizes death, Christians fast to show they have died to the world so that their souls might live, even as Jesus said, "Blessed are those who hunger and thirst after righteousness, for they shall be filled."[74]

While there is nothing particularly extraordinary about these comments on fasting, they do seem to represent a kind of general approach to fasting that can be felt in most of the orthodox Church Fathers. Fasting must be humble, and it is secondary to deeds of justice for one's neighbor. It is formally associated with church rituals like baptism and the station fasts, and these are done for the spiritual purposes of purification and combating the flesh. These kinds of actions please God, and he will bless those who do them from a sincere heart.

Tertullian: Fasting Is a Key Component in Christian Life
and Ritual, and Disciplines the Flesh to Obey the Spirit

Tertullian (ca. 160-225) is an important link to early Christian fasting attitudes and practices. He clearly valued fasting, both during his days as an orthodox Christian as well as during his time as an apologist for the even stricter fasting regimens of the Montanists. A variety of references to fasting will be examined below, with special attention paid to his influential treatise *On Fasting*.

- Various Incidental References: Fasting as a Key Component in Christian Life and Ritual

There are a number of incidental references to fasting in his writings from his orthodox years, in which he cites a variety of reasons and occasions for fasting. In his treatise *On Baptism* he mentions that candidates for baptism "ought to pray with frequent prayers, fastings, and bowings of the knee, and long watchings, and with confession of all their past sins, that they may shew forth even the baptism of John."[75] Although Jesus fasted after his baptism for forty days, his fast was for strength when under temptation, and the candidate for baptism now finds his position in the reverse, so that victory and rejoicing come with baptism after the time of penitence and temptation is over. He also urges people to "cherish prayer by fasts, to groan, to weep, and to moan day and night unto the Lord his God" as part of confession:

> Wherefore confession is a discipline for the abasement and humiliation of man, enjoining such conversation as inviteth mercy; it directeth also even in the matter of dress and food, to

lie in sackcloth and ashes, to hide his body in filthy garments, to cast down his spirit with mourning, to exchange for severe treatment the sins which he hath committed.[76]

He considered fasting an act of the operation of patience in the body, which would strengthen prayer and "open the ears of Christ our God."[77] Fasting ought to be hidden, in line with Jesus' teaching in Matthew 6, so the kiss of peace should not be withdrawn during a fast lest we show ourselves to be fasting (except in the case of the Paschal Day, in which case all are fasting and so the kiss of peace is not passed).[78] During "Fasts and Stations no prayer must be observed without kneeling, and the other usual modes of humiliation."[79] In describing why a woman cannot be a Christian and married to a heathen, he says that she would not be able to observe fasts and stations, as well as so many other Christian duties, as the Lord would want her to do.[80]

So in these references, we see that Tertullian advocated fasting as part of prayer, confession and repentance. Also, it is clear that the church of his day was incorporating fasting into rituals surrounding baptism, and practicing the station fasts mentioned already in the *Shepherd of Hermas*.

- ### Tertullian's *On Fasting*: Fasting Disciplines the Flesh

The first extant extended Christian treatise about fasting is Tertullian's *De jejunio* (or *De ieiunio*), translated *On Fasting*, bearing the subtitle "In Opposition to the Psychics."[81] The treatise was written around A. D. 208, after Tertullian had sided with the Montanists against the Catholics. The Montanists were practicing various more rigid fasting rituals, including prolonged stations, "xerophagies," that is, dry diets that kept food unmoistened, abstinence from "winey flavour," and abstaining from the bath.[82] Tertullian begins with a frontal attack on gluttony and lust, which he believes are related due to the proximity of the belly and the sexual organs.[83] The "psychics" he attacks are those Catholics that he views as "materialists, men of the flesh."[84] Rufe writes, "To the Gnostics, 'psychics' were Christians who did not have the saving knowledge (γνῶσις) that freed the spirit imprisoned in the material body. To Tertullian, 'psychics' were Christians who had not embraced the strict self-discipline (ἐγκράτεια) deemed essential for salvation."[85]

Tertullian's orthodox opponents taught that the regulations of the OT were no longer binding, that the times of fasting were for when "the Bridegroom was taken away" (likely referring to the pre-Easter fast), and that other fasts (such as Wednesday and Friday stations) were matters of individual choice.[86] However, Tertullian's description of his opponents' position, which is intended to portray them as gluttonous and carnal, actually seems to have the effect of making them appear moderate and his own position in fact the novelty, the charge from which he is trying to vindicate himself.

For support, Tertullian begins with Adam, who became a "psychic" when he ate and fell: "He ate, in short, and perished; saved (as he would) else (have been), if he had preferred to fast from one little tree."[87] The curse of God then rested on food, and even if no other discussion of fasting ever occurred, this would be sufficient for Tertullian to "have habitually accounted food as poison, and taken the antidote, hunger; through which to purge the primordial cause of death."[88] This excessive statement suggests a problematic assignment of meritorious value to abstention from food, as if the material world were the spiritual problem of humanity.[89] But it also shows that the idea of fasting beginning in paradise with Adam and Eve has very ancient roots in Christian tradition.

According to Tertullian, God allowed a widening of allowable foods after the flood, because man had proven himself unable to keep even the lightest commands. The law of Moses then restricted more food usage, as God revealed to his people, whom he was restoring, more of the nature of their need for abstinence.[90] Moses and Elijah are held up as examples, as are other OT instances of fasting.[91] In the NT, Anna is a positive example, as is the fasting of Jesus in the wilderness after his baptism and before his temptations:

> By the virtue of contemning food He was initiating 'the new man' into 'a severe handling' of 'the old,' that He might show that (new man) to the devil, again seeking to tempt him by means of *food*, (to be) too strong for the whole power of hunger.[92]

As evidence for xerophagies, he cites Daniel and his friends abstaining from wine, as well as Paul's instruction to Timothy to take a little wine for his stomach (1 Tim 5:23) as a reverse evidence of Timothy's devoted abstinence: "from which he was abstaining not from rule, but from devotion—else the custom would rather have been beneficial to his stomach—by this very fact he has advised abstinence from wine as 'worthy of God,' which, on a ground of *necessity*, he has *dissuaded*."[93] He uses some strained argumentation from Peter's experience in Acts 10 over which hours to end a station fast,[94] concluding in favor of a longer fast that requires more rigor. The rigors of fasting would help prepare one to face suffering and martyrdom, "the soul herself withal now hastening (after it), having already, by frequent fasting, gained a most intimate knowledge of death!"[95]

Tertullian finally seeks to place the Montanists in moderate ground, rejecting the charge that he was guilty of the Galatian heresy by assigning that to the Jews. He notes that Montanists practice their xerophagies only two weeks of the year, excepting Sabbaths and Lord's days. He says they are "abstaining from things which we do not *reject*, but *defer*."[96] He cites Rom 14:17, asking the Catholics who they are to judge another's servant. Since the eating of food is of no great consequence to Paul, it should be thought a good thing to abstain.

Self-indulgence is a great sin, and even the pagans observe fasts, in devilish imitation of the truth. Devotees of Isis and Cybele fast similarly to the Montanists, which Tertullian admits:

> It is out of truth that falsehood is built; of religion that superstition is compacted. Hence *you* are more irreligious, in proportion as a heathen is more conformable. He, in short, sacrifices his appetite to an idol-god; *you* to (the true) God will not. For to you your belly is god, and your lungs a temple, and your paunch a sacrificial altar, and your cook the priest, and your fragrant smell the Holy Spirit, and your condiments spiritual gifts, and your belching prophecy.[97]

As Tertullian concludes, he contrasts his way with the epicureans, and says that the Montanists do not hesitate manfully to command,

> "Let us fast, brethren and sisters, lest tomorrow perchance we die." Openly let us vindicate our disciplines. Sure we are that "they who are in the flesh cannot please God;" not of course, those who are in the *substance* of the flesh, but in the *care*, the *affection*, the *work*, the *will*, of it. Emaciation displeases not us; for it is not by weight that God bestows flesh, any more than He does "the Spirit by measure." More easily, it may be, through the "strait gate" of salvation will slenderer flesh enter; more speedily will lighter flesh rise; longer in the sepulchre will drier flesh retain its firmness.[98]

He ends with the note that athletes eat robustly, but the Christian's wrestling is not against flesh and blood. So perhaps dining sumptuously for bodily strength would help over-fed Christians be able to physically battle lions and bears—but when they meet them (in the arena of martyrdom), they would have been better off having practiced emaciation.

No doubt Tertullian's words and images are chosen for rhetorical effect, and one hopes that he does not believe in the literal truth about lighter flesh rising faster in the resurrection. Although one can see that Tertullian was flirting with heresy, one can also see from this discussion that his orthodox opponents did indeed practice fasting, though they did not enjoin it with as much discipline as the Montanists.

Basil the Great: Fasting is a Positive Virtue That Christians Should Welcome

St. Basil the Great (ca. 330-379), also known as Basil of Caesarea, was one of the famous fourth century Cappadocian fathers and archbishop of Caesarea. He is noted not only for his doctrinal contributions, but is also heralded as one of the most important figures in eastern monastic movements. He also wrote fasting homilies for Lent that have been influential in history, *About Fasting*, Sermons 1 and 2.[99] Although his writings on fasting stress themes of abstinence, Basil strives hard to turn the focus of fasting from the negative to the positive. He sees fasting as a positive Christian virtue, one that purifies body and soul. He believes that any spiritually minded Christian should welcome such an act, regarding it as an integral part of sanctification, which for Basil, is basically the process of salvation.

- Basil's Monastic *Rules*: Monks Should Fast for Positive Virtues

Basil wrote a good deal on asceticism and composed rules for monastic life, the most important of which are known as *The Longer Rules* and *The Shorter Rules*.[100] The *Longer Rules* consists of fifty-five questions with rather extended answers, while the *Shorter Rules* consists of 313 questions with rather brief answers.

Basil requires complete abstinence from all that is harmful, but as food needs differ from person to person, much latitude is allowed. But the stomach should not be full, and eating should be for necessity and not for pleasure. Monks should eat as little as possible to get by, and be satisfied with water to drink (*Longer Rules* 19).[101]

Basil rejected extreme forms of asceticism, yet sought to promote the virtues of abstinence and self-control, not to "protect one from what is evil but rather to purify one's disposition, mortify the passions and free the spirit from servitude to the flesh."[102] In actual practice for monks who followed these rules, Basil allowed for just one meal per day, so that "of all the twenty-four hours of the day and night barely this one may be spent upon the body. The rest the ascetic should spend in spiritual exercises."[103] While Basil frowns on competitive forms of asceticism, it is clear that he advocates austerity in bodily pleasures for the sake of spiritual attention.

Basil's *Longer Rules* do not concern themselves with fasting specifically, but the *Shorter Rules* 126-40 address the topic. In answer to the question, "How can a man avoid taking pleasure in eating?" Basil responds: "By taking as his criterion what is fitting and having it always as his guide and teacher as to what things should be taken for use, whether they are pleasant or unpleasant"(*Shorter Rules* 126).[104] From this it appears that monks were to try to avoid deriving pleasure from food, a rather tall order—although perhaps the pleasure to be avoided would be more of an excessive attachment, since Basil acknowledges that foods may indeed be "pleasant," urging rather a focus on fitting portions. When asked, "If a man wishes to practise abstinence beyond his strength so that he is hindered in fulfilling the commandment set before him, must we permit him so to do?" Basil responds:

> The question does not seem to me to be rightly framed. For abstinence consists not in refraining from material foods, whereby the severity to the body condemned by the apostle results, but in complete giving up of one's own will. But how great is the danger of falling from the Lord's commandment owing to one's own will is clear from the apostle's words: "Doing the desires of the flesh and of the thoughts, and we were by nature children of wrath."[105]

Since Jesus commanded that his disciples "appear not unto men to fast," the question is put to Basil of what someone should do, "when he is seen against his will." Basil responds:

> This precept applies to those who study to do the commandment of God to be seen of men, that they may cure the fault of men-pleasing. For that the commandment of the Lord, when done for God's glory, is by nature unfitted to be hidden from those that love God, the Lord showed when He said: "A city set on a hill cannot be hid. Neither do men light a lamp and set it under a bushel, etc."[106]

From these it is clear that Basil promoted fasting for its positive virtues, although he did not want to see abstinence become an end in itself. Jesus himself, he believed, commanded fasting, and therefore it should be practiced with proper motives. Monks in his tradition were expected to be disciplined in body and spirit, in order that they might more readily be pleasing to God in doing his will.

- Basil's Homilies *About Fasting*: Welcome the Sanctifying Virtue of Fasting Between the Times

Basil's authentic, extant sermons on the subject of fasting are known as *De jejunio 1* and *De jejunio 2*.[107] (There is a third homily on fasting in the Basilian corpus, but it is universally regarded as inauthentic.)[108] Unfortunately they are not readily available in English, and so a fresh translation has been undertaken, and can be found in the appendix. These English translations will be referred to as *About Fasting 1 and 2*. The only available English translation that the author has found, and that of only the first homily, is a translation by Reginald Cardinal Pole, who appended a translation of it to his *Treatie of Iustification* in 1569.[109] Needless to say, the English there is rather antiquated in style, although it was done well.

Basil's homilies focus on the sanctifying virtues of fasting, and in the following discussion the main themes he presents will be examined. He establishes the need for fasting, and calls his parishioners to willingly participate in the Lenten fast. Basil traces the origins of fasting to paradise, and cites numerous biblical examples as models. He names spiritual, physical, domestic and societal benefits of fasting to encourage his people to engage in the practice. And finally, he keeps a theological focus on the eschatological basis for fasting.

The Need for the Sanctifying Virtue of Fasting. Basil approaches fasting as a sanctifying, virtuous act. Preached at the beginning of Lent on a feast day, Basil urges that the time of joy should merge seamlessly into the time of fasting. So the season remembers Christ's suffering and passion, but that is a positive thing, one that works salvation in our souls, in anticipation of our glorification. Basil stresses the positive role of fasting like a preacher who knows he has to turn a disagreeable subject for his congregation into a palatable one. He cites Jesus' command in Matt 6:16-17 not to look gloomy-faced, and urges his congregation to happily embrace fasting:

> Therefore let's agree, as it has been taught, that we won't be looking gloomy on the days that are approaching, but we will cheerfully, agreeably look forward to them, as is fitting for saints. No one is passionless when he is receiving a victory crown! No one is gloomy when a victory monument is being erected for him. Don't make being healed gloomy![110]

Similarly, the second sermon begins with Basil comparing his role as a priest to a general giving a rousing speech to his troops before battle, and a trainer urging his athletes to exert themselves in the games: "And so it is now with me. The soldiers of Christ have been ordered to war against invisible enemies, and the athletes of godliness are preparing themselves for crowns of righteousness through self-control. So the word of exhortation is indispensable."[111] By Basil's day, the Lenten fast was widespread and considered obligatory, though only five days long.[112] He says that "all around the world the proclamation is being announced. There isn't any island, land, city, nation, or remotest border where they haven't heard of the proclamation."[113] Yet it appears that church leaders felt it necessary to remind the faithful of their duties, since many obviously observed the fast less than whole-heartedly. Basil calls heaven to witness against them, urging them not to be deserters in this spiritual warfare: "The angels are writing down the names of those who fast in each church. See to it that you don't forfeit the angelic register through a little pleasurable food, and make yourself liable as a deserter, since you have been enlisted as a soldier by the scriptures."[114]

The Origins of Fasting. The origins of fasting are not to be found in the Jewish law, but fasting has the most venerable of histories, being the first command in Paradise: "Fasting is as old as mankind itself. It was given as a law in paradise. The first commandment Adam received was: 'From the tree of the knowledge of good and evil do not eat.' Now this command, 'do not eat,' is the divine law of fasting and temperance."[115] Abstaining from the tree of the knowledge of good and evil was a command to Adam and Eve to fast, before sin ever entered the human race. Humanity could have been like the angels, partakers of divinity. But with their failure to keep the appointed fast came the curse of pain and toil, and Basil quips: "If Eve had fasted from the tree, we would not have to keep this fast now."[116] Commenting on this theme of fasting to restore paradise, Franco Beatrice writes:

> We must conclude by saying that also the interpretation of ascetical fasting as a remedy for the Fall and as the best means of re-opening Paradise is an integral part of the Asiatic theology which was deeply rooted and widely diffused in broad sectors of the early church.[117]

In fact, Augustine would refer to this passage in Basil and the broader theme of fasting to regain paradise in his struggle against the Pelagians, because he found it useful to defend the doctrine of original sin.[118]

Biblical Examples of Fasting. Basil engages a good deal in what Musurillo referred to as citing "exempla," characters from sacred history that are used to illustrate the desired fasting principles, positively or negatively.[119] Noah, although he got drunk, is excused, because he was ignorant of the potency of wine, and after the great flood man's food regimen was altered away from the ideals of paradise. Moses fasted forty days and received the divine law, but it was for naught, as the people ruined the results of this fast with one night of drunken debauchery.[120] Esau threw away his birthright for a single meal, the glutton! By contrast, Hannah conceived the prophet Samuel because of fasting. Likewise Samson's parents conceived him in fasting, and he was nurtured to manhood and great strength through fasting regimens of the Nazirites. Elijah received his beatific vision of God after fasting, and he and Elisha performed great exploits related to their fasting and austere lifestyles. The three Hebrew children escaped the fiery furnace because fasting had turned their bodies into inflammable substances.[121] Likewise, lions could not eat Daniel, because they "weren't able to sink their teeth into him. Fasting is like sharpening the edges of a man by dipping his body in iron—it makes him tougher than lions! They couldn't open their mouths against the saint." So "when he was thrown down in their den, he taught the lions to fast!"[122]

The rich man and Lazarus provide sharp contrasts of luxury and poverty and the results. Speaking of the rich man: "You should be afraid of the example of the rich man. That which is delightful throughout life cast him into the fire. It wasn't unrighteousness, but delicate living that accused him, roasted him in the flames of the furnace." And referring to Lazarus, "What was it that caused Lazarus to wake up in the bosom of Abraham? Wasn't it fasting?"[123] John the Baptist renounced the normal pleasures of this life, and Paul fasted and suffered many things for the sake of the gospel.[124]

But above all, Jesus fasted, teaching us to follow his example before facing temptations: "But above all that has been said, our Lord took flesh and fortified it with fasting on behalf of us. Then in that condition he welcomed the assault of the devil, teaching us to anoint and to train ourselves with fastings before struggling with temptations."[125] While he was fasting, he could welcome the attack of the devil, and in his ascended, resurrected body he could show what real food, real nourishment was all about.

In these illustrations, Basil shows his keen awareness of biblical history, as well as his rhetorical skill and communicative flair.[126] Basil connects fasting with the spiritual power evidenced by these biblical characters, and calls his parishioners to imitate them.

The Spiritual Benefits of Fasting. The spiritual benefits of fasting commend the practice to any Christian. Basil chides his listeners for their willingness to prefer their stomachs over their souls. Fasting is like medicine that can kill the noxious worm of sin. Faces are darkened to obscure hypocrisy, like actors who wear masks. Rather, Christians should "run to greet the cheerful gift of the fast."[127] The Spirit and the flesh are adversaries, and "just like when one army defeats the other, the flesh is handed over to the conquering spirit, and the spirit is changing the rank of the flesh to slavery."[128] All of the passions need to be kept in check by fasting, because anger, lust, and greed can have the same general effects as drunkenness: "For as smoke drives away bees, intoxication drives away the spiritual gifts."[129] So fasting is seen as spiritually purifying, enabling the worshiper to enter into the presence of God in a holy state: "The Lord admits the one who is fasting inside the walls of holy places, but he doesn't approve of extravagance, he regards that as profane and unholy."[130] Fasting must be done with the right motives, and be accompanied by righteous living. If the believer approaches fasting that way, spiritual blessings and joy can be expected:

> Let's fast in an acceptable manner, one that's pleasing to God. A true fast is one that is set against evil, it's self-control of the tongue. It's the checking of anger, separation from things like lusts, evil-speaking, lies, and false oaths. Self-denial from these things is a true fast, so fasting from these negative things is good. But on the positive side, let's delight in the Lord, being in pursuit of the words of the Spirit. And let's delight in taking up the laws of salvation, and in all the doctrines that restore our souls.[131]

The Physical Benefits of Fasting. Fasting in this life is good for the body as well as the soul, keeping a person from being overburdened with food, making him like "the boat in stormy weather that goes right over a dangerous rock."[132] Even animals are healthier when on a plain diet, and people should consider fasting a healthy way to live.[133] The water that replaces wine during the fast is superior, because "No one ever got a hangover from water. No head ever ached because it was burdened with water."[134] Fasting heightens the anticipation of food, making regular meals taste better.[135] Fasting even brings a healthy complexion and pleasant demeanor, and the inner senses come alive.[136]

Domestic and Societal Benefits of Fasting. Fasting has domestic benefits as well. The household servants get to rest when the members of the house are fasting, so give them a break, Basil urges.[137] Wives and husbands are less suspicious of each other when they see each other fasting—after all, if one can abstain from eating, surely one can abstain from sexual immorality that would destroy the marriage.[138] From the familiar refrain of Isaiah 58, Basil urges his listeners to fast consistently with matters of justice.[139] The fast benefits the city as well: "But how is our public life in this society? The entire city has come together, and the entire region adopts good conduct, puts to sleep the shouting, gets rid of quarrels, and silences insults."[140] In fact, in rather grandiose fashion, Basil envisions that fasting could be the means to world peace and the end of social ills!:

> If only everyone who needs a counselor would take her in, there would be nothing preventing a deep peace from abiding in each house. Nations wouldn't be attacking each other, and armies wouldn't be engaging in battle. Neither would weapons be forged, if fasting ruled. There would be no point in holding court, prisons would be unpopulated, and evildoers wouldn't

have a place to hide. If slanderers were found in the cities, they would be thrown into the sea.[141]

The Eschatological Dimension of Fasting. In the conclusion of his first homily, Basil highlights the christocentric, eschatological place of fasting for the Christian. He asks the congregation, "So, do you know whom you are about to receive? He who promised us, that 'I myself, and the Father, we will come and make our home with him.'"[142] In addition to the Father and the Son, the Holy Spirit wants to come in, so the people should be sober, because "drunkenness chases away the Holy Spirit."[143] He urges that the fasting days should be as joy-filled as the current feast day, and he hopes that feasting will have the same dignity as fasting. But the people should remember that they participate in the upcoming fast days "as competitors in these preliminary contests," as the Christian looks forward to the final Day of Judgment.[144] Previously, Basil had already mentioned that fasting prepares us for the heavenly banquet table in the Kingdom of God. Conversely, there is an eschatological warning for gluttons. The rich man (Luke 16) was condemned to hell for his luxurious lifestyle, while Lazarus went to Abraham's bosom because he knew what fasting was like.[145]

To conclude his second homily, he says that "Wisdom" has prepared a spiritual feast, a "wineless bowl." So fasting becomes a spiritual feast, and then he alludes to Jesus' words in that theologically important fasting passage in Matt 9:15, Mark 2:19, and Luke 5:34: "Once we have thoroughly taken our fill, may we also be found worthy of the exhilaration that comes in the bridal chamber of Christ Jesus our Lord!"[146] The fasting of this age will consummate in the spiritual feasting of the eschatological age, when the bride of Christ enters his bridal chamber.

Believers are lodged between the times of Christ's passion that is being remembered and the final day of recompense. This age, for Basil, is a time for fasting and spiritual feasting, both positive virtues working together to sanctify the believer. This attitude recalls the paradise from which we have fallen, the salvation that has been brought about in Christ, and looks forward in anticipation of the consummation of the ages.

Augustine: Fasting to Defeat Temptation and to Create Capacity for Love and Good Works

Augustine of Hippo (354-430) was the perhaps the most important Latin church father. He mentions fasting in numerous places in his writings, and also devotes an important homily to the subject. Robert P. Kennedy says that for Augustine, fasting has two basic functions, (1) ascetical and (2) spiritual or ecstatic.[147] Ascetical fasting has to do with fighting temptation and gaining mastery over desire. Spiritual fasting aids the mind in transcending earthly realities for heavenly ones, creating a greater capacity for love and good works. While fasting is a profitable discipline, there may be community diversity in its practice. It is not an end in itself but a means of developing "our capacity for contemplation of God and service to the church."[148]

- Various References: Fasting Aids the Christian in the Struggle Against the World and to Be Like Christ

Augustine clearly believed in abstaining from worldly pleasures. He mentions in his *Confessions* 10.31 that he fights against the sweetness of earthly pleasures with fasting, because he has come to view food as a necessary medicine for sustaining life rather than existing for enjoyment. In what is perhaps his longest sermon, *Discourse of Augustine the Bishop Against the Pagans* (which may have lasted three hours), he filibusters on New Year's Day 404 to keep his congregation in church and away from the pagan festivities going on in the streets outside.[149] Apparently, it was customary to observe fast days in the church during pagan feast days: "We regularly say that fasting is to be practiced during these festive days of the pagans, precisely as a kind of prayer to God for the pagans themselves," but unfortunately it seemed that Christians were just as willing to participate.[150] He says the Lord was figuratively fasting in not taking the godless into his body, as he was fasting from the fruitless tree that he cursed.[151] In an echo of *Did.* 1.3, he urges his people to fast for the Gentiles. He chastises them for going without food while they gamble on games, when the church asks such a small thing of them as fasting on January first. This custom apparently was divisive in the congregation, as some wished to regard it as a feast day.[152] Some Christians were so caught up in pagan frivolities that the faithful congregation ought to fast on behalf of the large number of these wayward brethren as well. Christian feast days should be more like a letting up of fasting, rather than like the pagan revelry around them.[153] Toward the end of his fiery sermon, he ties prayer, almsgiving and fasting together, saying that they will reach Christ if done in sincerity, because Christ made himself poor for us, he fasted for our sakes, and prayed for us and forgave our sins.[154]

Augustine annually preached a "solemn exhortation" at the beginning of the Lenten fast, to feed the minds of his people as they set about chastising the body and making a cross of the pleasures of the flesh.[155] As Moses, Elijah and Jesus fasted forty days, so Lent is celebrated for forty days; but what is signified in Lent should last through the whole of the year. All year one should abstain from sin, but during this time one should abstain even from some of that which is good, such as food and marriage partners. Ascetics might fast on other days of the year as well, and they should add to those fasts during Lent. Delicacies should not be merely rearranged by eating or drinking unusual things, because that would be a mere pretense of self-denial.[156] But above all, one should fast from quarrels, and do justice in line with Isaiah 58.[157] This theme of doing justice and fasting is echoed again and again, and when these virtues are practiced, prayers will fly more readily to heaven.[158]

In a sermon dating from A.D. 420-25, Augustine says that almsgiving is:

> ... a practice which with holy and faithful men customarily goes along with fasting, so that what is subtracted from the one who has may be added to the one who has not. This is the way to cheat your soul to your own profit; to place firmly in heaven what you take away from the flesh.[159]

Here Augustine ties the ascetic value of fasting to the classic acts of righteousness of Matthew 6, and the early church's connection of fasting with deeds of social justice is continued. This use of the acts of righteousness is a repeated theme in Augustine's work, especially his Lenten sermons. For instance, he says,

> And so let us perform our alms and deeds of kindness all the more lavishly, all the more frequently the nearer the day approaches on which is celebrated the alms, the kindness that has been done to us. Because fasting without kindness and mercy is worth nothing to the one who's fasting.[160]

The almsgiving ties in with the theme of social justice, and together sincere, virtuous lives of righteousness show one to be acceptable to God, and thus prayers go unhindered to heaven—and so the link with Isaiah 58 and Matthew 6 is made complete.

Augustine explains the calendar cycle of Lenten fasting and Easter baptism, like Tertullian, as being a kind of inverse of Christ's experience.[161] Since in baptism a Christian strips off the old, flesh-bound life, it is most appropriate (though any day of the year might be acceptable) to be baptized on Easter, the day of Christ's resurrection. There is no special merit in the day, but the majority of people seeking baptism converge on that day due to the greater joy of the feast. But it must be remembered that Christ's baptism differs from John's; Christ received John's baptism, Christians receive Christ's. So Christians do not necessarily need to fast after baptism, as Christ did. Rather, like Christ, we should fast when faced with temptation, and the period of Lent, and before one's baptism, symbolizes that. Fasting during Lent is a humbling of oneself. The bridegroom has been taken away, and we have to mourn

(Matt 9:15-17; Ser. 210.4). He echoes Tertullian's "let us fast and pray, for tomorrow we shall die."[162] During the fifty days of Pentecost the fast is lifted for the joy of the resurrection.[163] He urged more frequent fasts for those who were able. He also noted that total abstinence from food is impossible, but the same is not true of sex. He says, "I don't think it's asking too much to suggest that married chastity can do for the whole paschal solemnity what virginity can do for the whole of life."[164]

Apparently the act of fasting could be viewed as a kind of punishment, perhaps in connection with the idea of penance for sin. In discussing the reality of original sin in even infants, he mentions the example of Ninevite children being required to enter into fasting and prayers of repentance, and finds Jerome (and all of orthodox history) in agreement with him.[165] In describing the kind of righteousness that is possible while away from the presence of the Lord, he goes to the acts of righteousness of Matthew 6, almsgiving, fasting and prayer. He says:

> By fasting he meant, of course, the whole chastisement of the body. By almsgiving he meant every instance of good will and every good deed, whether in giving or in forgiving, and by prayer he suggested all the forms of holy desire. The chastisement of the body holds in check that concupiscence which ought to be not merely held in check, but ought not to exist at all and will not exist in that perfection of righteousness in which there will be no sin whatsoever.[166]

Augustine cites Basil's sermon on fasting (which he notes that he translated himself from the Greek to gain more exact fidelity to the original), and notes that the command to Adam not to eat from the tree implied fasting.[167] Because Eve did not fast, we fell from paradise. Now we must fast so that we may return to it. He uses this passage from Basil to show that Basil was in agreement that the healthy do not need a physician, but the sick, and that because of the original sin in paradise, humanity is fallen.[168]

In his list of heresies, he mentions the Aerians, followers of a bishop Aerius who fell in with the Arians and added some of his own teachings. He taught that "the solemnly prescribed fasts should not be observed, but that each one should fast as he wishes so that he does not seem to be under the law."[169] A monk, Jovinian, taught that all sins are equal, and that once one has been baptized into regeneration, fasting and abstinence from foods were of no value. He also taught that chaste marriage was of equal merit with celibacy, which was considered heretical and stamped out.[170]

Augustine makes an analogy between sexual desire and the desire for food, saying that a Christian can put up with the desire for food so long as it does not overtake him. Nevertheless, it should be fought against by fasting and eating less than is desired, because it is a fallen desire that wars against what is good in the spirit. Sexual desire is even more hazardous, because one might still enjoy conversation and rationality while enjoying food, but engaging in sex often causes couples to be totally given over to bodily passions. Augustine thinks this is something wiser Christian couples would even want to give up, if they could.[171]

Franz Cremer notes that Augustine's comments on the synoptic fasting query places the Christian in a temporal continuum, after the mournful fasting of the old covenant, and in the new covenant that fasts in joy in anticipation of knowing and being like Christ. Cremer says that Augustine's approach to fasting in these passages can be characterized by the contrast between "Trauer und Freude," or "sadness and joy."[172] Christ has turned our mourning into gladness with his appearing, so for Augustine, Christian fasting could no longer signify mourning in the redemptive-historical sense. This appears to be a creative theological exegesis of the text, one that over-realizes the eschatology inherent there. But at least there is present in Augustine an awareness of the eschatological turn of the ages, which for him connects to the joy of being like Christ.

On the whole, these passages show Augustine to be committed to fasting, yet clearly in the context of Christians willingly giving themselves over to Christ. Ritual acts like fasting are valuable, but they must be understood as means to an end. Worldliness is all around the Christian, and fasting will help to learn to avoid it. There is perhaps an underlying aversion to the material world that affects his understanding of fasting, which results in some devaluation of the goodness of the creation as given to us by God. While the tone seems a bit more negative than that of Basil's examined above, it is clear that Augustine wants to use fasting to promote Christ-likeness. The next sermon to be examined makes that even more clear.

- *On the Value of Fasting*: Christians Caught Between Heaven and the World Must Tame the Flesh

Among the voluminous works of Augustine is a sermon, *On the Value of Fasting*.[173] This sermon might be dated to Lent or some other fast day, perhaps around AD 411 or 412.[174] In *Value of Fasting* 1 he calls fasting a "strengthening of the spirit, this cheating of the flesh and profiting of the mind."[175] The angels do not observe fasting, for in heaven they are filled with God. People in the flesh must eat food, but the incarnation came about for the purpose of giving heavenly food to humanity: "Christ instructed us to hunger for this food, when he said, 'Blessed are those who hunger and thirst for justice, since they shall be satisfied (Mt 5:6).'"[176] In being hungry, people stretch themselves, are enlarged, increase their capacity, and in due time are filled (a reference to eschatological bliss). This is the perspective of Paul, who may seem to be so great, yet he considered himself not yet to have attained, but was striving after the goal (Phil 3:13-14).

Value of Fasting 2 goes on to say that there are people of faith who occupy a middle ground, between the angelic realm of perfect obedience and fleshly, carnal people who think the only good is earthly delight. By this middle course he means not some specialized caste of holy Christians, but rather, the calling of all Christians (though his neoplatonic approach is clearly in view). The flesh drags the believer down toward the earth, but the spiritual mind is being drawn up toward heaven (and here he cites Wis 9:15):

> For the body which is being corrupted weighs down the soul, and the earthly dwelling oppresses the mind thinking many things (Wis 9:15). So if the flesh, inclining to the earth, is a load on the soul, and a burden weighing down the soul as it tries to fly ahead; the more you delight in your higher life, the more ready you are to lay down your earthly burden. There you have what we are doing when we fast.[177]

He compares the flesh to a horse he must ride to "Jerusalem," and it must be tamed by regulating its rations. Otherwise the horse might gain control, and run off the course, which is the way of Christ.[178] While the flesh wars against the spirit (Gal 5:17), that should not be understood to mean that the flesh itself has an evil origin (as the Manichees think), since God made them both and everyone loves his own flesh.[179] Rather, "there is a kind of marriage between flesh and spirit."[180] From Adam we derived the flesh, and because it is fallen, something to be overcome. But the flesh is subordinate to the Lord in all cases, though not in all cases to the individual person. So God uses the flesh to train a Christian, and likewise the Christian trains the flesh to be obedient, like a slave. Temperate people abstain even from lawful pleasures, so as not to cross the line into those that are unlawful.[181]

At this point in the sermon, Augustine begins to digress into a lesson about church unity. Pagans, Jews and heretics might fast, but unless fasts are properly directed toward God, they are rejected, and fall under the words of Isa 58:4-5.[182] This points toward the unity and supremacy of the body of Christ, and the fasting of the church ought to promote that unity, though sometimes pagan worship puts Christian worship to shame.[183] The heretics have rejected Christian unity, but Augustine calls them back like a loving son who dutifully tries to rouse his father from a dying slumber even when he prefers to die. Since God will never die, we cannot divide up his inheritance among his children.[184]

- Augustine's Monastic Rule: Subduing the Flesh to Restore Internal Order

After his conversion, Augustine engaged in a lifestyle that might be described as monastic for a time in Thagaste, and later as Bishop of Hippo wrote rules for a monastery there, which have continued to guide Augustinian communities to the present.[185] In his *Rule* 3.1 he urges fasting and abstinence practices for the community: "To the extent that your health allows, subdue your flesh by fasting and abstinence from food and drink. If anyone is unable to fast, let him at least take no food between meals, unless he is sick."[186] Along with his neoplatonic philosophical bent, Augustine's experiences with worldly pleasures in his youth affected him deeply, and his reaction to this in his maturity no doubt drives a good deal of his desire for asceticism.[187] The verb translated above as "subdue," from the Latin *domo/domare*, means "discipline" your flesh, and is used primarily of breaking in an animal for riding.[188] It is a moderate word without harshness, and "implies understanding, moderation, courage, perseverance, and, above all, a striving for unity and harmony."[189] This kind of discipline flows from Augustine's previous rules on self-giving and prayer, to stretch his followers to greater capacities. Sister Agatha Mary writes:

> To dispossess ourselves of rank, money, goods, and the like is one thing; but dispossession of nourishment above a basic minimum is to place ourselves entirely at God's disposal. As Augustine says, it is not for us to go beyond the degree of tolerance that our body has, but voluntarily to live on the borderline is an act of great courage. It is in this area that the asceticism of the eastern monastic tradition finds expression in the West.[190]

The order of creation was disturbed in the fall, and self-denial helps Christians to restore proper order in their hearts.[191] Reading takes place all through meals, because "Food is not for the mouth alone; your ears also should hunger for the Word of God."[192] Special food might be given to some due to illness, but on recovery this should not continue, lest they become enslaved to pleasure. When putting up with privations, the members should consider themselves richer, "For it is better to need less than to have more."[193] It is worth observing that while Augustine urges fasting, he did not prescribe specific days, or forbid certain foods, but rather left the details up to local communities to apply.[194]

So even in his *Rule*, Augustine clearly grounds fasting practices in his understanding of the body in the world. The need for restoration of order and mastery over the primitive desires seems to dominate in this conception of sanctification as struggle against the world and the flesh. It is clear that fasting could play a significant role in such a theology.

Leo the Great: Fasting as the Link Between God and Neighbor

Leo the Great (d. 461) was Bishop of Rome from 440-61, and he garnered a good deal of authority for the papacy. He preached a number of sermons related to fasting coinciding with the fasts of the church calendar that have been translated into English.[195] Leo's work forms something of a bridge between the previous Church Fathers and medieval Roman Catholicism, and so it is very much worth examining his writings on fasting.

Leo takes the three themes of almsgiving, prayer, and fasting from the Sermon on the Mount (Matt 6:1-18) and orders their sequence logically into prayer, fasting, and almsgiving. These three actions form a paradigm for Leo for understanding Christian duty—to God, self, and others. In Sermon 12.4 he writes:

> For by prayer we seek to propitiate God, by fasting we extinguish the lusts of the flesh, by alms we redeem our sins: and at the same time God's image is throughout renewed in us, if we are always ready to praise Him, unfailingly intent on our purification and unceasingly active in cherishing our neighbour. This threefold round of duty, dearly beloved, brings all other virtues into action: it attains to God's image and likeness and unites us inseparably with the Holy Spirit. Because in prayer faith remains stedfast, in fastings life remains innocent, in almsgiving the mind remains kind.[196]

So then fasting is a kind of bridge: an aid to prayer in our relationship with God on the one hand, and an incentive to charity on the other. Fasting, then, occupies a central place, and the individual is purified internally for the obligations to God and neighbor, bringing the Christian's entire duty into focus. The one who fasts truly abstains from sins of the mind as well as pleasures of the body. By doing so, "he will be made pure and holy by true fasting, and will be fed upon the pleasures of incorruptible delights, and so he will know how, by the spiritual use of his earthly riches, to transform them into heavenly treasure" by sharing with those in need.[197] The Lenten fast "is imposed on all the faithful without exception; because no one is so holy that he ought not to be holier, nor so devout that he might not be devouter."[198]

Reginald Cardinal Pole used Leo's emphases during the Counter-reformation as a foundation for understanding the relationship between faith and works. In his *Treatie of Iustification* he argues for the need of grace on the one hand, and the need for penance and good works in the salvation process on the other. To his treatise he appended fresh English translations of patristic sermons: Augustine's *Of Faith and Works*, Chrysostom's *Of Praying unto God*, Basil's *Of Fasting*, several sermons by Leo on fasting, and Cyprian's *Of Almesdeedes*. These sermons were used to support Pole's thesis of the need for joining faith and works in justification. While fasting itself plays only a minor role in the text of the treatise, it is obvious that Pole felt that fasting was an integral part of demonstrating true repentance (or "doing penance" as the Catholic literature tends to render the term). Christ's admonitions from the Sermon on the Mount linked prayer, fasting, and almsgiving as "acts of righteousness," so it is not surprising that these components factor into such a discussion of justification, especially from the Catholic side which tended to emphasize the role of works in righteousness. Whether or not one agrees with Pole's particular approach to linking faith and works in the context of sacramental theology, one can at least appreciate the moderate and serious discussion of this important issue from his perspective. His work lacks some of the unseemly polemics so common to that period, as he attempts to steer a middle course as best he could. It also demonstrates that some of the Protestant positioning against Catholicism involved caricature of their positions, even as the Catholics tended to caricature the position of the Protestants as antinomian.

Alexandre Guillaume has thoroughly studied Leo's theology of fasting, and his work can be found in the French publication of his dissertation, its later expansion, and an abridgement.[199] Guillaume analyzes Leo's theology of fasting practice as proceeding from an attribute of God he designates *pietas*, that is, a covenantal, filial bond of devotion the Father has with the Son, which can be reciprocal with men as well.[200] The five main points Leo makes about fasting can be distilled as follows:

1. Christian fasting differs from the fasting of Jews and Manichees.

2. Fasting without the exercise of charity would not be true Christian fasting.

3. Fasting stands in the central place in the work of charity, as the hinge of purifying self, between relations with God and neighbor.

4. Fasting, as the source of almsgiving, is itself a work of charity, as it causes one to identify with the needs of others.

5. The efficacy of fasting depends on its expression of charity.[201]

Guillaume sums up Leo's view of fasting by saying that it is an expression of charity, an act of worship, a participation in the sacrifice of the cross, and a work that renders glory to God's divine charity.[202]

While Leo builds his approach to fasting on Scripture and previous church tradition, he clearly takes it some distance further in his thinking. The commendable aspect of fasting as an act of charity gives Guillaume hope for renewal of appropriate fasting practices in the present, which is reflected in recent papal statements as well as Vatican II.[203] But one can also see in Leo no-so-subtle shades of emphases on fasting that will guide medieval Catholic practice into something the Reformers came to reject. Most notably, these include the binding of all people to follow certain fasting practices and the view of fasting as an act of worship that earns a person saving merit before God. There appears to be a minimizing of the spiritual benefits of voluntary, sacrificial fasting in the daily life of the normal believer, since fasting was becoming so encouched in ritualized behavior. By the time of Leo, there is a theology of fasting, but its context has been split into two main arenas: the life of the faithful in the rituals of the church on the one hand, and the austerities of ascetic monks on the other which will be examined in more detail in the following chapter. This important development of fasting as prescribed behavior in the church needs more examination, and to that we now turn.

The Development of Official Church Fasting Practices: Formalizing Fasting into Seasonal and Liturgical Ritual

The teachings and traditions of the early church were formalized through various official church pronouncements. Often church councils are remembered for their important doctrinal controversies and decisions about those things that are central to orthodoxy. But it must be noted that church councils also often dealt with issues related to church practice, such as rituals and liturgy, that were very much considered by them to be part of orthodox Christianity. And so fasting practices came to be formalized through the gradual processes of church pronouncements that codified some traditions and rejected others. It is likely that as this happened, the voluntary aspect of fasting was largely lost for the bulk of the laity, replaced by seasons of prescribed and defined fasting practices.

Eucharistic Fasting: Requiring Purity to Partake of Christ

Christians in the early centuries developed their approach to the Eucharist with fasting concepts in mind. Occasionally small groups of Christians practiced the Eucharist with various elements (such as milk, honey, cheese, oil, salt, vegetables), the main reasons having to do with a bit of a blurred line between regular and ritual Christian meals, typical available foods, and symbolic meanings that might be attached to them.[204] Tied more closely to fasting practices in asceticism were some early Christians who practiced "ascetic Eucharists" of bread and water, a practice that was rejected in favor of the traditional elements of bread and wine. Some of these were heretics, like Marcion, or more orthodox ascetics, like Cyprian, who rejected the drinking of wine.[205] This tension can be seen in different recensions of the *Acts of Thomas*, where the earlier Greek edition has him asking for water for the Eucharist, but the later Syriac texts change this to wine, in line with later ecclesiastical mandate.[206]

That fasting was associated with the dispensing of the Eucharist can be seen in the discussion of the canons of the councils.[207] Augustine had commented in A.D. 400 that reverence for the Lord's body prompts fasting before the Eucharist, and that there was no reason to change what was by then an established custom. So, by the beginnings of the 5th century, fasting before the reception of the Eucharist was essentially church law, which also had the practical effect of limiting the celebration of the Eucharist to mornings.[208] Fasting from midnight before reception of the Eucharist became universally binding in the Roman Catholic Church. Combined with the emphasis on the awesomeness of the divine presence and the authority of the priest in offering the sacrifice, this tended to produce hesitancy among the faithful to participate. These factors "progressively obscured the notion of the sacramentality of the communion of all those present at the Eucharist," observes modern Catholic canonist Joseph Dieckhaus.[209] As will be shown in the next chapter, these age-old traditions would finally give way to reform in the 20th century, especially in the wake of Vatican II.

Fasting in Canons of Early Church Councils: Establishing Universal Seasonal Fasts

The many references to fasting in the Church Fathers received some formal codification in the early church councils. It was understood that fasting was a practice with biblical and apostolic warrant and a long history of practice. The councils' references to fasting largely concern aspects of Lent, baptism and Eucharist, and characters who were violating what were considered standard practice.

- Nicea: The Formalizing of a Forty-Day Lent

Numerous Church Fathers, including Eusebius, mention that the Council of Nicea (A.D. 325) dealt with the establishment of a common paschal date, although the official acts of that council are not extant. It is generally agreed that the tradition of forty days of Lent prior to Easter (the "Quadragesima" or similar terms are used in various languages) was given ecumenical authority here, having grown from shorter observances in previous times.[210]

- Gangra: No Fasting on Sunday, and the Church Reserves Its Rights for Traditional Fast Days

The Council of Gangra (A.D. 325-81) condemned the practices of a bishop Eustathius and his followers, who promoted (among other things) "fasting on the Lord's Day, despising the sacredness of that free day, but disdaining and eating on the fasts appointed in the Church; and certain of them abhor the eating of flesh."[211] Canon 18 anathematized anyone who, under the pretense of asceticism, fasted on Sunday. This was seen as an act of rebellion, because fasting carried with it connotations of mourning, but Sunday was to be a celebration of the resurrection.[212] Conversely, Canon 19 condemns those who disregarded the "fasts commonly prescribed and observed by the Church, because of his perfect understanding of the matter."[213] This phrase appears to be sarcastic, and the condemnation highlights the fasting practices involved as schismatic.

- Laodicea: Regulating Lenten Fasting

The Synod of Laodicea (A.D. 343-81) ruled in Canon 45 that no one could be received as a candidate for baptism after the second week of Lent.[214] This highlights the practice of catechumens fasting before their Easter (or Easter Eve) baptism during Lent, and basically codifies a kind of procedural rule for the practice. Canon 49 of this synod also stipulates that bread is not to be offered during the liturgy during Lent, except on Sabbath and Lord's Day, emphasizing the fasting going on during this period.[215] Canon 50 explicitly commands continuing the fast on Maundy Thursday so as not to dishonor the Lenten season. Apparently some had a practice of breaking the fast on that day to commemorate the Last Supper of Jesus with his disciples. This canon also defined the fast of Lent as "eating only dry meats," a statement in itself a bit unclear, but apparently intended to forbid animal flesh that once flowed with blood.[216]

- Carthage: Ministers Must Observe the
  Eucharistic Fast, and More Regulations for Lent

The "African Code" of the Council of Carthage (A.D. 419), Canon 41, states "That the Sacraments of the Altar are not to be celebrated except by those who are fasting," except for Maundy Thursday.[217] The Council in Trullo, or Quinisext Council (A.D. 692), used similar language, "that the holy mysteries of the altar are not to be performed but by men who are fasting" in Canon 29, even on Maundy Thursday, noting however that there were customs to that effect.[218] This highlights the practice of eucharistic fasting in the church. In Rome, there was a local practice of fasting on Saturdays during Lent (the day before Easter excepted), which was condemned in Canon 55, though this practice apparently did not change much.[219] Some churches in Armenia and elsewhere were following different practices on what was allowed during Lent, and so Canon 56 included eggs and cheese as foods forbidden, so that "the whole Church of God which is in all the world should follow one rule and keep the fast perfectly."[220] Canon 89 says, "The faithful spending the days of the Salutatory Passion in fasting, praying and compunction of heart, ought to fast until the midnight of the Great Sabbath: since the divine Evangelists, Mathhew and Luke, have shewn us how late at night it was [that the resurrection took place]."[221] This stipulated that the fast of the day before Easter should extend until midnight, so that essentially a vigil is kept for the coming of day of the resurrection.

- Trullo: No Fasting on Saturday or Sunday,
  and More Regulations for Lent

Trullo also affirmed the authenticity of "The Apostolic Canons," which had been handed down from the fathers. Since Trullo is considered ecumenical by the Eastern Orthodox, so they also accept the authority of these canons. In "The Apostolical Canons" fasting is mentioned in a couple of places, and expansion of these is found in other canon law. Canon 66 forbids fasting on Sabbath and the Lord's Day. Canon 69 requires that fasting be observed for Lent, the "Quadragesimal fast of Easter," and includes the "day of Preparation," the one Saturday that would be an exception to the rule not to fast on Sabbath days.[222]

- Conclusion: The Fasting Calendar Summarized

As the net result of the formalization of fast days in the patristic era, fasting practices became ritualized into the seasonal cycles of the calendar of the church. The old "station fasts" of Wednesday and especially Friday were regarded as traditional markings of Christ's betrayal and death, with Friday becoming more binding over time. Saturday fasts were practiced by some, but could not succeed in the long term and were condemned in the East. Sunday, the day of Christ's resurrection, was never to be a fast day. The "Ember Days," fasts to mark the beginnings of the four seasons, did gain traditional and authoritative status, although their dates could change and practices could be altered. But the most universal and binding fast was the paschal on the Friday before Easter. This fast in preparation for Easter, along with the days of Lent that preceded it, emerged definitively as the central Christian fast.[223] People would generally fast before baptism or ordination, and perhaps other special occasions. Beyond these, Christians might celebrate local or occasional fasts in their given communities before particular saints' feast days, or engage in voluntary submission to more rigorous ascetic behaviors. The fact of fasting was clearly established as a regular part of Christian life for the Catholic faithful for centuries, while the details were often left to be hammered out through the long processes of church canon law or simply subject local custom.

The establishment of fasting in the context of the formal church calendar has potentially both positive and negative effects. From the positive side, the church provides a seasonal reminder to believers of the need to remember Christ's passions, and identify with him through self-denial. As the Lenten fast proceeds to the Easter feast of the resurrection, the believer is reminded of the glorious fulfillment of the covenantal promises of God in Christ, and lives in hope of the final consummation. As such, the calendar can perform the very needed function of a regular, cyclical reminder of the Christian's place in this world between the times, and a kind of ritualized lesson in the eschatology of the nature of the age. But from the negative side, formalization of ritual practices tends to obscure the underlying theology, and focus seems to shift from what these actions *mean* to how to perform them correctly. Two more key elements are the loss of the voluntary nature of fasting and the increasing connection of works of self-denial with the earning of justifying merit before God. These are the tensions that grow through Catholicism and monasticism in the Middle Ages, coming to a head in the Reformation. Those themes will be dealt with in the following chapter.

§ 4
The Development of Fasting from Monasticism Through the Reformation to the Modern Era

Christian Fasting From Excesses To Decline

As has already been seen, Christian fasting practices began expanding from their basic biblical roots in the early centuries of the church. While this development was not always subversive, it did have the tendency of formalizing the practice into corporate rituals, with the result that voluntary fasting on the part of the people of the church was largely lost. Voluntary fasting was, however, taken up by those who embraced the submission of monasticism, and their austerities in asceticism colored the general perception of fasting for later Christianity. As a result, the Protestant Reformers largely reacted against fasting in Catholicism, divided as it was mainly into the two categories of ritual performance and monastic asceticism. With the onset of the modern era, Christian society further minimized the role of fasting until the practice was virtually forgotten by Protestants, and practiced in formal rituals in Catholicism that even the Catholic leadership began to question. This chapter traces the development of fasting from monasticism through the Reformation and Protestant traditions into the modern era, tracing the rise of excesses and the later decline of the practice. This will set the stage for an examination of the renewal of a theology of Christian fasting in the next chapter.

The Catholic Backdrop to Fasting Before the Reformation: Fasting as Monastic Asceticism and Churchly Devotion

The fasting traditions of the church handed down from the fathers and formalized in church pronouncements formed the basis for fasting practices by Catholics in the Middle Ages. The sacramental and seasonal fasts were observed universally as a matter of church policy, as discussed in the previous chapter. A development in the sacramental approach to fasting was to see fasting as a possible application of the sacrament of penance, thereby associating fasting more closely with the forgiveness of sins.[1] Ascetic fasting also continued to be practiced, and was developed primarily through the monastic movement, discussed below. Thomas Aquinas, the pillar of Christian systematizing and himself a monk, taught about fasting in the context of Catholicism, and his work will be examined in some detail as well. These factors of monastic asceticism and churchly devotion provide something of the backdrop for understanding the Protestant reactions and developments of their own with regard to fasting, which will be examined later.

Fasting in Monasticism: Attempting to Regulate Asceticism

The following section will show how fasting factored into the regulation of monastic asceticism, although controlling these behaviors within tempered orthodox theology proved to be a difficult task. Monasticism began as something of a grass-roots movement, but astute church leaders brought it into the mainstream of church life. Fasting played a significant role in the ascetic life of monasticism, and examples abound of its use. However, doctrinal and practical hazards related to the abuse of fasting also emerged, whether from heretics or the gradual corruption of theology within Catholicism.

• The Rise of Monasticism: Mainstreaming Asceticism

The rise of the monastic movement in early Christianity incorporated fasting as an integral component of the rhythms governing the ascetic life. The word "asceticism" derives from the Greek word ἄσκησις, which most literally has to do with the disciplined practice of athletes, but for Christians came to mean the "partial renunciation of bodily needs to obtain spiritual benefits."[2] Its Greek root occurs only once in the NT, in Acts 24:16, where Paul told Felix, "I also *do my best* to maintain always a blameless conscience both before God and before men" (NASB).[3] But the concept nevertheless came to play a large role in the understanding of the Christian life for many early Christians. Typical forms of ascetic renunciation that were thought to have roots in the NT included selling one's possessions and living in poverty or communally (as in Acts 2:44-45); dedicating oneself to virginity or sexual abstinence (inspired by texts like Matt 19:12, where Jesus speaks of "eunuchs for the sake of the kingdom of heaven," or 1 Cor 7:32, where Paul says "one who is unmarried is concerned about the things of the Lord"); and rigorous private disciplines that often included prayer and fasting in various forms. Traveling evangelists, widows in service to the church, dedicated virgins, and ascetics who withdrew to relative isolation from society all are found from the church's earliest times. With regard to ascetic fasting, the purpose "was to subjugate the powers of the flesh and to deliver the mind from distractions."[4] Meat and wine were prime suspects for leading to bodily sin, and abstinence from them came to be a regular call to virtue. Plus, asceticism encouraged the idea of purifying the body from sin by fasting, and so fasting came to be thought of as within the orbit of a broad doctrine of salvation as a process.

Already by the third century, church leaders had begun to consider how to regulate such behaviors more centrally and provide guidance for the flowering ascetic, monastic movement. This gave rise to several codes of conduct (often known as "Rules") being written, such as those by Basil and Augustine (already examined in the previous chapter), Benedict (discussed in more detail below), and Francis.[5] The goal was to incorporate the nascent para-church movement into the universal church's life.[6] While it is outside the scope here to deal with the many facets of monasticism, it is appropriate to try to understand how fasting factored into the monastic ideal and try to assess at least some of that impact.[7]

- Examples from Monasticism: Idealizing (and Sometimes Moderating) Austerity

Thomas O'Loughlin observes that "monastic fasting must be seen as a variant and development of fasting within Christianity as a whole."[8] The scriptural examples of fasting inspired imitation, and the earliest Christian documents already examined show that fasting was quickly becoming part of regular Christian experience. Christians held up ascetic ideals as examples and participated vicariously in the lives of others. Some of the ascetics became heroic figures in early Christianity, and "where the monk's austerities could not be imitated, they could be admired."[9] It should not be surprising, then, to see monastic fasting taking examples of fasting and habits that were already forming generally into more structured forms.

Antony: Fasting in the Archetypical Ascetic. Among examples of monastic fasting, Antony (ca. 251-356) stands out as "the undisputed pioneer of the monastic tradition and the most famous teacher of later generations," and "all later sources on early monasticism refer to Antony as the father of monasticism."[10] Athanasius' classic depiction of Antony shows him eating bread and salt, with water, once a day in the evenings, and frequently foregoing these.[11] Antony saw his ascetic life as a daily martyrdom, and combined fasting with wearing a hair shirt and refusing to bathe.[12] Fasting, combined with prayer, was seen as a means of thwarting demonic temptations.[13]

Ephrem and Eastern Monasticism: Championing Ascetic Orthodoxy. In the East, ascetic life took hold in monastic communities in Greek-speaking areas as well as Syria and points further distant. Fasting practices in the East drew inspiration from Basil's rules, and received similar teaching about fasting and self-control from prominent figures like John Chrysostom and Ephrem the Syrian (4th century), Diadokos of Photiki and Mark the Hermit (5th century), and John Climacus (6th century).[14] Ephrem (ca. 306-373), who championed orthodoxy against many heresies that were flowering in the East, wrote at least ten hymns on fasting that were featured in the liturgical year.[15] Hymn 1 features Jesus defeating Satan in the desert as an answer to the fall of Adam. Hymn 4.11 Moses and Elijah as forerunners of Christ experiencing the same fasting duration and supernatural power. Hymns 7-9 refer to the exemplary biblical fasts of Esther, the Ninevites, Daniel and his three friends. In addition to the negative example of Adam and Eve, the hypocritical fast of Ahab and Jezebel against Naboth is recalled in Hymn 3. For Ephrem, the many good uses of fasting were ultimately transcended by the purification it fosters that allows a clearer vision of God: "Beau et utile est le jeûne pour celui qui se purifie afin de contemplar Dieu."[16]

John Cassian and Latin Monasticism: Fasting to Counter the Principal Vice of Gluttony. Among the Latin fathers, John Cassian's (ca. 360-ca. 435) writings from the late fourth and early fifth centuries "present the fullest treatment of fasting and were looked to as basic teaching until modern times."[17] Cassian governed communities of monastic life in Egypt for some time and wrote his *Conferences* (Latin, *Conlationes*) and *Institutes* in that context.[18] In the midst of dealing with liturgical calendar questions about fasting around the time of Pentecost, Cassian teaches that fasting is not an "essential good," or intrinsically right, because its opposite, eating, is not intrinsically wrong. Therefore, fasting, like other behaviors, should be practiced in accord with what is essentially good and promotes true good.[19] But, since gluttony is the principal vice that led to Adam's fall, fasting should be encouraged to help the body to learn to abstain from gluttony as well as the other vices of lust that are related to it. Jesus, who by virtue of his sinless divinity was not affected by the vices of sinful flesh, still fasted when tempted by the devil, to show the means of conquering sin in the flesh.[20] Gregory the Great followed and modified Cassian's approach to the deadly sins, and retained fasting as the *sine qua non* of ascetic commitment, from which everything else flowed.[21] Cassian's approach to fasting and vigils were that moderation was required, because one could err on the side of too much as well as too little abstinence.[22] So while Cassian obviously presided over monks practicing rigorous disciplines that often included austere fasting, in the final analysis it was intended as a tool for more important matters of the spiritual life.[23] Maximus the Confessor (7th century) similarly urged fasting, among other disciplines, as a tool against sin.[24]

The Rule of St. Benedict: *Fasting Austerities Moderated. The Rule of St. Benedict* was composed sometime before 528 when Benedict of Nursia (ca. 480-ca. 547) moved from governing monasteries in Subiaco, Italy, to Monte Cassino, where he lived until his death.[25] Its organization of monastic life has stood as the rule for all these centuries for Benedictines as well as adherents of some other orders. While it does present a disciplined life, it is not particularly strenuous with regard to fasting. Its food ration allows for two cooked dishes and available fruits and vegetables at two meals per day, at the sixth and ninth hours, plus bread. More can be allowed by the abbot's discretion, though care should be taken, since "nothing is more contrary to being a Christian than gluttony."[26] Wine is allowed, though "those who have received the gift of abstinence will know they shall be especially rewarded by God."[27] Monks are to fast until the ninth hour on Wednesdays and Fridays from Pentecost through the summer, provided there is not too much hard labor or heat.[28] During Lent, monks should voluntarily plan to abstain in some way that is communicated to the abbot, though "a monk's life should always be like a Lenten observance."[29] One can see from these rules an encouragement of a voluntarily disciplined life, without extreme rigor in fasting practices.

- Hazards to Orthodoxy in Asceticism: Fasting Abused

While many fasting practices could be held up as examples for the orthodox, there were also doctrinal hazards emerging. Evagrius Ponticus, like Antony, urged fasting for spiritual combat with demons, stressing that gluttony was the first of the evil thoughts and led to lust and avarice, from which the other deadly sins proceeded. But Evagrius's fasting practices were also connected to his gnostic dichotomy between the body and mind, and one could see in some strands of monastic fasting an unhealthy deprecation of full humanity.[30] The Manichees practiced fasting in the context of asceticism and monasticism, and developed elaborate purification doctrines that essentially tied the spiritual life to the diet.[31] So it is clear that fasting was by no means a monopoly of the orthodox, or immune to divergent applications.

It seems entirely likely that abstinence from meat was influenced by some of the dominant philosophical strands at the time. The Neoplatonic approach, derived from Pythagoreans, taught that meat was a heavy food that dragged down the soul, was expensive, was too stimulating, and the living body would become somewhat defiled by contact with what was dead.[32] However, stoic philosophies also influenced Christians to view food as a matter that was indifferent. When these philosophies mixed with a Christian community with roots in biblical practices, a somewhat conflicted approach arose that can be seen in literature related to fasting through the years.[33]

As time passed, the emphasis on fasting and asceticism in general as a form of penance, coupled with a view of the body that saw it as a corrupted vessel containing a perfectible soul, increased the tendency toward extremes in self-inflicted pains.[34] Saints like John Chrysostom and Bernard of Clairvaux were praised for their holiness, while virtually ruining their health through constant fasting. Perhaps this is evidence of a view of fasting that is focused more on the effect on the human body than on the person's overall relationship to a God who created a good world. In the eleventh and twelfth centuries, self-flagellation (the practice of beating oneself, often rather cruelly) became a widespread movement among ascetics, whose fasting practices were intensified by the self-infliction of pain. It is not entirely surprising to see Giles Constable look back at practices that so superceded merely the restraining of indulgence and say, "we tend to regard self-inflicted punishment as a sign of spiritual and psychological disorder and not, as was believed in the Middle Ages, of a proper and praiseworthy attitude toward oneself and God."[35]

Thomas Aquinas: Fasting as Churchly Devotion, Toward the Virtue of Temperance

When it comes to systematizing theology in the Roman Catholic Church, Thomas Aquinas (1225-1274) is the unrivaled touchstone. In his *Summa Theologiæ* he addressed fasting on several occasions and once in an extended treatment. His teachings tend to reinforce the basic approaches to fasting handed down by the Scriptures and earlier fathers of the church, but as one would expect, his treatment is systematically ordered. As will be seen, he advocates fasting in the context of church traditions on the grounds that it is a tool for temperate virtues and therefore helpful against temptations.

- Christ's Fasting: An Example for Defeating Temptation in the Flesh

Thomas discusses fasting in relationship to the temptation of Christ in *ST* 3a. 41. Christ was tempted by the devil as the new Adam in order to conquer death, not by power so much as by righteousness. Since the world and flesh held no sway over his sinless nature, it was left to the devil to tempt him. But since the devil could also not succeed against Christ's impeccable nature, the temptation story is given not only as a demonstration of Christ's victory, but also as an example to us, since all of us must know how to face temptation. Thomas says that fasting is a weapon against temptation, that those fasting should expect temptation, and that Jesus undertook fasting to become hungry and face temptation to show that manhood is capable of withstanding the power of the devil. Citing Hilary, he says that "the devil was to be conquered, not by God, but by the flesh," and from Chrysostom he draws the conclusion that "in fasting he went no further than Moses and Elijah, lest his assumption of our flesh might seem incredible."[36]

- Fasting and Sacraments: Solemn Occasions
  Suggest Solemn Observance

Thomas also mentions fasting in regard to the sacraments. In *ST* 3a. 72, 12 he answers questions about the appropriateness of fasting before baptism and confirmation. Since these are solemn occasions, and usually performed on or around Easter, it is most fitting for fasting to accompany them, except in cases where this cannot be conveniently observed.[37] In *ST* 3a. 80, 8 he discusses fasting and the Eucharist. He follows Augustine in arguing that no food should enter a Christian's mouth before the sacrament. This is taken to mean a requirement of fasting from midnight until the sacrament is taken in the morning of that day, although exceptions for illness are allowed. Such fasting seems to go against the institution of the Lord's supper at a feast, but Thomas says it is in accord with Paul's admonitions about solemnity and not eating and drinking in the Lord's house. The priests administering the sacrament are also to fast afterwards for a few hours, although various customs may apply in local circumstances.[38]

- Fasting as a Tool for the
  Virtue of Temperance

Thomas's most extensive treatment of fasting occupies a section of his discussion of temperance, where questions 141-154 relate to temperance, intemperance, shame, honor, abstinence, fasting, gluttony, sobriety, drunkenness, chastity, virginity, and lust, in that order. *ST* 2a2æ. 147 deals with fasting through eight points of inquiry:

1. whether it is an act of virtue;

2. and of which virtue;

3. whether it is a matter of precept;

4. whether anybody is excused from its observance;

5. on the times of fasting;

6. whether it requires no more than one meal in the day;

7. on the hour of the meal;

8. on the foods to be abstained from.[39]

Fasting Itself Not a Virtue, but Used for Virtues. As to whether it is a virtue, Aquinas says that Isaiah 58 makes it clear that fasting by itself is not necessarily a virtue. But since Paul lists it as a virtue in 2 Cor 6:5, it can be a virtue, provided "it is set on some moral value."[40] The chief motives for fasting are to bridle the lusts of the flesh, to free the mind for contemplation of God, and to make satisfaction for sin (and here he cites the call to repentance of Joel 2:12). In addition to the problems of hypocritical fasting as in Isaiah 58, too much fasting can negate its very purpose. Here he cites Jerome, who says "it makes no difference whether you are sapping yourself for a long or for a short time; by excessive lack of nourishment and by eating and sleeping too little you are offering a sacrifice of stolen goods."[41] Fasting requires courage to endure hardship, and is an act of the virtue of abstinence. It can be metaphorically understood as abstaining from all things harmful, so that "fasting properly speaking is from all manner of lusts, since any act ceases to be virtuous, as we have pointed out, when it goes with any vice."[42]

Fasting is a Matter of Liberty, but Everyone Needs It. As to whether or not fasting is a precept, it is noted that not fasting is no sin, that it is not a sacrament, and is a matter of liberty. However, the fact that it is a matter of liberty suggests that it is intended to be practiced, even if how it is practiced may differ somewhat from place to place. So, in an insightful statement, he defends the practice of ecclesiastical fasting seasons:

> It is not binding under precept in the abstract, but in the concrete to each one who needs its remedy. And since for the most part we need it, according to St. James, *in many things we all offend*, and to St. Paul, *the flesh lusteth against the spirit*, the Church is rightly pragmatic in appointing some common fasts to be kept by all. Not, however, by turning a work of supererogation into one of obligation, but by giving a determinate shape to a common duty.[43]

Yet, liberty should allow for exceptions, and "a person may lawfully follow his own judgment in not carrying out the command," provided he counsels with justly constituted authorities.[44] Children are exempted from fasting until they are twenty-one, and qualifications can be made for labor and pilgrimages, as well as the poor who live hand to mouth.

Fasting for the Bridegroom: Choose an Interpretation, Regardless, It Promotes Fasting. Thomas then discusses the synoptic reference to the children of the bridegroom not fasting, and offers three interpretations from tradition. Chrysostom said the "children" were the weak, and so they were exempt from fasting, as beginners. Jerome saw it as a freedom from observances of the old law, as Christians were to be "breathing the freshness of grace." Augustine said that the passage could be divided into two kinds of fasting, that of those who mourn, and that of those who enjoy the presence of Christ and are "caught up by spiritual things, and this fasting is for the righteous."[45] While Aquinas seems to recommend all three interpretations, there does seem to be an ascendance in the interpretations from questionable, to biblical theology, to grand spiritualization.

Church Fasting Seasons Defended. Thomas defends the church's seasonal fasts as the common custom of church tradition. In preparation for Easter, the church inverts the sequence of Christ's baptism and fasting, in order to be buried with him in death before being raised again to life. Several imaginative numerological explanations of the number forty are offered from Gregory and Augustine, but in the end, it is Christ's fasting that is the reason for the forty days. Thomas shows great awareness of Jewish fasting practices, and although the church keeps similar times throughout the year, in echoing the *Didache*, she is careful not to observe the same days as the Jews, who are still observing the old covenant, and not breathing the newness of the Spirit.[46]

Reasons for Precise Fasting Regulations. Aquinas goes on to discuss what meals are allowed and what constitutes breaking a fast. He distinguishes two kinds of fasts, the first being absolute (allowing no food or drink at all), which should precede the Eucharist. The second kind, the "faster's fast," is broken only by partaking in what is not allowed, hence there is some latitude involved in the definition. So during church fasts, one square meal per day is allowed, but small amounts of "comfits" (basically snacks) or medicines do not violate a fast, "unless of course people cheat and wolf a lot or make a meal of them."[47] Christian fasting should last until the ninth hour (3 P.M.), because that echoes the time Christ gave up the ghost, although exactness of time is no great matter. Fasting from meat, milk and eggs may seem inconsistent, since fish and other foods might be made just as tasty and filling. However, Thomas believes that for the majority of people and times, meat and animal foods are considered more desirable, and so they are appropriate as the content of foods to be fasted from. Besides, he believes, they produce substances in the body that build up seminal matter and increase the pressure of lust, making abstinence from these foods particularly relevant to the purposes of fasting against temptation. However, local customs may prevail.[48]

Developments in Fasting in Protestant Traditions: Reacting Against Catholicism, but Allowing for Its Practice

In the section below, fasting in the Protestant tradition will be examined by looking at statements by key leaders in the Reformation, as well as leaders in the Anabaptists, the Church of England and Methodism. It will be seen that the Reformers strongly criticized several aspects of Catholic fasting in their polemics, but they still allowed for certain forms of fasting. There is little evidence that the Anabaptists paid much attention to fasting at all. The Church of England sought its middle way between Catholic fasts and the Protestant emphasis on freedom of the conscience. Wesley urged fasting as a form of personal spiritual discipline and churchly devotion for the sake of the ministry, as perhaps the strongest advocate and practitioner of fasting among the main Protestant figures. Yet taken as a whole, it will be seen that the trajectory of moving away from perceived Catholic excesses in fasting likely led to something of a decline in fasting in general in Protestantism, especially as it progressed into the modern era.

The Reformers: Fasting Cannot Garner Merit, but Can Have Appropriate Uses

The Protestant Reformation reacted negatively against the Catholicism of the time, especially those doctrines and practices that seemed to highlight human merit with regard to salvation. In such a context, one might expect the Reformers to look dimly on fasting, as it had come to be associated with penance and forgiveness of sins, as well as church rituals that they were beginning to reject wholesale. While this negative theme certainly does emerge in their specific discussions of fasting, what is perhaps more surprising is how the Reformers all acknowledge the positive role fasting can and should play in the life of the Christian and the church. The following discussion will show that despite strong warnings against the negative use of fasting, the Reformers consistently advocated fasting as a positive Christian behavior, when guided by what they believed to be biblically based theological norms.

- Martin Luther: Fasting is Too Associated with Merit, but Perhaps It Could Have a Role

Martin Luther (1483-1546), who was himself trained in the ascetic rigors of Augustinian monasticism, grew very suspicious of any human work or attitude that smacked of garnering merit before God. As will be seen, he viewed fasting skeptically, and he often railed against abuses he saw of the practices in Catholicism. However, he still makes several positive comments about the human need for disciplining the flesh, and he clearly believes fasting could play a role in the genuine believers' life. He even suggests some ways the church and state could promote fasting, provided it was clear what the bases for such fasting would be.

Fasting is Too Associated with Merit. Luther was concerned with protecting the purity of a subjective faith over and against placing personal trust in any works. The Christian is to place faith in Christ to receive the benefits of a passive justification. But this does not rule out the need for active works and discipline of the flesh but rather, they must be seen as proceeding from justification. In his "Treatise on Good Works" 18-19 he writes:

> The highest and first work of God in us and the best training is that we let our own works go and let our reason and will lie dormant resting and commending ourselves to God in all things, especially when they appear spiritual and good.
>
> 19. After this comes the discipline of the flesh, the killing of its gross evil lust and giving it rest and relaxation. We must kill the flesh and subdue it with fastings, watchings, and labor. And it is from this that we learn how much and why we should fast, watch, and labor.[49]

Luther strongly criticizes those who perform fasting because they think it will earn them some merit. Christ "is not my fasting, praying, waking, and toiling. No, my fasting is a work which has its source in me."[50] Luther despised what fasting had become because it was done to seek merit before God, atone for sin, and reconcile God as an imposed act of penance, which he saw as trampling Christ underfoot and hitting him on the mouth.[51] The source of true righteousness could not be anything emanating from within a person, like fasting or almsgiving, but rather must come from outside, from Christ. Clearly he believed the Roman Catholics had fallen into this error. "They tried to make God gracious to them on the basis of the cowl and the tonsure, fasting and prayer."[52] He emphasized that Christians are free from all human traditions, and fasting is not a divine requirement. Paul condemned abstinence from foods and observing Sabbaths and special days (Col 2:16), and believers should beware of falling into such rituals. In citing the synoptic fasting query, he says:

> Why do we fast frequently? We are "sons [of the bridechamber]," He says (Matt 9:15). This was a good and a true fasting, not like the fasting mentioned in Matt 6:16. Nevertheless, he rejects it. Fasting does not justify, but faith in Christ does.[53]

Interestingly, Luther does not address the fact that Jesus went on to tell the disciples that when he was gone, then they would fast.

Fasting could also too easily be an individualistic practice that neglected the community. Even monks like Paul of Thebes and Antony were viewed as saints, but they lived by themselves and were of no value to the church. "What if they pray and fast so often, if in the meantime no one is providing any service?"[54] Luther urged his people, "But godliness goes toward the advancement of the Word and the Christian religion. If there is still some godliness left over, then tire your body or work with your hands."[55]

Some refrained from certain foods like meat, eggs or butter, or scheduled fasting on certain special days according to the calendar and saints' days: "All these people seek nothing beyond the work itself in their fasting."[56] Echoing Augustine's pet peeve of substituting one food for another, he says, "Some fast so richly with fish and other foods that they would come much nearer to fasting if they ate meat, eggs, and butter. By doing this they would obtain far better results from their fasting. For such fasting is not fasting, but a mockery of fasting as well as of God."[57]

Fasting Could Have a Possible Role. For Luther, fasting was up to the individual as to when and how it was to be done, as "these matters should be regulated by the ebb and flow of the pride and lust of the flesh."[58] In the same vein, he tells his listeners:

> Or, can we not continue to pray, fast, and so on, as long as the right way is present? My answer is that if there is present a right Christian love and faith, then everything a man does is meritorious; and each may do what he wills [cf. Rom. 14:22], so long as he has no regard for works, since they cannot save him.[59]

He sees fasting as part of the exercising of the body, which Paul says in 1 Tim 5:8 is of some usefulness, but Paul "neither condemns nor encourages the manner in which each trains his own body."[60]

But Luther worries that this freedom will cause indifference, and that those who have never experienced fasting will conclude that it is not necessary.[61] In 1532, he wrote about the fasting instruction in the Sermon on the Mount:

> It is not His intention to reject or despise fasting in itself, any more than He rejects almsgiving and praying. Rather He is supporting these practices and teaching their proper use. In the same way it is His intention to restore proper fasting, to have it rightly used and properly understood, as any good work should be.[62]

"Real fasting" is a punishing of the body, compelling the five senses to learn to live without the comforts of life.[63]

Clearly Luther wished to forge a middle road of encouraging fasting as discipline, but discourage any association it might have with merit in itself. He recounts the growth of Christian fasting practices from the Jews, through the early practice of the church, and the addition of more and more fast days as well as monastic observances.

> The ancient fathers may have meant it well and have observed the fasts properly, but the filth soon overwhelmed and ruined it and made it worthless. And that is just what it deserved. As it was a mere human plaything to have these many special fasts, so it soon degenerated into shameful abuse.[64]

Luther could envision two kinds of commendable general fasts besides individual discipline. First, the civil government could call for a fast to regulate a moderate consumption of food, to save resources "from the kind of incessant guzzling and gobbling that we Germans do, and to teach people to live a little more moderately."[65] Second, he felt there could be general fasts before Easter, Pentecost, and Christmas, and even every Friday evening, as "an outward Christian discipline and exercise for the young and simple people, by which they can learn to keep track of the seasons."[66] By practicing these kinds of fasts, "the Christian Church would have plenty of fasting to do, and no one would have the right to accuse us of despising and completely rejecting the practice of fasting."[67]

In sum, Luther, viewed fasting skeptically, as potentially being viewed as a meritorious human work that could undermine justification by faith in Christ. Nevertheless, it might have some value in training the body and ordering the community. But from Luther's perspective, the role of fasting clearly needed to be downgraded from the practice of his day as he observed it.

- John Calvin: Seeking a Middle Way for Fasting
  by Avoiding Abuses and Encouraging Humility

Like Luther, John Calvin (1509-1564) desired to seek a middle way for fasting—approving the action if done with right motives, concerned lest the action itself be viewed as meritorious. Taken as a whole, his opinion of fasting actually seems more genuinely positive than Luther's, and somewhat less polemical. Commenting on Isa 58:5 he says, "fasting is neither desired nor approved by God in itself but only insofar as it is directed to its true end. He did not want it completely abolished, only its improper use—that is, because they believed the worship of God to consist in it."[68] The following analysis shows Calvin's desire for this middle way in his rejection of fasting abuses and encouragement of the practice when done in genuine humility, and for the right purposes.

Fasting in The Institutes: *Proper Purposes and Misconceptions.* In his *Institutes* 3.3.17, he sees the fasting of Joel 2 as a reasonable paradigm for publicly calling for fasting and weeping unto true repentance in the face of calamity. This kind of public fast is commendable on occasion, while "the life of the godly ought to be tempered with frugality and sobriety that throughout its course a sort of perpetual fasting may appear."[69] As he discusses in *Institutes* 3.7.1-5, the body ought to be brought into the process of self-denial. But one must beware not to let the conscience become ensnared in indifferent matters related to food, so that greater and greater abstinence is required to avoid the thought of wrongdoing.[70]

The *Institutes* 4.12.14-21 presents a more extended section relating fasting to the means of grace in the life and discipline of the church. He includes this section for the express reason, that "very many, while they do not understand how useful it is, regard it as not very necessary; others also, considering it is superfluous, completely reject it. And, since its use is not well understood, it can easily lapse into superstition."[71]

Proper fasting, for Calvin, has its three central objectives as weakening and subduing the flesh, aiding in prayer, and testimony of self-abasement before God. While subduing the flesh is a private discipline, fasting as an aid in prayer or sign of repentance can be either private or corporate in nature, and in *Institutes* 4.12.15 he suggests that pastors ought to call for such as occasions arise. He cites the biblical examples of the apostles in Acts, Anna, Nehemiah, and Paul, to show fasting is an aid to prayer, and experience teaches that "with a full stomach our mind is not so lifted up to God that it can be drawn to prayer with a serious and ardent affection and persevere in it."[72] He applies OT examples of fasting as a sign of corporate penitence in the face of disaster, reasoning that they could be applied rather directly to the church in times of crisis. This kind of fasting is not a ceremony that has been done away in Christ, but rather "an excellent aid for believers today."

While Christ excused the apostles for not fasting, Calvin reminds us that Christ also said days would come when Christ is taken away. He defines fasting as more than restraint and abstemiousness, and not only the general mark of sobriety and frugality of life that should constantly be a Christian's experience. Specifically, there are temporary fasts that consist of definite times and purposes for fasting, and abstention from foods in both quality and quantity.[73]

Now that Calvin has clearly laid out proper kinds of fasting, he goes after misconceptions related to it. He says that "it would be much more satisfactory if fasting were not practiced at all, than diligently observed and at the same time corrupted with false and pernicious opinions."[74] In line with Joel 2 and Isaiah 58, fasting must accompany true humility from the heart and not be merely an outward expression. Also, the idea that fasting is a work of merit or worship should be avoided, because it is rather a means to an end (and here he cites Augustine's refutation of the Manichees in support). Also, fasting should not be too rigidly enforced, lest seeds of superstition are sown and fasting itself comes to be praised as virtuous.

Calvin believes that the general observance of Lent was an example of the degeneration of fasting in the church. Rather, Christ followed in the line of Moses and Elijah, establishing the authority of the gospel over the law. Since Lent was based on this forty-day period of fasting, the church was mistakenly making a precept of fasting ritual: "Christ did not fast to set an example for others, but to prove, in so beginning to proclaim the gospel, that it was no human doctrine but actually one sent from heaven."[75] Even worse, this period of fasting in Lent degenerated into a time when people mocked God with feigned abstinence. Echoing Jerome and Augustine, Calvin strongly decries the substitution of certain acceptable delicacies in the place of eating meat. The Catholic fasts had been turned to more sumptuous, dainty feasts, leading to a harsh conclusion: "I say only this, that both in fasts and in all other parts of discipline the papists have nothing right, nothing sincere, nothing well-ordered and arranged, to give them occasion to boast, as if anything remained among them deserving of praise."[76]

Some of his comments on the synoptic gospels also reflect this distancing of fasting from merit or true worship in itself, while still allowing for its proper place. In commenting on the fasting of Anna in Luke 2:37, he takes pains to point out that not everything in a saintly person needs to be emulated by all, but that different people will be called to different acceptable vocations of good works. Fasting is not required, but prayer is. Fasting may be an aid to prayer, but should not be mistaken for worship in itself. "We must keep the distinction, that prayers are a direct service to God, but fasting only consequentially."[77] Similarly, Christ's fasting for forty days was not given as an example to be followed in the Lenten season (which he mocks here), but rather it set him apart from common men and validated his heavenly message, like Moses and Elijah before him.[78]

Fasting in Commentaries on the Gospels: Brief Comments Toward the Middle Way. In brief comments on Matt 6:16-18, he reiterates his understanding of fasting as "a work of indifferent value," inferior in itself to prayer and almsgiving in the near context. Fasting can please God to a point, "as long as it is directed to an end beyond itself, namely, to prompt us to abstinence, to subject the lasciviousness of the flesh, to incense us to a desire for prayer, to testify to our repentance, whenever we are moved by the judgment of God."[79] Commenting on the synoptic fasting query of Matt 9:14-17, Calvin notes how easily people wish to make into law those means that they find agreeable to themselves. John's disciples were "ensnared in these coils of Satan," and although their fasting regimen may have been a good thing, it could not be imposed on Christian liberty. Like Luther, Calvin does not even mention in this section the possible appropriate use of fasting after the time of Christ's earthly ministry, but merely notes that it is a sign that when things are well, we can be assured that harder times will come.[80]

While Calvin clearly was advocating the same basic theology of fasting in his commentaries that he was in his *Institutes*, it is somewhat striking how little is actually said. Those things that are said mention that fasting can be a positive thing, but the emphasis here appears to have turned to the more negative. While both Luther and Calvin have said some positive things about fasting, it would not be surprising for their followers to lose this sense of balance that, at least by their words, they were hoping to promote. In short, later Protestants could easily lose the positive words about fasting amid the negative polemic against Catholicism.

- Ulrich Zwingli: Liberty of Conscience Over Fasting

If Luther and Calvin were seeking a middle way for fasting but couched it in negative polemics, Ulrich Zwingli (1484-1531) focuses rather on the polemics while allowing, at least in word, a theoretical basis for fasting. Zwingli took an especially dim view of the fasting of the Catholic church, although some of his comments indicate that it could have a positive purpose.

On True and False Religion: *Avoid Pretense and Fast Simply.* In his work *On True and False Religion* he discusses fasting on a few occasions, particularly as an example of works done for wrong motives. In discussing almsgiving and fasting in relation to Matthew 6, he criticizes the use of fasting that would be for show, or would substitute different delicacies, or for weight loss, or saving money, or as a good work in itself. But he does say that, in contrast, fasting "ought to be done simply for the purpose of hearing of the voice and bidding of the Spirit."[81] Fasting is listed as a possible pretense before God along with murmuring prayers and feeding the hungry, if done without faith.[82] In arguing for his symbolic understanding of the Eucharist, he cites Origen, who places the Eucharist in a category with fasting as something which enhances one's religious experience, and Hilary, who said that those who were without Christ were fasting in his absence, while true believers had the resurrected Christ in their hearts.[83]

Liberty Respecting Food in Lent: *Fasting Cannot Be Mandated Over a Free Conscience.* Zwingli came over time to reject Lenten fasting as a practice that was not obligated by Scripture and therefore could not be enforced on the Christian populace. In a sermon entitled *Liberty Respecting Food in Lent,* dated April 16, 1522, he declared the observance of Lent as incongruous with the general practice of the Christian gospel, and the ensuing dispute actually caused street fighting.[84]

Zwingli argued that foods themselves do not defile a person, and that the NT endorses the eating of all kinds of foods (citing Peter's experience in Acts 10). Paul saw foods as indifferent and matters of expediency (1 Cor 6:12, 8:8, 10:25), and no one should be judged in regard to observance of a holy day (Col 2:16). Forbidding foods may even be a sign of false teaching (1 Tim 4:1; Titus 1:5; Heb 13:9).[85] Therefore, food itself is neither good nor bad, and the only true sin comes in abusing it too much, not in eating or not eating at certain times. Forbidding certain foods at certain times is an edict of men, not of God, and therefore not binding on the conscience.

However, Zwingli does allow for free exercise of the practice, saying, "Let each one fast as often as the spirit of true belief urges him."[86] He notes how Jesus allowed his disciples to break the Sabbath practices as observed by men in Mark 2:23, and that Paul preaches freedom of conscience in indifferent matters (1 Cor 3:21, 7:35). Rather than fasting like naughty children who refuse to eat broth when meat is not set before them, Christians should fast when they are moved by conscience.

> In a word, if you will fast, do so; if you do not wish to eat meat, eat it not; but leave Christians a free choice in the matter. You

who are an idler should fast often, should often abstain from foods that make you lustful. But the labourers' lusts pass away at the hoe and plough in the field.[87]

The rest of the sermon argues similarly for Christian liberty, concluding that no governors of the church have a right to set up fasting or abstinence as a common law, though Christians may accept such practices for themselves.[88] Zwingli had to defend his positions before certain church delegations, and clarified that he did not forbid people to observe Lent, but wanted to keep it from being imperiously prescribed. Those who wished to fast during Lent could fast all year as far as he was concerned, and he doubted that there would be any lack of people who advised fasting—he just wanted to keep them from running things. "While I forbid no man's fasting, I leave it free to him."[89]

Defense of the Reformed Faith: *Catholic Fasting Is Hypocrisy*. In Zwingli's *Defense of the Reformed Faith*, Article 16, he chastises Catholic hypocrisy, including the fasting practices of Lent, which he considered foolish. He says that the fasting query of Matthew 9 shows that where Christ is present, fasting is not needed. If someone becomes carnally minded, the Spirit might lead him by fasting and sorrow back to Christ.[90] In Article 26 he compares Catholics to the Jewish hypocrites who fasted and prayed ostentatiously, and Jesus rebuked them strongly.[91]

These few comments of Zwingli are enough to show his strong desire to emphasize the liberty of Christian conscience. While he allows for fasting as a possible expression of that free conscience, he clearly is moving in a direction away from fasting as a regular, prescribed practice. This has the effect of generally diminishing the practice of fasting while it is still endorsed, at least theoretically. In Zwingli we clearly see the pendulum swinging from the prescriptions of Catholic fasting to putting it in the realm of the freedom of the conscience. While this appears to be a proper and helpful corrective, the abolition of Lent and the general tenor of the polemics against Catholic fasting suggest an overall downgrading of the importance of fasting. Following this line of reasoning, then, it should not be surprising that fasting would eventually receive relatively little attention in certain strands of Reformed Protestantism.

- John Knox: Catholic Fasting Is Hypocrisy,
  but True Fasting Is Encouraged

Like Zwingli and Calvin, John Knox (1514-1572) came to reject the mandatory practice of Lenten fasting. But more like Calvin, Knox seeks to retain a genuine role for fasting in religious experience. In his *History of the Reformation in Scotland,* he records the condemnation of George Wischart, a martyr for the Reformed cause. In Article 17 of his condemnation, he was accused of being a heretic, condemning fasting and saying that people should not fast. His answer shows that he did not condemn fasting, and actually practiced it, which was confirmed by other testimonials.[92] But he desired a true fasting:

> My Lordis, I find that Fasting is commended in the Scripture; tharefor I war a sclanderar of the Gospell, yf I contemned fasting. And not so onlye, but I have learned by experience, that fasting is good for the health and conservatioun of the body. But God knowith onlye who fastith the trew fast.[93]

Knox wrote a fairly lengthy treatise on the occasion of the proclamation of a general public fast in Scotland in 1565, the first called there since the Reformation, and ordered by the assembly due to the extreme need for ministers and gathering of strength for the churches amidst Catholic persecution. This tract was published on several later fasting occasions as well.[94] Knox was concerned that the Papists understand that he was not advocating what he had previously condemned in them, and that on the other hand, people ignorant of the practice of fasting might understand its purposes.[95] He maintained his belief that the Catholic fasts were hypocritical and not true fasting before God. He cited familiar and obscure biblical examples of fasting and hypocrisy, urging a genuine fast that includes repentance of the heart. The message includes liturgical instructions, beginning with a confession to be read, followed by reading the preacher's own chosen Scripture text on which the sermon will be founded, followed by certain prayers, psalms, and Scriptures. The abstinence would start from Saturday night and extend through Sunday afternoon, broken only by bread and water, and include abstaining from other pleasures like games. This routine would last a week.[96]

It is clear, then, that Knox and his fellow Scottish Reformers believed in creating a positive role for fasting in both their individual and community lives. While rejecting Catholic fasts as hypocrisy, Knox took pains to teach and encourage the kind of fasting that Calvin had also advocated in his *Institutes.* The Reformed tradition encouraged fasting, especially for special, solemn, corporate assemblies, as evidenced in the discussion "Of Religious Worship, and the Sabbath-Day" in the *Westminster Confession of Faith* 21.5:

> The reading of the Scriptures with godly fear, the sound preaching and conscionable hearing of the Word, in obedience unto God, with understanding, faith, and reverence, singing of

psalms with grace in the heart; as also, the due administration and worthy receiving of the sacraments instituted by Christ, are all parts of the ordinary religious worship of God: beside religious oaths, vows solemn fastings, and thanksgivings upon special occasions, which are, in their several times and seasons, to be used in an holy and religious manner.[97]

Anabaptists and Mennonites: An Ascetic Tradition That Says Little About Fasting

Moving forward to the heirs of the "Radical Reformation," one discovers something of an anomaly. Interestingly, fasting receives little to no attention in the Anabaptist tradition. Considering their emphasis on personal piety, sobriety in customs, and renunciation of worldliness, fasting would seem to be a natural fit. Kenneth Davis has described Anabaptists as having a basically ascetic structure to their theology of holiness.[98] Considering this, it is remarkable that fasting does not seem to factor into that theology or practice in any large way. There are no references to fasting in the writings of Menno Simons or their other major leaders, although there are references to sober eating and drinking.[99] Van der Zijpp mentions only the Gnadenfeld-Alexanderwohl communities' joint confession of faith of 1787 apparently contained a statement about "right evangelical fasting according to the teaching of the Holy Scriptures," but little else is said.[100] There are a few records of special days of fasting and prayer being called in certain assemblies, and a handful of references to Mennonite and Amish communities who fasted occasionally in connection with seasonal communion services, or Good Friday. Some of these practices have died out, while some communities still observe them.[101]

Perhaps the primitivist approach to religion of Anabaptists, which often led to a rejection of established church tradition, led to a disinterest in fasting, which they might have associated with the traditions that persecuted them. Whatever the reason, it seems that fasting did not play much of a role in the shaping of the Anabaptist tradition, and certainly this tradition has been influential in modern evangelicalism. While it would be difficult to document, it seems reasonable to conjecture that this is one strand in the reasons for a relative lack of explicit references to fasting in modern evangelical thought and practice. Yet the basic theology of Anabaptist tradition would suggest at least the possibility of a welcome place for fasting, and perhaps that too could factor into an evangelical resurgence of interest in the practice.

The Anglicans and Methodists: Balancing Traditional Fasting and Spiritual Discipline in Protestantism

The Church of England sought to promote fasting as spiritual discipline. They retained fasting traditions that had been handed down from Catholicism, while doing so in the context of the Protestant ideal of a free conscience. While this attempt at balance may not always have been met with general enthusiasm, John Wesley and the early Methodists provide an example of this virtuous balance in practice.

- The Church of England: Fasting Traditions Promoted to a Free Conscience

The nature of the Reformation in England had the effect of retaining similar forms for fasting as traditionally practiced in Catholicism, even though some currents of thought led to more Protestant distinctions. Specifically, the liberty of individual Christians is valued highly, so that the traditional fasts are encouraged, but seen as voluntary.

This noble desire to uphold ancient church traditions on the one hand, while not overly binding conscience on the other, can be seen in Thomas Becon's "Treatise of Fasting." Becon was chaplain to Archbishop Cranmer during the reign of Edward VI and author of the first major English catechism. His fasting treatise purports to be the first discussion of religious fasting in the English language.[102] Becon defines true Christian fasting as being done freely and willingly, and it is not only abstaining from food and drink, but other pleasures as well, in contrition of heart with a mind bent toward godliness.[103] In support of fasting, he examines dozens of the typical biblical examples. He contrasts true fasting with the "popish and superstitious fast" that is done for mere custom, or even worse, to earn forgiveness and everlasting life.[104] Becon chastises the Catholics for substituting better tasting fish for a little meat, or eating large quantities at night, and compared them to the hypocrites Jesus condemned.[105] Becon follows Chrysostom's comments on Matthew in saying that true fasting requires anointing the head, washing the face, and doing it in secret. The anointing is spiritually interpreted as mercy for the poor, and the washing as a pure conscience.[106] Fasting reminds us that possessions are to be shared, as not eating will make us appreciate those who go hungry. The purity of heart in fasting is in line with Isaiah 58 and freedom from hypocrisy. And secrecy is not so much that no one else knows, as it is that the true heart motive is that the actions are done for God alone. As for the ends of fasting, the first is that of mortifying the flesh, so that it will obey the spirit, "as an hand-maid her mistress, or an horse his keeper."[107] The second reason to fast is to learn to give liberally to the poor. Third, fasting makes one "more apt to pray," and the biblical examples are once again reviewed.[108] Fourth and finally, fasting makes one more receptive to hearing the word of God in humility.

The desire to uphold tradition in fasting while freeing the conscience can again be seen in a pronouncement on fasting communion adopted in 1899.[109] Pains are taken to affirm that fasting is a healthy self-discipline and the reception of the Eucharist a very solemn occasion. Nevertheless, the Lord's Supper was initiated in the context of a meal, and the reasons for fasting before the Eucharist are probably more customary in nature, having to do with the rise of asceticism in the early church, and do not arise from Scripture. Therefore such rules are not binding, and the church is reminded, "Fasting, again, is a means to an end and not an end in itself."[110] On this particular matter, the Church of England desired to apply Paul's teaching not to let matters of eating or not eating be a matter of judgment, as in Rom 14:3 and 14:5.

So while the Church of England in theory seeks to free the conscience, and to a great extent does so in general practice, it still advocates the seasonal fasting rituals of the Roman Catholic Church.[111] A comparison of the canon law of the two bodies on fasting shows that beyond similar Lenten practice, the Church of England actually retains more fasting days than the Roman Catholic Church, since the latter has substituted days of prayer for fasting on traditional ember days (fasts at the beginning of the four seasons of the year, as well as before ordinations, certain feast days or those called by bishops) and rogation days (the Monday, Tuesday and Wednesday before Ascension Sunday).[112] In a tract from 1833, Edward Pusey said 108 possible fast days appeared on the Church of England's calendar, although Pusey himself was noting how little they were actually observed.[113]

- Wesley and the Methodists: A Revival of Disciplined Fasting

John Wesley (1703-1791), founder of the Methodists, both practiced and advocated fasting in strong ways. Wesley's comments make it clear that he did not believe the Church of England of his day was actually practicing the kind of fasting that it officially advocated, at least not in accord with biblical truth or vital habits of the disciplined life. The many statements by Wesley in his journal about fasting, discussed below, show that he and the early Methodists associated with him regularly practiced fasting. Additionally, his sermons and other writings advocate a balanced, but passionate, approach to fasting as a spiritual discipline.

Wesley's and the Early Methodists' Experience: Fasting as a Living Discipline. With regard to his personal practice, Wesley recorded in his journal in December 1, 1725, how he resolved to fast every Wednesday in a month when he felt he was struggling with careless sins during his Oxford days.[114] He came to regularly practice this Wednesday fast, and in a letter of Oct. 11, 1732, said he had been practicing this for six months.[115] He said that his Holy Club of Oxford Methodists began observing the fasts of the church, "the general neglect of which we can by no means apprehend to be a lawful excuse for neglecting them."[116] This suggests that the early Methodists felt their fasting practices were both traditional, and because of the lack of common practice, revivalist.

Wesley recorded on March 30-31, 1736, how he and his companions in Savannah were experimenting with a diet that consisted only of bread and "were never more vigorous than while we tasted nothing else." While every kind of food is a good gift from God, those who need help in purity should "use every help, and remove every hindrance."[117] On Friday, August 17, 1739, Wesley records that many of his society agreed to "obey the Church to which we belong by observing all Fridays in the year as days of fasting or abstinence."[118] Wesley and his companions practiced their Wednesday and Friday fasts regularly throughout their ministry, patterned after the early church, and his diaries suggest a great level of self-denial in relation to food, sleep, and other things.[119]

In Wesley's *Appeals* he makes it clear that there were those who wrongly felt they were righteous for going to church, taking the sacraments, and observing certain fasts, like that of the Anglican memorial to the execution of King Charles on January 31. Such religion could prove vain, if done without love, a form of godliness without the power, since an inwardly motivated religion of the heart was necessary.[120] He defended his Methodists when they were accused of undermining church law by pointing out that they were actually keeping church law more scrupulously than others, as evidenced by their attention to the fast days.[121]

There are dozens of passing references to fasting in his journals, giving evidence that he and his companions observed national, church and personal fasts at a very dedicated level.[122] Wesley commended the duty of fasting in a letter, writing that "Our Lord annexes a peculiar promise even to secret fasting."[123] He speaks of consecrating a solemn fast during a mission in Bristol, after which the work revived.[124]

Yet later in his life, Wesley would note that few of his Methodists were practicing the regular fasts. A sermon from 1790, "Causes of the Inefficacy of Christianity," notes the decline. He decries the lack of self-denial evidenced by the abandonment of their previous fasting habits, including even ministers on days of giving the sacraments. He strongly asserts here that according to Scripture, "the man that never fasts is no more in the way to heaven than the man that never prays."[125] In the 1797 *Form of Discipline*, he wrote:

> The neglect of this is sufficient to account for our feebleness and faintness of spirit. We are continually grieving the Holy Spirit by the habitual neglect of a plain duty! Let us amend from this hour... . Begin next Friday, and avow this duty wherever you go.[126]

Sermons on Fasting: Not an End, But a Precious Means. When preaching on the Sermon on the Mount, he showed keen awareness of the Pharisees' practice of fasting twice a week. He urged his people to avoid the hypocrisy of those who wished to be seen by others, like the Pharisee who commended himself to God in Luke 18.[127] Yet, Christians ought not let their righteousness fall short of the Pharisees, and while fleeing hypocrisy, should be sure to pray and fast diligently, availing themselves of the means of grace and doing good.[128] In another discourse, he notes how some go to extremes of fasting, others to neglect:

> Those have spoken of it as if it were all in all; if not the end itself, yet infallibly connected with it: these, as if it were just nothing; as if it were a fruitless labour, which had no relation at all thereto. Whereas it is certain the truth lies between them both. It is not all, nor yet is it nothing. It is not the end, but it is a precious means thereto; a means which God Himself has ordained, and in which therefore, when it is duly used, He will surely give us His blessing.[129]

In his sermon, he shows himself aware of ancient Jewish fasting practices and early church references as well as biblical teachings and examples. He says that the natural grounds of fasting are sorrow and burdens for sin, and as an aid to prayer, where believers might avert the wrath of God's judgment, or seek his blessings. He urges Christians to practice fasting regularly and as much as desired, while being careful not to set aside normal Christian duties.[130] Christians should fast before God and not for men, not fancying any notion of merit in the bare act, and with diligence to afflict the soul as well as the body, praying and doing good deeds as fitting accompaniments.[131]

The Decline of Fasting Practices in Western Christianity to the Modern Era

It is generally agreed that there is a lack of attention given to fasting in the modern era. In 1968 Arthur Wallis commented, "For nearly a century and a half fasting has been out of vogue, at least in the churches of the West."[132] Similarly, Richard Foster remarked that in his research on spiritual disciplines, he could not find a single book that had been published on the topic of Christian fasting between 1861 and 1954.[133] While there are minor exceptions to Foster's statement, the substance seems basically accurate.[134] Additionally, examples of the decline of attention being paid to fasting can be seen below in monastic practice, Protestant practice, and the gradual elimination of national fast days. The points discussed below suggest a decline in these specific aspects of fasting practice, and this relative lack of attention might suggest a more general decline in interest in Christian fasting.[135] Some possible reasons for this decline will be offered below.

The Decline of Fasting in Monasticism

Adalbert de Vogüé, a great French scholar of the history of asceticism and himself a Benedictine monk, notes the decline of fasting in monastic tradition and seeks to trace the reasons. The decline from strict observance of ancient rules is obvious, but the reasons remain elusive. He rejects some suggestions offered by his brethren, such as the notion that modern men are more feeble than their ancient counterparts, the need for more frequent food because more work is being done in monastic communities, and the need to eat frequently for fellowship in the common life. Instead, he finds the decline most in evidence in tracing the evolution of eating practices in Europe, arguing that the sole evening meal of antiquity encroached earlier into the day until there was a noon meal, and finally breakfast was added.[136]

This historical reconstruction may apply in a general way to the practices of monastic life, but lacks evidence for a more general understanding of eating practices in general society, and so it is less than entirely convincing. Still, it is interesting to note that an astute observer of asceticism in history and modern practitioner sees the fact of the decline of fasting as rather general and obvious. De Vogüé criticizes the commentaries on St. Benedict's *Rule* that praise the latitude offered the community: "By praising Benedict for having mitigated the observances of his predecessors, the monks absolve themselves implicitly for not being faithful to his."[137] There is evidence that despite monastic vows of poverty and commitments to self-discipline, typical monks often partook of diets that were anything but austere. English Reformer Thomas Becon caricatured a monk who was especially known for fasting, who in his regular meal ate what could have served "six godly fasters."[138] In Léo Moulin's intriguing article, "Monks Fasted but were Plump," he describes the regular ration in medieval monasteries as consisting of up to 4,700 calories per day. Their regular diets combined with regular fasting created an unbalanced approach to eating, which actually seems counterproductive to their own lifestyle goals of temperance:

> These practices promoted an obsession with food, and on the other hand, led to a sense of suffering (which has its merits) when they mortified the flesh by fasting. Leaving the table without having wholly satisfied one's hunger, not eating between meals, abstaining from meat—the most beneficial thing they could have done—these things were in fact a challenge which was no doubt more keenly felt than the twin burdens of chastity and obedience.[139]

Under such circumstances, it is not surprising that observers both inside and outside the monasteries might criticize monastic fasting practices. One might also speculate that the sharp Reformation critique of Catholic fasting could have found some resonance even within the walls of the monasteries, creating a sensitivity that could prompt changes in behavior.

The Decline of Fasting in Protestantism

As examined above, the controversies of the Reformation clearly put Catholic fasting practices in a dim light. While the Reformers themselves may have kept a place for fasting in their minds, they certainly put the Protestant churches on a general trajectory away from the ritualized, formalized and often trivialized approaches to fasting in Catholicism. When the Reformed churches quit practicing Lent, fast days became more occasional than regular in nature. With the emphasis on the freedom of the conscience, natural human tendencies to choose not to fast could certainly gain momentum, and so it should not be entirely surprising that Protestant churches practiced fasting less and less over time.

The Reformers sought to rescue fasting from what were seen as affronts to the gospel inherent in its contemporary practice. In this effort they sought a middle way between the apparent excesses of Catholicism and the danger of self-indulgence on the other hand. But this trajectory of reduction was followed until, over time, fasting was virtually eliminated by Protestants. De Vogüé also discusses the comments of Luther (whom he sees as simplistic) and Calvin (whom he appreciates much more for his synthetic thought), and concludes that they tended to minimize the role of fasting because of the excesses of their day. His trenchant comment here deserves note: "Desiring to purify fasting, we have killed it. Were not all its defects in the end less grave than the total effacement of it, which is our present state?"[140]

Wesley's comments examined above show that he believed that fasting had already declined greatly in England by his day. As already noted, the Anglican church in its calendar maintained a closer resemblance to Catholic fasting practices, and 108 possible fast days appeared on the church's official calendar when Edward Pusey wrote about the subject in 1833. But the church's allowance of generous liberty in the practice of fasts apparently resulted in fasting not being regularly practiced, and according to Pusey, "the Church herself had tacitly abandoned them."[141]

It is interesting to note that in Princeton Seminary's 1810 charter, "The Plan of a Theological Seminary," Article 5, Section 1, "It is also wished and recommended, that each student should ordinarily set apart one day in a month for special prayer and self-examination in secret, accompanied with fasting."[142] So here is an example of fasting being promoted as a spiritual discipline by a major Protestant institution, although one wonders how much of this older Calvinist piety was actually being practiced, and how much or it survived the school's reorganization of its charter in 1929.

As already noted, the lacuna in literature related specifically to fasting makes it difficult to assess Protestant attitudes toward fasting as the modern era progressed. As will be seen in the following chapter, there was a mushrooming of books related to fasting as a spiritual discipline by Protestant evangelicals beginning in the latter half of the twentieth century. This change in the published literature suggests in a general way that a lack of attention was being then being addressed. But one further point is yet to be addressed, and that is the phenomenon of the decline of national or societal fast days.

National Fasts and Their Modern Decline

It was only natural in politically Christian nations, as in the Israelite kingdom that served to some extent as their ancient model, for government and religion to coordinate social structures, especially as responses to disasters or wars. These responses often included official, national proclamations of fast days, with attendant moral requirements of special liturgies for corporate worship in prayer and fasting, as well as social requirements of shutting down of commerce. These practices began to decline in the modern era, apparently corresponding with the secularization and pluralization of Western nations.

- New England Puritan Community Fasts

The modern decline in community fasting practices stands in sharp contrast to the early days of Puritan New England, when some of Calvin's staunchest followers apparently took to heart his admonitions to pastors to call for days of fasting in the face of difficulty and for repentance:

> Records indicate that Plymouth called for at least sixty-nine fast days between 1620 and 1697, a figure that does not include the "frequent fasts" that were observed between 1654 and 1667 due to their lack of a pastor, and undoubtedly numerous other fasts that were simply not recorded.[143]

Difficult days prompted calls for prayer and fasting, while times of feasting and thanksgiving helped the community maintain a cyclical relationship between fasting and normal eating without the trappings of the more detailed church year.[144] In a fast day sermon first preached January 7, 1748 in Philadelphia, Gilbert Tennent stated that fasting was abused by the Catholics, and neglected by Protestants:

> Indeed the Papists do sometimes make a pretence of fasting, but ity may be truly said that many of their fasts are mock-fasts, feasts instead of fasts. It must also be confessed that many Protestants sadly neglect this duty of fasting to their great prejudice in religion. All those who would have their corruptions mortified must take pains and use proper means for that end. Fasting is among the most uselful means for it has a noble tendency to keep the body in subjection to the mind. But this duty is so contrary to people's keen appetites that they can scarcely be brought to believe in it, and it is still more difficult for the to practice it.[145]

It appears that these kinds of fasts took place into the nineteenth century, though they were practiced less and less over time. National fasts were observed in the United States through the Civil War period, but there is no record of any after 1865.[146]

- British National Fasts

Richard J. Janet has provided a thorough historical examination of the nature of and responses to general fasts proclaimed during the Victorian era in England. Up until this time, these specifically occasional, general fasts were a fairly regular part of civic life in England, as well as the American colonies. In the period examined five general fasts were proclaimed, in response to a cholera epidemic, the Irish potato famine, the Crimean war (two occasions), and the Indian mutiny. After these, however, the British government ceased calling for general fast days, though there were national observances of days of prayer, carrying less solemn requirements and legal overtones.

With incidents like the cholera epidemic and potato famine, it is easy to see continuity between biblical fasts in times of national threat or disaster beyond human control. As such, the fast functions as a time of repentance, solemn reflection on the wisdom of providence and seeking of guidance for a course of action. But war can be a trickier application, as the Crimean example suggests. Finding occasion for repentance and immediate danger in this occasion was difficult for the British, as their homeland was not threatened and it was an act of flexing military muscle abroad. The picture of Britain as a pious knight keeping a solemn vigil before going out on a noble crusade harked back to an era of Christian aggression that was disappearing, and the irony that Russian Orthodoxy also prayed for victory for their presumably despotic czar heightens the feeling of incongruity. The mixed results of the campaign stirred debate about the appropriateness of a second general fast day that was called, and one can see the erosion of Britain's moral certainty coupled with its growing confusion over it global position and national identity.[147] The Indian mutiny of 1857 likewise confronted Britain with a national military problem far from the homeland. While moral outrage seemed to prevail when "pagans" attacked the Christian government in India, it is interesting that this marks the last occasion for a general fast. To some it seemed that the fast was more utilitarian as a common expression of sympathy grief rather than as national repentance, though some still called for that in conjunction.[148]

Janet convincingly argues that the pluralizing of British society in the Victorian era was bringing about a different understanding of the interactions of church and state, and this led to the decline of general fast days. As an example, he cites prime minister Gladstone, who said in 1846, "The process which I am now actively engaged in carrying on is a process of lowering the religious tone of the State, letting it down, demoralizing it—i.e., stripping it of its ethical character and assisting its transition into one which is mechanical."[149] While people generally may have viewed prayer and fasting as having value, its role in national life was becoming marginalized. "In a modernizing, increasingly democratic and pluralistic state religious neutrality becomes the reflex response to agitation by minority sects or confusion generated by traditional public religion."[150] While there may have been some tendency in modern England to forsake supernatural explanations of events for more naturalistic, scientific ones, in the end the social forces of modern life probably had more to do with the end of general fasts than theology did. Janet concludes:

> It can be seen that fasts were challenged (and finally abandoned) because of their inevitable entanglement in the

political, social, intellectual and ecclesiastical controversies of a modernizing world. The change in English politics (toward democratic participation), society (toward egalitarianism, or, at least, civil liberties) and ecclesiastical structure (toward stricter denominational definition and discipline) meant the outdating of public fasts as universal expressions of religious belief called by the state and directed by the established church.[151]

Possible Reasons for the Decline of Fasting

Along with his historical observations, de Vogüé offers four plausible theological reasons why fasting may have declined into the modern era.[152] First, one must take into account the natural concept of the weakness of the flesh, which requires constant diligence for the maintaining of practices that require discipline. "Christian fasting has disappeared, because pastors and faithful have not reinvented it together in each generation."[153] Second, a "disincarnate spirituality" seems to prevail in the church, one that divorces spiritual realities from bodily, physical practices. Third, the approach that categorizes fasting as a penalty for sin impoverishes its positive value. Fourth, the idea that obedience is better than fasting can easily cause other good things to become substitutes for fasting itself, so that in time fasting is no longer practiced, though it may be held up in name.

Régamey, writing in 1959 (before the renewal of fasting which he hoped for in Catholicism was to some extent set in motion, as discussed in the following chapter), offered five possible reasons for the decline of fasting.[154] First, the dualism of body and soul, deeply embedded in Christian tradition, hampers a proper understanding of the role of fasting. Second, the popular notion that the form of fasting is not important for spirituality leads to an abstraction of the practice, until the concept of fasting becomes relatively meaningless. Third, he suggests that the weakened condition of faith in modern Christianity precludes Christians from a general willingness to follow in the way of the cross and discipline. Fourth, the development of naturalism has affected people so that they see fasting as a mystical element from an ancient worldview. Finally, the upheavals in the structures of modern life militate against cultural fasting practices on a wide scale. Together, he believes these factors have led to a practically complete neglect of authentic fasting practices in modern church life.

Perhaps it is not surprising in light of history, theology and human nature that fasting declined in the modern era. When one considers Catholicism, one is reminded of the excesses of ancient and medieval ascetics, the cumbersome intricacies and exceptions of canon law, and the popular redefinition of the practice.[155] Considering Protestantism, one is sent on a theological trajectory against Catholicism that reduces the importance of fasting, severs it from churchly and governmental authority, and marches into a modernity that stands in a largely antithetical climate to its practice. While there appears to be no substantial voice in the leadership streams of Christian thought that has decided definitively against fasting, relatively little specific, substantial attention has been paid to fasting as a practice.

So it appears that Catholic Christian communities largely obscured the underlying biblical theology of fasting over the centuries, and the Protestant Reformation tried to recapture biblical emphases. But in practice, the pendulum swung away from actually practicing fasting. Governments in Christian nations, like England that was examined in some detail, gradually saw their role move from promoting clear spiritual functions in society to more pluralized functions. So with churches and society promoting fasting less and less, with the excesses of monasticism in the background and modern materialism in the foreground, it would be more surprising if fasting had somehow continued to have a robust Christian expression. If there is to be some kind of renewal of fasting practices in contemporary times, Christians will need to sense a defensible underlying theology of fasting, and something of the possible spiritual effects of the practice. In the latter part of the 20th century such a renewal appears to have begun. An examination of that renewal, with attendant theological questions, will be undertaken in the final chapter.

§5
Toward a Contemporary
Christian Theology of Fasting

This chapter will suggest an integrative theological approach to fasting that is based on the scriptural and historical insights studied so far. These will first be set in the context of the renewal of fasting practices in certain Christian traditions, and then oriented toward an eschatological, christocentric understanding of the nature of the Christian age, in dialogue with some authors attempting similar or contrasting approaches.

With a view toward a contemporary renewal of ascetical theology and application, Margaret Miles has examined the history of asceticism rather thoroughly, categorizing its main forms into four major models.[1] The first kind was the individual, rigorous asceticism of the early desert fathers, who retreated from worldly life to attempt to regain their spirituality through austerity. The second kind was the monastic movement, which promoted asceticism within a renewed vision of communal church life. The third model came from Augustine, and emphasized the gathering and focusing of energy away from the flesh and toward the spirit. The fourth model, from Ignatius of Loyola, emphasized the intensification and concentration of consciousness, so that a unified person would make life's choices.[2]

Miles urges a critical eye toward evaluating and recapturing a renewed asceticism. She rightly urges us to "reject rationales for ascetic practice that are inconsistent with the Christian affirmation of the human body by the doctrines of creation, incarnation, and resurrection."[3] Additionally, the notion that we take upon ourselves the punishing of the body in expiating guilt should also be discarded as assuming God's own prerogative.[4] Since these two elements so often characterize perceptions of asceticism in general, it is little wonder that modern Christians have found little use for trying to value ascetic practices, including fasting.

On the positive side, Miles suggests what a "new asceticism" for our time might look like. She suggests that "First, any rationale for ascetic practice must assume that the human body is permanently and integrally connected with the soul."[5] This entails her second point, which is that ascetic practices must be as good for the body as they are perceived as being good for the soul. Third, "ascetic practices must be temporary," suggesting that they are designed to work on particular issues.[6] Finally, she allows for the perennial usefulness of some practices, such as fasting, in order to orient ourselves properly to our bodies and to the outside world and time, as well as other disciplines that might aid in overcoming the deadness of soul and body.[7]

This summary is helpful to the extent that it suggests the possible value of fasting in religious experience. But it will also be expanded through more specifically theological ideas that will be proposed below. In the following section Eastern Orthodox, Roman Catholic, and contemporary Evangelical Protestant fasting practices are examined. But further, a theological framework will help to integrate the scriptural teachings and the best of the historical models. Toward that end we now turn, beginning with an examination of the renewal of fasting before setting forward a constructive theological integration of fasting in the context of the nature of the age.

The Renewal of Fasting in Contemporary Christian Traditions

Christians have reawakened to the possibilities of fasting in recent decades. The Eastern Orthodox tradition offers a long-term witness to fasting, grounding the practice theologically in their doctrine of theosis, as explained below. The Roman Catholic Church has reevaluated many of its longstanding fasting practices, investing them with renewed meanings and freedoms since the reform-minded Second Vatican Council. And many Protestants of the evangelical variety have incorporated fasting into a broadened understanding of the role of spiritual disciplines in the life of the believer.

Fasting in Eastern Orthodoxy to the Present: Part of Tradition and Theosis

The Eastern Orthodox churches offer a living example of continuity in Christian fasting traditions. They place fasting within their doctrine of *theosis*, or divinization, as part of the sanctification (or for them, salvation) process. These aspects will be explored below, with attention to the contribution the Orthodox might make for developing an evangelical theology of fasting.

- Fasting as Part of Christian Tradition

Eastern Orthodoxy has held the teachings and practices of the Church Fathers in high regard through the centuries. Without the earthquake of the Reformation that so affected Western Christianity, the Orthodox communities have transmitted ancient practices into the modern era in a rather organic way. Whatever the actual fasting practices may be on a local level, it is clear that official Orthodoxy has sought to maintain continuity with the past. For the Orthodox, "tradition is not something limited to that found in the Early Church. It is that which binds the past and present and which survives today."[8] The characters in Scripture, the Church Fathers, the councils and bishops, are all part of the same community that is alive and worships today. This idea, "that the Church is always identical with herself," helps to shape the Orthodox approach to fasting.[9] It is not surprising, then, to see Orthodox treatments of fasting begin with Scriptures, move through patristic teachers of authority (especially the Greek fathers), and then make fairly direct applications for the church.[10]

- Fasting as Part of Theosis

Akakios says that to understand the importance of fasting for the Eastern Orthodox, one must understand the place of asceticism within its cosmology, and he notes these elements: "its view of human sin, salvation and restoration, and *theosis* (or divinization) and enlightenment."[11] Humanity's fall from paradise is not viewed so much in Augustinian understandings of original sin, as in "a dynamic process of deviation which led to disobedience and which changed the course of human growth from something natural to something unnatural."[12] As a result, salvation is also viewed as more of a dynamic process, a restoration to the right path for humanity that has deviated from it. In a collection of Orthodox essays on fasting, Lazar Puhalo says this:

> Fasting is a special keystone in our struggle to acquire the Holy Spirit and to become robed in the "wedding garment" of divine grace. To understand the fasts and to keep them is, therefore, fundamental to our salvation itself. To fail to keep the fasts in a true Orthodox fashion is to undermine our salvation and turn ourselves away from the Heavenly Kingdom.[13]

The transformation that takes place in the believer is theosis, the process of becoming like God; but more than like God, this is done through partaking in his nature, the Holy Spirit, so that there is a deep sense of one's unity with God in this saving, transforming process. [14] While its full realization awaits death, the process of theosis divinizes a person by degrees throughout life. The Orthodox resist the judicial approach to justification prominent in the Western Christian tradition, because there fasting has been viewed as part of a legal covenant between man and God.[15]

In clarifying theosis, or deification, for Western Christians, Bishop Kallistos (Timothy) Ware makes six points:

1. Deification is not reserved for a few, but is intended for all alike.

2. Deification involves a continual attitude of repentance, and does not expect freedom from sin.

3. The methods for deification are not extraordinary, esoteric or mystical, but normal and moral.

4. Deification is a social process of loving God and neighbor.

5. Love of God and neighbor must be practical, issuing in good deeds.

6. Deification presupposes life in the church and sacraments, where the coinherence of believers with the Spirit can be realized.[16]

In this context of theosis, fasting is not seen as a negative act, but rather it "constitutes a constructive adherence to a practical therapy by which spiritual illness is cured. It is not a rejection of certain foods or of the body, but a realignment of our attitude toward food and the body."[17] This emphasis on the therapeutic role of fasting prompts theological interest in medical and scientific approaches to fasting, so that fasting basically becomes a kind of medicine for body and soul.[18] In Orthodox fasting, the Christian is limited to those things that grew in Paradise when Adam and Eve were not yet fallen (i.e., abstaining from all animal products). Recalling themes in Tertullian, Basil, and Augustine already discussed, the Eastern believes Christian who fasts becomes "a living icon of the human person in the Paradise restored."[19]

These idealistic visions of the role of fasting have prompted traditionalist Orthodox leaders to maintain a robust and fairly rigorous approach to fasting at the various levels of church calendar and ascetic life in monasticism, often in a manner that would make St. Basil proud. Ware says these rules "will astonish and appall many western Christians."[20] All the traditional fasts of the ancient ecumenical church are maintained, as well as the observance of stations on Wednesday and Friday, and even Monday in some monasteries. The rules are somewhat stricter in food choices allowed during fasting times than in Roman Catholicism. However, traditionalists also lament the modern deemphasis on fasting among the Orthodox, demonstrating that perhaps the ideals held up so strongly by conservative officials might not be as widely practiced as they would wish, or perhaps even lead us to believe.[21]

- Contribution to a Fasting Theology

What might evangelicals learn from Orthodox fasting practices? First, we can appreciate something of the value of tradition that often we have lost. If the church is an organic unity of believers throughout the ages, then our theology and practice should be done in conversation with that tradition. This does not need to undermine Scripture's authority or place the traditions of men above the Word of God, but rather evangelicals can enrich their understanding of God's work by renewed appreciation of the great traditions of Christianity. Second, the Orthodox emphasis on the body as essential in the sanctification process contributes to a renewed awareness of us as whole beings devoted to God. Admittedly, evangelicals will have serious differences with the Orthodox over the role of works in salvation, as the Orthodox see fasting and other practices as contributing to the lifelong process of salvation. But evangelicals need not abandon the doctrine of justification by faith to appreciate the contribution an awareness of embodied spirituality can bring. These insights will be explored further below. Now we turn to the Roman Catholic tradition, where fasting has seen renewed emphasis and revitalization in the contemporary era.

Developments in Fasting in Modern Roman Catholicism:
Moving from Legalistic Forms to a Theology of Community Worship and Solidarity

In addition to the work of de Vogüé discussed in the previous chapter, and other scholarly works to be discussed below, there appears to be a growing popular interest in the discipline of fasting among Catholics in the past few decades.[22] Régamey wrote of a hope that fasting could be revitalized by more reliance upon the guidance of the Spirit, which would produce more genuine and rigorous fasting in the context of community.[23] As mentioned in the previous chapter, Alexandre Guillaume wrote of hope that fasting as an act between prayer and charity, following a renewed form of Leo the Great's theology, could revitalize fasting in the modern church.[24] This revitalization of fasting in the Roman Catholic tradition corresponds to sweeping changes that precipitated around the time of the Second Vatican Council. Not only were there changes in the liturgical requirements related to fasting, but more importantly, Catholic theologians and church leaders began examining the theological frameworks that underlay their own fasting practices. These emphases will be examined below, with special attention to the main emerging theological themes.

- Canon Law and Vatican II: From Law, Structure, and Ritual to Theology, Community, and Worship

In the modern era, Roman Catholic fasting practices have come under some scrutiny. Some of the rational hair-splitting over details has been modified to keep larger issues to the fore, and an attempt is being made to recover early church tradition in a context relevant to modern circumstances.

Marcellino Zalba writes of fasting in the Roman Catholic Church as having two primary theological emphases.[25] First, fasting must start from the need to share one's property with others (rather than beginning with the thought of managing concupiscence). Pope Paul VI connected this facet of fasting to the responsibility for social justice among the nations: "Nations who enjoy economic plenty have a duty of self-denial, combined with an active proof of love towards our brothers who are tormented by poverty and hunger."[26] Secondly, fasting helps integrate the body into the life of faith, which is a summary of the value tradition has placed upon it, as already seen clearly in Augustine and Aquinas.

In the collection of canon law done some fifty years before Vatican II, canons 1250-54 related to fasting and abstinence. These basically fell into two categories, the "law of abstinence" and the "law of fasting." The law of abstinence forbade eating meat of mammals and birds and meat broth, but not animal products (eggs, milk, etc.) or fish and seafood. Everyone above seven years of age was subject to the law of abstinence, and everyone twenty-one to sixty to the law of fasting. Questions are submitted to local usage. The law of fasting permitted only one full meal per day, but this was not interpreted to mean the forbidding of small portions throughout the day, and such were subject to local custom. The single meal could be interchanged from noon to evening. The law of abstinence was to be practiced on all Fridays, and the law of both fast and abstinence on Ash Wednesday, Fridays and Saturdays of Lent, Ember Days, and the vigils of the feasts of Pentecost, Assumption, All Saints, and Christmas. The law of fast applied on all other days of Lent. Sundays were generally exempt from fasting, except on holydays during Lent.[27]

The early twentieth century collection of canon law brought a modern sense of order out of what may have been previously a rather chaotic approach. However, this order came under scrutiny within the Roman Catholic Church, so that even its own experts in canon law felt it needed a greater sense of theological grounding and less emphasis on the letter of the law.[28] One can observe the almost dizzying discussions of rules and exceptions to fasting practice, and it is easy to imagine losing a sense of its significance.[29]

With the reforms of Vatican II came a revision in canon law, which affected the canons regarding abstinence and fasting in several ways.[30] Canons 1249-1253 fall under the heading, "Days of Penance." The age of those bound by the law of abstinence was raised to fourteen, and those subject to the law of fasting are described as adults up to sixty (though parents are to see to it that their children observe an authentic sense of penance in their own ways). Additionally, bishops could now substitute other forms of penance in place of laws of abstinence or fasting, "especially works of charity and exercises of piety." Bishops can also substitute abstinence from meat for some other food.[31] Pope Paul VI's Apostolic Constitution Paentimini brought these changes into effect, and the Pastoral Statement of the National Conference of Catholic Bishops, *On Penance and Abstinence*, interpreted them for Americans.[32] The bishops preserved the tradition of fasting and abstinence from meat on Fridays in Lent, but for other Fridays, they terminated "the traditional law of abstinence as binding under pain of sin."[33] Great pains were taken to remind the faithful that they were not doing away with the need for penance or abstinence, but were encouraging people to apply the practices from a free conscience, and perhaps with wider applications to good works besides merely abstaining from eating meat. The guiding norms for such practices were laid out as solidarity with the church's past, and the need to "preserve a saving and necessary difference from the spirit of the world."[34]

In the twentieth century, the Roman Catholic Church began to alter its strict official approach to the Eucharistic fast. While in practice exceptions to the rules had grown to be interpreted rather widely, it was observed by a doctor of canon law in 1941 that it "obliges with a severity unknown in any other purely ecclesiastical discipline, not involving validity," although he noted that changes in attitude had already been set in motion.[35] In order to increase Eucharistic piety by making the celebration more flexible, Pope Pius XII issued the apostolic constitution, *Christus Dominus*, in 1953. This promulgation brought about "the most far-reaching changes in the law of the Eucharistic Fast since Apostolic times" for the Roman Catholic Church.[36] This allowed concessions for the sick and hard working, and a three-hour fast before celebrations of the Eucharist at times other than morning.[37] Pope Paul VI further reduced this in conjunction with Vatican II to simply one hour, which is the standing norm in the *Code of Canon Law* of 1983, with even exceptions to that for the infirm or those caring for them.[38] The emphasis on the communion of the entire body of Christ in the Roman Catholic Church since Vatican II has resulted in these changes. While it may seem small, this alteration of centuries old, inflexible practice at its best could represent a shift in the Roman Catholic Church from law to theology, from structure to community, and from prioritizing ritual to prioritizing worship. However, for those who still see Catholic spirituality in terms of works-righteousness, these shifts might represent only a shift from strict laws to more lenient ones.

- ## Contemporary Catholic Emphasis: Fasting as Solidarity

And so, fasting has officially become for contemporary Catholics not only a means of identifying with the sufferings of Christ, but also a means of showing solidarity with the church of the ages, as well as those who need its ministry. These are the overriding themes of the papal sermons delivered for Lent in the decades following the publication of Vatican II.[39] These sermons largely elaborate the imagery of the parable in Matt 25:35-40, where the righteous serve Christ in the needs of the poor and afflicted. The sermons address such contemporary issues as hunger, refugees, the environment, and political disorders. While fasting *per se* is not the emphasis, clearly themes of abstinence have been enlarged into this concept of brotherhood and solidarity in humanity. John Paul II urged the church in 1979: "Going without things is to free oneself from the slaveries of a civilization that is always urging people on to greater comfort and consumption."[40] With regard to hunger, he asks in 1985:

> Within the same family, can some members eat their fill while their brothers and sisters are excluded from the table? To think of those who suffer is not enough. In this time of Lent, conversion of heart calls us to add fasting to our prayer, and to fill with God's love the efforts that the demands of justice towards neighbour inspire us to make.[41]

- ## Contribution to a Fasting Theology

One can only hope that these theological strides in the fasting practice of Roman Catholics will result in effecting the idealistic changes they envision. Perhaps even Protestants can find inspiration and some direction here for our own long neglect of fasting practices. It has become almost axiomatic for Protestants since the Reformation to characterize Catholic fasting as legalistic behavior. The changes in at least the official Catholic stance toward fasting since Vatican II show that they have seen this issue themselves, and made moves in the direction of correcting it.

It must be understood that legalism and ritualism are not matters restricted merely to church structures and hierarchies. Rather, these problems proceed from human hearts that prefer to aggrandize themselves through religious practices. Like the Pharisee of Luke 18:12, or the hypocrites of Matt 6:16-18, there will always be people who use fasting to bolster their opinions of themselves and their worth before God and others. The church must always warn against such things, and in promoting fasting, be on guard lest we encourage the very kinds of behaviors that have taken the Roman Catholic Church centuries to address.

Also, the renewed Catholic emphasis on fasting as subordinate to community life highlights the need to engage spirituality at a corporate level. Fasting is not merely about individual asceticism, but rather Christians are reminded that they are part of one another. Worship becomes more vital, and service becomes more heartfelt, when one of the purposes for fasting is Christian solidarity.

A final caution that might be offered here is that Catholics and evangelical Protestants are probably not yet ready come to agreement on the issue of viewing fasting as a penitential practice. The language of the *Catechism of the Catholic Church* continues to suggest that fasting is part of a complex of works that demonstrate penance, thereby bringing the believer into unity with Christ. The catechism describes fasting, prayer, and almsgiving as acts of "interior penance" that "express conversion in relation to oneself, to God, and to others."[42] Even Catholic commentator Monika Hellwig says that this emphasis on penance in the catechism needs further revision: "By constantly addressing the issue of serious sin and loss of grace, the text achieves a burdensome and depressing effect which cannot be helpful to catechesis."[43] Clearly biblical fasting was often associated with repentance, at least in the old covenant. But in the age since the coming of Christ, can any fasting or other penitential practice procure forgiveness of sins? For Protestants who believe the order is reversed, and forgiveness is a free gift in Christ and repentance is part of believing, there may still be appropriate reticence about adopting a Catholic fasting theology wholesale. Nevertheless, it is hoped that the insights noted above can be integrated into a relevant evangelical Christian theology of fasting.[44] As Daryl Charles says, "It is not insignificant that at present the Roman Catholic Church is emphasizing listening to Scripture in ways that are unprecedented, just as Protestants are simultaneously discovering tradition as they have never known it."[45]

Reawakening to Spiritual Disciplines Among Contemporary Evangelicals

A renewed desire to engage in spiritual disciplines has awakened among evangelical Protestants in recent decades, and this renewal has sparked increased interest in fasting. At the forefront are two prominent books: Richard Foster's *Celebration of Discipline* and Dallas Willard's

Spirit of the Disciplines.[46] Both books offer discussions of fasting in the context of spiritual disciplines. They are theologically grounded and offer practical direction, with Willard heavier on the former, Foster on the latter. Willard notes that the renewed emphasis on spiritual disciplines in his ministry "was only a part of something much larger that was happening in the flow of American Protestantism and the culture associated with it."[47] He attributes the change to a "widespread shift of religious consciousness and sentiment," noting the contributions of reactions to the excesses of pop culture and the positive contribution of Christian psychology. Willard regards liberal Christianity as having become largely impotent spiritually, and conservative churches awakening to the fact that they often give lip service to biblical authority without functioning practically that way.[48]

Numerous other works (of varying quality) that discuss fasting as a discipline have been published in and around their wake in the latter half of the twentieth century, most of them being more pastoral and practical in orientation, often with a revivalist spirit about them.[49] Several minor theses and dissertations have been written that could reasonably be related to this movement, exploring the origins of fasting and generally encouraging Christians in the practice.[50] A few works by evangelical Protestants react in a basically negative manner to fasting, regarding it with ambivalence as a religious practice from the Old Covenant.[51] All of this publishing activity by Protestant evangelicals follows a dearth of almost a hundred years, from the decline of public fast days following the Civil War era until basically the 1950s, when interest apparently began to flower.

It is clear, at least from the writings of Willard and Foster, that this evangelical resurgence has been aware of and borrowed from the broader heritage of church tradition, including monasticism.[52] The fasting advocated in the spiritual disciplines movements generally has nothing to do with the church's liturgical calendar, although occasionally those traditional themes may be drawn upon for inspiration. Rather, the fasting advocated seems to be of a more individualistic, ascetic variety. Generally fasting is viewed as abstaining from food for an entire day or even multiple days, advocating a rigorous austerity with regard to fasting might have made the early monks proud.[53]

Willard works hard to establish the link in spiritual disciplines to the imitation of and obedience to Christ. The "secret" to true spirituality "involves living as he lived in the entirety of his life—adopting his overall life-style."[54] So for Willard, the imitation of Christ is the adoption of the disciplined way in which he lived his earthly life. This noble ideal calls Christians to a life of humility in order that they, like Christ, may experience true dependence on the Father and share in some way in the power of his resurrection. The result is a Christian theology that is truly practical, embodying holiness in actual human life.

Amid all the good that this renewed emphasis on spiritual disciplines appears to be doing, there also seems to be a hazard of a formulaic approach to sanctification. Foster makes important qualifications about the need for grace and avoidance of legalism.[55] When asked what he expects to happen to a person who faithfully practices the spiritual disciplines, Dallas Willard responded:

> They will increasingly manifest the fruit of the Spirit—love, joy, peace, patience, kindness, goodness, faithfulness, gentleness, self-control (Gal 5:22-23)—and this will be obviously easy for them; and there will be manifestations of divine power in conjunction with who they are and what they do.[56]

It must be kept in mind that the desired spiritual results of such disciplines are the blessings that come ultimately from God for his own good purposes and glory in our lives. If these qualifications are kept in mind, Christians can avoid pursuing spiritual disciplines from improper motives. Tradition has shown that many problems spring from the desire to promote ourselves before others as "spiritual," in violation of the spirit of Jesus' words about fasting in Matt 6:16, "to be seen fasting by men."

Is it possible to develop the insights and practices of the spiritual disciplines movement beyond the basically ascetic approach to a thoroughgoing theology of fasting? If so, this theology should be set in an overarching framework of what it is that God has done and will do in Christ, and what he is doing through Christians when they fast. Such a theology will affirm the various contributions of the spectrum of positive fasting practices as component parts of a larger whole. To that end we now turn, in developing a theology of fasting in the context of God's work in Christ in the Christian era of redemptive history.

Fasting and the Nature of the Age

The primary focus of Christian fasting must be on the person and work of Christ. This comes from the fact that central NT passages related to fasting specifically use fasting as a way of highlighting Christ and his messianic work, as discussed in previous chapters and integrated below.[57] This is consistent with, and helps to inform, an eschatological understanding of the nature of the age, one caught between fulfillment and anticipation of fulfillment. In such a context, the biblical examples of fasting can find proper expression, and Jesus' teachings can be implemented. A christocentric, eschatological approach to fasting will allow for a full integration of the biblical theology of fasting that has already been examined in the first two chapters.

In addition to the biblical theology, the study of fasting in Christian history and the contemporary movements to renew fasting examined above call for a further, integrative, theological understanding of the possible value of fasting in a contemporary, evangelical Christian context. Reviewing the results of the previous two chapters' study, one can see that from the earliest days of the church, Christians have practiced fasting. Early Christians imitated biblical characters that fasted, and sought to follow Jesus' instructions about fasting in their lives. Leaders as important as Basil and Augustine wrote about the spiritual and physical benefits of fasting, urging their parishioners to practice discipline of the flesh. Even after all the abuses of fasting by medieval monasticism and church formalism, the Protestant Reformers unanimously affirmed that fasting could find a proper role in Christian practice, and their followers sought ways to implement these ideals. The Church of England sought to balance fasting traditions with the Protestant emphasis on a free conscience, which if practiced, could result in a powerful testimony to Christian unity and spiritual discipline. John Wesley was the epitome of practicing such a balance, and he promoted fasting in both private and churchly devotion. Although fasting seems to have declined in the modern era, the spiritual disciplines movement calls evangelicals to renew a practice that has biblical warrant and thorough support from every wing of Christian tradition.

At a broadly conceived level, this theology of fasting can begin with an understanding of the nature of the age in which Christians find themselves.[58] This theology takes Jesus' response to the synoptic fasting query of Matt 9:14-15/Mark 2:18-20/Luke 5:33-35 as its central integrating motif: "You cannot make the attendants of the bridegroom fast while the bridegroom is with them, can you? But the days will come; and when the bridegroom is taken away from them, then they will fast in those days" (Luke 5:34-35, NASB). The fasting Jesus responded to there was from the old covenant, in anticipation of eschatological fulfillment. Jesus was that fulfillment, the "bridegroom," and his companions in his presence could not fast. Yet he foresaw the present era as a time when the bridegroom would be taken away, and he said this would be a time for fasting. So we find ourselves in an age of fulfillment, while still being in an age of anticipation. In his profoundly integrative recent work, *Covenant and Eschatology*, Michael Horton writes:

> We proclaim as a present reality the "new creation" of which Jesus Christ is the firstfruits, and yet we cannot point to the present state of the world or any part of it (including the

church) and indicate univocally what this means. This fuels the now-not yet dialectic in our own Christian experience and activity. Capable neither of resting nor of waiting, we are driven by the historical fulfillment and the eschatological hope to act in the liminal space in which faith, hope, and love are simultaneously inflamed and threatened.[59]

While we profess our faith that the bridegroom has come, we acknowledge his absence as we await him again. So the Christian era is an age of fasting and feasting, of holding the tension of unfinished business, while confessing in faith to the outcome. The "already but not yet" character of the age calls for both expressions in the rhythm of our spiritual seasons, which can move from dry to satisfied, to dry to satisfied again. In this way, fasting both reflects and contributes to the eschatological understanding of Christian thought and practice.

So, as laid out below, a Christian theology of the nature of the age will be centered first on Christ. Christ represents the apex of God's revelation (Heb 1:2), and this makes any attempt to know God or reflect his ways necessarily christocentric. As Dallas Willard suggests, our approach to Christian living will be characterized as "Christ-centered piety."[60] In fasting, he can be remembered, imitated, and anticipated, and these three aspects will form the basic outline for the theology of fasting in the first section.[61] Spiritual blessings from properly motivated Christian fasting may be anticipated, as "your Father who sees in secret will repay you" (Matt 6:18, NASB). Second, recalling the insights of Basil, Augustine, and the Orthodox traditions, Christian fasting requires a view of sanctification that embraces the human body as the arena of personal sanctification. In this way, Christian fasting requires a view of spirituality that must embrace the whole person, and fasting can help engage the self in the rhythmic seasons of life lived in human flesh. Finally, the spiritual body that is Christ's church will need to balance the renewed awareness for fasting as Christian solidarity and the Protestant emphasis on the freedom of the conscience. This will encourage discipline without mandating the exact methods the Spirit will use, and Christians who fast will remember one another's needs while remembering their Lord.

A Christocentric Approach to Fasting: Remembering, Imitating, and Anticipating Him

The practice of fasting can play a role in a balanced understanding of the nature of the age. Not only do we have explicit teaching that should guide our understanding of our time, but we also have a tangible practice that at least potentially links us to both ancient and contemporary communities of faith that wait for God's redemption. There is continuity with the Old Covenant in that both fasting and feasting mark our experience. But since Christ has come, their significance has been reversed. Where once the faithful feasted in hope, we may feast in realization of hope fulfilled. Where once the community fasted in mourning, we may fast because of Christ's absence and in anticipation of the return of our beloved.

Michael Horton describes this shifting of the tenses of the eschatological horizon as a "trialectic." He writes, "the present activity of the Spirit involves the application not only of the work of Christ in the past, but the work of Christ in the future. Together, these points of origin define the work of Christ in the present, in the power of the Holy Spirit, to the glory of the Father."[62] Such an approach becomes intrinsically christocentric, locating Christian religious practices within the overarching theological context of what God has done in Christ.

Taking as our cue the NT theology that uses fasting as a messianic motif, a basic christocentric approach to fasting in this age can be laid out as follows. First, as the Christian tradition has practiced since basically its inception, fasting can help us to remember Christ, especially his incarnate humiliation and the work of his passion. Second, fasting can help us to imitate Christ in his discipline of the flesh and connection to spiritual realities. And third, fasting will remind us of our need for Christ during this time between his appearances, and of our dependence on the Spirit as we anticipate his presence again.

- Christian Fasting Remembers Christ

As suggested in the previous chapters here on fasting in biblical theology, one of the main functions of fasting in the biblical literature is to point out Jesus as the fulfillment of the eschatological hopes of Israel. His forty-day fast in the wilderness (Matt 4:1-4; Luke 4:1-4) especially demonstrated that point, linking him in the messianic, prophetic line as the one who would come. Keith Main is right to point out that Jesus is pictured by the NT as the fulfillment of the mourning fasts of Judaism, but he assumes that this christological fulfillment basically means the end of fasting as a practice.[63] Yet when Christians remember the joy of Christ's presence, are we not also reminded of his absence at the present time? Is it not possible to do both, to hold this eschatological tension together, by recognizing that the historical Christ event both fulfilled all things, and also inaugurated an age that still experiences sorrow?

As previously discussed, Church tradition memorialized that forty-day time period for fasting in Lent, placing it on the calendar so that it climaxed through Christ's passion to his resurrection, when the fast was broken. Additionally, the traditional half-day fasts on Wednesday and

Friday, which came to be known as the station fasts, were infused with memorial meanings of his passion, marking the days of his arrest and crucifixion. Similarly, the Eucharistic fast was necessarily linked to Christ's passion, as we are told that its inception came from the command of Jesus, "Do this in remembrance of me" (Luke 22:19; 1 Cor 11:24). And just as the resurrection follows the passion, Christians also celebrate the Lord's Supper in remembrance of his death "until he comes."[64] It is clear that Christians from the earliest days and throughout history have in the liturgical calendar and in their celebration of the sacrament viewed fasting as memorializing the work of Christ, while building toward eschatological realization.[65]

In this framework, we see that the church at least implicitly, if not always explicitly, saw itself functioning in a similar way to the people of the Old Covenant, in that the liturgical seasons reflect the theological understanding of redemptive history. Willem VanGemeren writes of the purpose of seasonal holidays in the Old Covenant:

> Through the framework of the feasts and festivals, the Israelites transmitted their redemptive history. They passed on from generation to generation the stories of the exodus from Egypt, the miraculous happenings in the wilderness, the revelation of the law and covenant, and the conquest of Canaan. Through these celebrations they developed a consciousness of being God's people and of having been specially blessed.[66]

Church tradition has sought to do a similar thing for Christians, only in the New Covenant context of remembering Christ's work. While perhaps the Catholic traditions had a tendency to inflate fasting practices, it should also be recognized that Protestants have had a tendency to truncate them.[67] Fasting practices could contribute to a renewed sense of participation in redemptive history in the future, if the churches would continue to foster a christocentric approach.

- Christian Fasting Imitates Christ

But since Jesus' salvific mission was unique, should imitation of him be central to Christian spirituality? Does this somehow reduce him to a teacher or example at the expense of him being a redeemer? When this question was posed to Dallas Willard, his cogent return was this:

> The question is, how can you trust Jesus as Redeemer and not trust him in what he says to do? And of course what he says to do is what he did. People who say they trust Jesus as Redeemer and do not bend every effort to obey him are self-deceived.[68]

Memory of Christ should trigger imitation of Christ. The believer will want to be as much like his or her Lord as possible. Fasting, at least to some extent, helps the believer to identify with Christ in his humanity, in his willingness to renounce the privileges of his natural high rank to become humble and lowly. In commenting on Paul's theological approach to obedience, Herman Ridderbos writes, "The religious, theocentric character of the new obedience surely finds its most pregnant expression in the concept of sanctification."[69] The sanctifying work of God must be understood primarily as his work of making his children to be like his Son, Jesus Christ, a work which has already been decreed and vicariously applied, and now is being worked out in anticipation of the consummation.

Often fasting practices have been geared toward a restoration of Eden, a focus on humanity in its created goodness. But perhaps an even deeper, more authentic focus of human restoration is to identify our fallen humanity with the one true savior who took upon himself our fallen humanity. What is the believer to model in this age between the times? Are we to recapitulate the unstained innocence of paradise, transcending the fallen world through a superceding form of sanctification? Instead, it would be better for Christians to find their model of sanctification in the one who lived in the fallen world among us, yet without sin. All of the effects of fallenness came upon him, even to the point of sharing in death with humanity.

So as Christians fast in imitation of Christ, it may not be primarily about doing exactly what Christ did when he fasted, as if we were setting ourselves up as messianic figures. Rather, it must be seen as signifying something larger. The Christian takes on humility in imitation of Christ, who "learned obedience from the things which He suffered" (Heb 5:8, NASB). When Christians fast, they experience some measure (albeit even a small measure in comparison) of the nature of that needed humility that comes from willing submission, and by doing so they might learn something of the obedience of Christ. This kind of imitation of Christ reminds believers that we, like Christ, are incarnate beings, dependent on food and drink for pleasure, normalcy, and even our physical lives. Yet fasting reminds us of how much we need something else even more—we need to depend on the living word of God, the one who is the source of all that is truly alive. Fasting reminds us that there is more to life than food, and like Christ, we are learning to live that sanctified life in the body.

It is in this context of humility and dependence on the Father that Christians can display the consistent connection between humble, sorrowful prayer and fasting. Jesus' fasting in the desert (Matt 4:1-4; Luke 4:1-4) can indeed be seen as an example of personal humbling that believers can follow, at least to some extent. While he did not fast in repentance from sin, his fasting was certainly connected to the resistance of temptation from the devil. Jesus made the point in that context that "Man shall not live on bread alone" (Luke 4:4), and Christians through the ages have taken that statement as an instruction to fast. But this imitation is also qualified by the fact that Christ also knew how to enjoy the good gifts of God in life, so much so that he was thought of as "a gluttonous man and a drunkard" (Matt 11:19).[70] His disciples were not known for their fasting, even though Jesus instructed them in how to fast and assured them that days were coming when they would fast (Matt 6:16-18, 9:15).

In this way, Christians find themselves in a long line of saints from the Hebrew Bible like Hannah (1 Sam 1:7-8), David (2 Sam 12:16-23), Nehemiah (Neh 1:4), Esther (Esth 4:16) and Daniel (Dan 9:3) fasted and prayed when they felt sorrow, showing their dependence on God and seriousness in humbling themselves to beseech him. Such times certainly come to believers in the new covenant as well, and there does not seem to be any legitimate theological reason why fasting could not continue in a similar role. While Christ came to bring joy and comfort to those who mourn, Christians should not forget that human experience is indeed one of mourning. Anything less would be a tacit denial of the ongoing presence of sin and death and their effects, symptoms of an over-realized eschatology. Christ identified with those who mourn, so Christians should imitate Christ and "weep with those who weep" (Rom 12:15).

So fasting is more than just imitating the concrete actions of Jesus (though that may be a commendable part). The imitation of Christ involves the believer in a patterned representation of the work of Christ. William Isley writes:

> Most broadly conceived, the Christian's imitation of his master is to participate in the pattern of redemptive history. Both Hebrews 3 and 4 and Paul in 1 Corinthians 10:1-13 understand Israel's wilderness wandering as a type of the Christian life. Christ, God's Son called out of Egypt (Mt. 2:15/Hos. 11:1) and our representative, successfully resisted temptation in the wilderness and through his cross and resurrection accomplished our exodus. We now follow him into the wilderness to be tested and journey towards the promised land, the final resurrection and the coming of the new heaven and the new earth. It is a time for fasting in which we express sorrow over our, humanity's, sinful state. It is most likely not without significance that the book of Revelation's descriptions of the consummation of the ages employs figures

of a wedding feast (19:9) and the abundance of food and drink which had been found in the primeval paradise (22:1-3). Then there shall be no reason to fast for there shall be no mourning (21:4).[71]

Horton sees this aspect of Christian practice as the "community theatre" of the "divine drama":

> Equipped with a set, a script, performers, and props, the divine drama takes on concrete form not only as a redramatization, but as the enactment of that redemptive-historical reality. Unlike the performers of *King Lear*, contemporary actors in the covenant renewal ceremony actually participate in the reality that is indicated by the performance.[72]

While Horton most centrally applies this to the performance of the sacraments and church discipline, it seems reasonable to extend the theology to wider religious practices that are entailed in our pursuit of sanctification, such as fasting. Then it is clear that fasting must also reflect the third aspect of this eschatological perspective, as discussed below.

- Christian Fasting Anticipates
  Christ During His Absence

If Christian fasting is done in imitation and remembrance of Christ as suggested above, then it follows that this also anticipates something. Anna, an old covenant saint at the dawn of the new covenant, fasted and prayed in anticipation of the messiah she met just as she, and the old covenant she represented, were getting ready to pass away (Luke 2:37). So too, Christians now may fast in anticipation of the end of the ages, longingly awaiting the new creation when all will be made right. Like Basil said, "Once we have thoroughly taken our fill, may we also be found worthy of the exhilaration that comes in the bridal chamber of Christ Jesus our Lord!"[73] As Isley noted above, the depictions of creation's consummation in Revelation are more oriented toward feasting, signifying the end of mourning. Surely that is related to the fact that the presence of God is in clear manifestation for his people there, and that Christ himself is among them (Rev 21:22-23, 22:4-5).

But since this is the time of his absence, then we must understand fasting now as a sign of our need of his presence. We long for him, and fasting reminds us of our anticipation of his return.[74] "Fasting helps us to focus on and to experience that reality of hopeful living between the times by reminding us of the not yet. Jesus is not yet with us. He has not yet returned; so we should be longing for his return."[75]

But more than just anticipating Christ's personal return in the eschaton, anticipating Christ in this time between the times must mean that he can manifest himself to us through his Holy Spirit, who is in us and among us. So when Christians fast and pray, we may anticipate the Spirit moving and guiding as a token and genuine blessing of the coming presence of Christ. Is that not the picture of the apostles praying in Acts 13:2-3? This body of believers, living so close in temporal proximity to the realized eschatology of the first advent, still fasted in anticipation of God moving. The divine response was to guide the believers in their ministries, and so the disciples repeated this pattern as they went out among the fledgling Gentile churches (Acts 14:23). In the Sermon on the Mount, Christ said that his disciples should fast in secret before the Father, "and your Father who sees in secret will repay you" (Matt 6:18). Clearly this suggests that, like prayer or almsgiving, fasting with proper spiritual motives will lead to spiritual blessings from God. So while fasting may at times seem mournful, Christian fasting is also never completely separated from the anticipation of God's Spirit breaking into our experience even now. As our attentions are lifted from sole concentration on material needs to the often unseen, secret world of God's kingdom, the believer anticipates connecting with the God who can operate beyond our normal experience. This points us forward on the larger trajectory of anticipating the consummation of all things, an eschatologically future reality that we are in organic connection with even in the present.

Now that a christocentric framework has been set out, fasting also raises some anthropological issues that remain to be discussed. Specifically, the implications of fasting on the Christian view of the body need to be explored, and to that we now turn.

Christian Fasting and the Body

Fasting quite naturally raises the question of the body's place in Christian spirituality. Familiar verses like Rom 12:1 remind Christians to "present your bodies a living and holy sacrifice, acceptable to God," and 1 Cor 6:19 reminds Christians that "your body is a temple of the Holy Spirit" (NASB). Although the question of the body's place in spirituality has perhaps been implicit in much of the discussion above, some explicit interaction may be necessary. It will be shown that Christian fasting can be a means of embracing the body in the process of sanctification, rather than rejecting it in favor of some kind of mental picture of a disembodied spirituality. This can provide a healthy corrective to excessive or abusive forms of asceticism in which the body is punished for sins, as well as the other side, that of neglect of fasting and the role of the body in sanctification and spirituality in the modern era. Dallas Willard reminds us that true spirituality includes bodily behaviors, and "whatever is purely mental cannot transform the self."[76] The following approach will then show that the embodied, spiritual Christian can use fasting to reflect the rhythms and seasons of life.

- Christian Fasting Embraces the Embodied Nature of Spirituality

Was fasting, as part of the ascetic impulse in Christian tradition, related to a deprecation of the human body? There is certainly some truth to that charge, as the abuses of asceticism mentioned in the previous chapter have shown. Yet the whole picture may require a nuanced understanding of the Christian theology of the body. A response to Veronika Grimm's view of Christian fasting as a renunciation of the goodness of creation appears below. This is followed by a more positive integration of the works of Shaw, Bynum and others who emphasize the role of the body and spirit together in Christian asceticism. But beyond that, this leads to a constructive theology of the potential role fasting can play in an embodied spirituality for Christians.

A Response to Viewing Christian Fasting as a Renunciation of the Goodness of the Body. Veronika Grimm promotes a rather dim view of Christian fasting in her recent, academically important monograph on fasting.[77] She suggests that early Christianity misunderstood Jewish fasting and adopted body-soul dualism from the surrounding cultures that merged into a heightened asceticism. According to Grimm, Jewish fasting was for a diversity of purposes, with ascetic purposes rising in prominence in the inter-testamental period.[78] For Grimm, the NT allows for fasting even though it does not generally advocate the practice. But with Paul a new element is introduced, and that is abhorrence of sexuality—a conclusion drawn from a psychologically driven reading of his epistles. She says that Paul, in contrast to the balanced Jewish view of the flesh as neither inherently good nor bad, "felt the power of sin 'in the flesh,' which for him meant in the sexually charged body."[79] She says that Paul himself does not advocate fasting, but his negative view of the flesh and body informs later Christianity. Throughout the Christian tradition asceticism gains renewed vigor in the attempt to quench the power of the fleshly appetites, and fasting becomes an important part of the quest. Much of this impetus is seen as emerging not from Christianity's Jewish roots, but rather from the Greco-Roman culture as the empire's power base shifted from pagan to Christian.

Grimm's analysis of Jewish material is helpful, but her negative opinions of the NT and early Christian material are clearly overstated. She argues that the apostles are relatively indifferent to food's role in their theology, only worrying about whether food practices cause dissension.[80] She mentions that there is teaching about food in some of Paul's disputed epistles, but she never really integrates the positive nature of texts like 1 Tim 4:1-5 into the discussion of Paul or early Christianity. This text warns against false teachers who forbid marriage or advocate abstaining from eating certain foods, and concludes: "For everything created by God is good, and nothing is to be rejected, if it is received with gratitude; for it is sanctified by means of the word of God and prayer" (1 Tim 4:4-5, NASB).

Also, Grimm's psychoanalysis of Paul is less than convincing. The fact that Paul highlighted singleness and mentioned fornication frequently as a sin to shun does not necessarily mean he had an aversion to sexuality as Grimm suggests. The actual Pauline texts that Grimm cites provide several statements that contradict her thesis on Paul. For instance, she describes the mental anguish of Rom 7:22-25, but she leaves out the joyous declaration of deliverance of Rom 7:25 by means of an ellipsis.[81] She also mentions the importance of 1 Corinthians 7 as if it is restrictive, without calling our attention to the fact that Paul tells couples not to sexually deprive one another (7:5), and that if singles lack self-control it is better to marry than to burn with lust (7:9). Apparently Paul himself was not "burning" in his struggle, as Grimm's analysis of Romans suggests, nor does the text support her idea that his singleness derives from his aversion to sexuality as a whole. It seems more consistent to say that Paul cared deeply about morality and believed his calling, with the Spirit's aid, was to fulfill his vocation in singleness.

Grimm is certainly right that elements of platonic dualism crept into the Christian tradition, and she demonstrates some of that in her discussion of the Church Fathers. But Grimm's main thesis is called into question, not only because of her reliance on a dubious turn of emphasis toward sexuality in Paul, but also by her latent assumptions about Christianity as a rejection of the beauty of the world and the human body.[82]

One should not assume that Christian asceticism somehow implied an essentially negative view of the body and humanity, or of creation in general. In fact, there would appear to be a growing number of voices that see fasting and ascetic practices by Christians generally as having a positive goal for the human body. Margaret Miles says that in the best of asceticism, "The body is a prize that the spirit and the flesh must struggle to possess."[83] Samuel Rubenson comments:

The close relation of body and soul in the Bible and the dogma of the incarnation of the divine in Jesus Christ contributes to an understanding of the body as sanctified, a temple of the Holy Spirit. On the other hand, it excludes any kind of asceticism that is based on contempt for and negation of the body. Even the most rigorous ascetic practice characteristic of early Eastern monasticism has as its goal the sanctification and transformation of the body.[84]

If that is the case, then perhaps fasting (and asceticism generally) do not need to be viewed as primarily negative practices, that necessarily disparage a healthy view of the body. Now we turn to integrating some more positive approaches into the theology of an embodied spirituality.

Integrating More Positive Approaches to Fasting and the Spiritual Body. Teresa Shaw has provided an important historical analysis of fasting and virginity in the history of ancient Christianity. While she is not specifically advocating a particular normative theological view of fasting, her understanding of the role of the body in early Christianity provides a helpful corrective for the too facile assumption that Christians are plagued with a heritage of platonic body-soul dualism. In some contrast to Grimm, Shaw suggests that the kind of dualism found in early Christianity is one in which the fleshly appetites are controlled *by means of the body itself.*[85] In other words, fasting and sexual abstinence for the early Christians were not so much issues of mind over matter (as in traditional dualism), but rather release of the body itself for its fullest pursuit of pleasure in God. The life of the early Christian ascetic is one that looks back to the unfallen state of paradise and forward to the restored body of the new creation:

> Fasting and virginity are, according to the several texts examined in this chapter, ways of imitating the original blessed human condition in paradise before the fall and life in the paradise to come. By fasting and sexual abstinence one also imitates the ways of the angels.
>
> ... [I]n Christian ascetic theory both eating and sexual activity take on the weight of the fall and its consequences of mortality, hierarchy, labor, and pain in human life. Thus the one who takes up a life of chastity and dietary renunciation becomes identified with original purity and immortality, and the ascetic body anticipates—or even returns to—the condition of original creation.[86]

Whether or not all of the specifics of this understanding are correct, the main thrust of Shaw's argument, that early Christian ascetics had the former paradise of Eden and the future paradise of the resurrection in view, is clearly substantiated by her work in the historical texts (and as seen in previous chapters above in Tertullian, Basil and Augustine).[87] Shaw goes on to show that in the early Christian ascetic tradition, fasting (along with chastity as a prime example of ascetic renunciation) in the body becomes a "medicine of the soul." Christian theology absorbed not merely the negative aspects of a body-soul distinction from the Greco-Roman context, but also the more positive aspects of contemporary medical theories that linked body and soul in close interaction.[88] If such an analysis is correct, one can see that the ascetic Christians of the late classic and medieval periods may not always have been denouncing the body. In their own way, they were honoring it and seeking to restore it, even if their methods may appear to our modern eyes to have sometimes moved toward the dysfunctional.[89] If the basic insights of sanctifying the body can be reintegrated into our theology today, we could advocate a Christian fasting that values the body while avoiding the hazards of pathological renunciation (such as viewing physical pleasures as evil, as done by the false teachers Paul denounced in 1 Tim 4:1-5, or the eating disorders that so plague contemporary life).

Mary Timothy Prokes makes the point that "*Christian faith is embodied faith,* deriving from the incarnate Word, Jesus Christ, and the Revelation that he lived out bodily, but principally through his passion, death and resurrection."[90] As human beings, we are necessarily embodied; in Christ's incarnation, he *became* human, taking our flesh upon himself. It is entirely reasonable then, that Christian theology should reflect on the embodied nature of human life for Christian practices. It is the Christian in the body that must become holy, be transformed into the image of Jesus Christ. Samuel Powell writes:

> [M]embership in this body of Christ (1 Cor 12:27) and participation in the body of Christ (1 Cor 10:16) imply something about the holiness of the individual Christian's body (1 Cor 6:19-20). So, the physical bodies of believers are clearly subjects of holiness, as the many exhortations of Paul's letters remind us. The physical body of Jesus Christ is of capital importance in holiness, both because of its central role in the doctrine of the atonement and because of the exemplary value of Jesus' life for Christians. The church as the body of Christ looms large in any discussion of holiness, not only because it is the church as such that Christ wishes to make holy, without spot or wrinkle, but also because the church is the living

context in which the Christian becomes holy. Finally, the sacramental body of Christ is important for holiness because thereby Christ is incorporated into us and we into him. In short, the centrality of the body to the concept of holiness is plainly a teaching of the new Testament.[91]

While it is not my purpose here to develop a thorough Christian anthropology, it is enough to note that fasting can and should be conceived as a bodily act of spirituality.[92] The act of renouncing food for a time is not necessarily a renunciation of physicality itself, but rather it can be a means of sanctifying the body, of symbolically presenting it as a vessel for God's divine presence. Adam and Eve were created in God's image, with bodies that were part of a creation that was deemed "very good" (Gen 1:26-31). Though our humanity, and thus our bodies, are fallen and subject to sin, Christ took on our flesh, and bore our sins in his body (1 Pet 2:24). He ascended to heaven, and Paul says in the present tense that "in Him all the fullness of Deity dwells in bodily form" (Col 2:9, NASB). It should come as no surprise, then, that believers are called to offer their *bodies* as "a living and holy sacrifice, acceptable to God" (Rom 12:1, NASB). As we anticipate the resurrection and glorification of our bodies, we can exercise our bodies for spiritual discipline and growth. As Paul said in 1 Cor 9:25, "And everyone who competes in the games exercises self-control in all things. They do it to receive a perishable wreath, but we an imperishable" (NASB). With this purpose in mind, Paul said he beat his body and made it his slave for the sake of the ministry (1 Cor 9:27). Hopefully, fasting can play a role in the future of evangelical theology's appropriation of embodied spirituality. Perhaps that can be done by understanding something of how fasting engages the Christian person in the embodied, temporal nature of life, and to that discussion we now turn.

- Christian Fasting Engages the Self in Transformation of Temporal Life in the Flesh

The eschatological formulation for understanding redemption history helps Christians to understand their place in the seasons of life in the flesh. Such a doctrine necessarily entails praxis that reflects the continuities and discontinuities of embodied life in the Spirit. Horton writes, "In the redemptive-historical model, doctrine is a creature of time, not a denizen of the disembodied *res cogitans*. Doctrinal or ethical formulations ignore the discontinuities and new, specific situations in redemptive history at their own peril."[93] In the situation Christians find themselves, theology as well as life in the world requires a mature ability to alternate between the poles of realization and anticipation.

The spiritual disciplines movement has recognized this dynamic to some extent. Willard differentiates between "disciplines of abstinence" and "disciplines of engagement." Together, these are "the outbreathing and inbreathing of our spiritual lives, and we require disciplines for both movements."[94] In acts of abstinence (like solitude, silence, fasting, frugality, chastity, secrecy, and sacrifice) the Christian is trained for "sober and moderate use of all God's gifts" and learns to combat temptations to excess.[95] Acts of engagement (study, worship, celebration, service, prayer, fellowship, confession, and submission) lead to growth and development.[96] There is here a tacit recognition of the eschatological nature of the age, an innate awareness that life is lived in cycles and patterns. What the historic Christians did by embedding patterns in the church's liturgical calendar, contemporary evangelicals may be seeking to do through practicing spiritual disciplines.

In the section below, the classic therapeutic function of fasting as an ascetic discipline will be suggested. This will be done by noting that we live in an age that demands a certain measure of discipline, even renunciation, due to its focus on physical excess. Then, a few suggestions will be made as to how fasting might contribute to transformation in the practical arena of life in the flesh in a sensate age.

The Sensate Nature of the Age. Paul clearly taught that rules about abstinence, in themselves, could not produce spirituality, criticizing them in Col 2:23: "They have the appearance of wisdom with their self-imposed worship and false humility, by an unsparing treatment of the body, but they are thoroughly useless when it comes to restraining the indulgences of the flesh". Coupled with the reminder that "every creation of God is good and no food is to be rejected if it is received with thanksgiving" (1 Tim 4:4), a Christian might conclude that there is no need, and hence no place, for fasting in the battle against sin in the flesh.

But on the other hand, it is also clear that the NT urges Christians to develop virtues like self-control, which is listed as a fruit of the Spirit (Gal 5:23), and to avoid such vices as those listed in Gal 5:19-21.[97] It is clearly reasonable that the long tradition of Christian fasting to counter vice has some merit, provided that the trust for the empowerment comes from God and not the deed itself. With these thoughts in mind, fasting should be considered as a means of lifting the believer's mind from earthly things to engaging the whole self in pursuit of God's spiritual blessings.

What are some contemporary cultural focuses that fasting might address? One item for reflection is that while our theology has traditionally not focused on the body, our cultural context is marked by an almost overwhelming fixation on the body. Medicine and fitness have become gigantic business enterprises, largely trying to fix some of the problems caused by the rise of other business like the prepared food, restaurant, tobacco and alcohol industries. Indeed, the dauntingly large majority of references to fasting in academic databases today (that are essentially repositories of Western culture's literature) are strictly medical or biological, and texts that deal with the spiritual implications of fasting are few and far between.[98]

Plus, Christians can hardly view the gratification of the sexual urge that is mass marketed so dominantly as a healthy approach to human behavior. After amassing mounds of historical data on major civilizations, sociologist Pitirim Sorokin decades ago pronounced that Western culture is in the decadent stage of the "sensate" phase of culture.[99] This analysis is followed by evangelical Harold O. J. Brown and appears to be basically sound.[100] Material wealth and pleasure are the driving forces of our culture, and even those spiritual and "ideational" values we have left are often driven to cooperate with the sensate ideals. Thus our churches and institutions are forced to run like businesses, Christians dress, eat and drink like everyone else, and we largely suffer the same maladies of body and soul as the world. As Christians awaken to the renewed need for fasting, perhaps it is because, as Margaret Miles suggests:

> We feel the longing to be 'truly alive,' and we are learning to look for deadness in precisely those aspects of experience identified by the Christian tradition... . We are beginning to look at our own materialism and that of our culture, as well as our ways of constructing self-esteem. We are learning to recognize deadness in exploitive sexuality.[101]

In an article wonderfully titled "To Hell on a Cream Puff," Frederica Mathewes-Green addresses the topic of gluttony, which she ironically says will "make you soft and huggable. It's the cute sin."[102] She rightly concludes that "Gluttony is not wrong because it makes you fat; it is wrong because it is the fruit of self-indulgence."[103] Food is a powerful force, largely because we must have food to physically survive. But the overtones of what food can provide—comfort, pleasure, escape—can become tools in the hands of the enemy.

Fasting as Transformation. Fasting cuts across the cultural grain and says, "I refuse to constantly acquiesce to my body's control. I believe that the Spirit has other values, and I wish to hear them." This does not seem too different from the situation addressed by Paul in Phil 3:17-21, in which Christians are enjoined not to follow those whose god is their appetite and who mind earthly things, but to focus on their heavenly citizenship and the future transformation of their bodies.[104] This kind of fasting focus is found up to and through the Reformation in the Christian tradition, although it was largely forgotten in the modern era and has only been recently reawakened in the last few decades. Kathleen Dugan reminds us that the monastic ideal of fasting had to do with finding fullness outside of the decadence of the later Roman Empire: "They lived in a moment of history that was fraught with indications of social decay and moral bankruptcy, and they responded by seeking wholeness and new life."[105]

Perhaps as the Christian tradition has so long suggested, fasting can play a practical role in combating our material addictions. Dennis Okholm, an evangelical professor from Wheaton College who is also an oblate of the Roman Catholic order of St. Benedict, suggests that ascetic practices, like fasting, need to again be used by Christians in order to help overcome some of the attachments people develop to the material world in this age.[106] To put it as bluntly as he does, we need to develop fasting as a therapy for gluttony. To this end Okholm offers six guidelines:

1. Associate fasting with meditating on Scripture.

2. Rely on community.

3. Aim at moderation and temperance.

4. Tailor the regimen to the individual.

5. Remember progress occurs one step at a time.

6. Attend to the body by honoring, but not worshiping it.[107]

In a similar, though more abstracted vein, Bernard Tyrell has linked fasting to psychotherapy from a Roman Catholic perspective, which he calls "Christotherapy," though his "spirit feasting" and "mind fasting" is more metaphorical than literal.[108] Still, these examples show that fasting has potential as a tool in the hands of Christians who wish to counteract the obsessive grip of the sensate nature of the age in which we live.

Christine Gardner has recently highlighted the growing role of fasting in evangelicalism.[109] From Lenten fasts to Bill Bright's "Fasting and Prayer" conferences to World Vision's youth-oriented "30 Hour Famine," fasting is riding a wave of growing popularity. Interest in the spiritual disciplines is high, and mentioning fasting in conversation almost always gets surprisingly interested responses.

In such an age, the abuse of fasting is a constant danger. Christians certainly need to be reminded that the Bible warns about fasting that becomes hypocritical. Isaiah and Jeremiah denounced the fasts of Israel as hypocrisy when social justice did not accompanied them (Isa 58:3-6; Jer 14:12). Jesus warned his disciples not to fast for the purpose of being seen by others to emphasize their own piety (Matt 6:16-18), and he set up the

Pharisee who boasted that he fasted twice as a counter-example to true righteousness (Luke 18:12).

The editorial that accompanies Gardner's article challenges readers to consider the problems associated with some of the popular fasting emphases.[110] The main cautions given are: results are not the point (that is, pragmatism that promotes apparent spiritual success based on unreliable, quantifiable statistics); America is not equivalent to the church (referring to the frequent refrain that we need revival in our country), and the priority of feeding the hungry and putting outward action to our intentions. Additionally, there are those who abuse their bodies through eating disorders, having unfortunately associated weight loss with a false bodily image of skinny perfection. In such a climate, Christians may be more likely to think of fasting in terms of weight loss for the sake of appearance rather than as a means of expressing our desire for fellowship with our Lord. Dugan writes, "When fasting becomes a symptom of pathology in persons afflicted by eating disorders, the very question of fasting's value is endangered."[111] She offers this trenchant conclusion:

> In particular, the attention given to the body in our times would seem to necessitate a spiritual response to all the negative images that abound. And the healthy rediscovery of the role of the body in the spiritual life heralds a new stage in Christian awareness (and a welcome one). I return to a thought in the beginning of this paper—that fasting in Christianity is only truly itself when it realizes the sacredness of the body. Like its foundational insight, that humanity was created for Incarnation, I often think that this still remains only partially accepted and understood by most Christians. If we *did* understand it, then we would regard the body and human life as holy, good, and capable of wonderful transformation. Fasting is the door to that transformation.[112]

The quotation above proceeds from Dugan's own pilgrimage as a Catholic woman who has long practiced spiritual disciplines and has been maturing in theological reflection. We evangelicals are not used to viewing the body as "sacred," yet some of our favorite biblical passages suggest that. In Rom 12:1 Paul urges believers to present their *bodies* as living sacrifices to God, which certainly could be understood as a sacred act.[113] Paul calls believers' bodies the "temple of the Holy Spirit" in 1 Cor 6:19, and temples would normally qualify for the description of sacred places. To be sure, evangelicals will want to affirm that this sacredness is derived from the believer's relationship with God, and not inherent in the self. While fasting may not be the *only* or even *primary* door to spiritual transformation, evangelicals would do well to consider the possibility that fasting can help us to reconnect to a more holistic approach to spirituality.

Christian Fasting and the Body Which Is Christ's Church

The Eastern Orthodox have strongly emphasized the unity of the church in their fasting tradition, and Roman Catholics since Vatican II have emphasized the church's solidarity in fasting practices. Evangelicals also need to see that individual Christians can never remove themselves from that fact that they are part of a spiritual community, that their bodies are participants in a greater body, the church of Jesus Christ. What fasting does for the individual Christian, then, will also be reflected and have impact on that larger body. From the other direction, the church as a body affects its individual members. Leaders who set the corporate tone of the church influence how the church body functions. So some consideration should be given about how fasting fits into the communitarian aspects of the functioning of Christians in the body of Christ. Below, two summary considerations are offered: that Christian fasting should cause believers to consider others who share (or even potentially share) in the body of Christ, and that the church can and should encourage proper forms of Christian fasting at the corporate level with respect to the Spirit's leading and calling of various Christians.

- Christian Fasting Reminds Us of One Another

Taking Jesus' words in Matt 6:18 about not being seen fasting as a cue, fasting might be relegated to a privatized realm.[114] Yet one need only reflect on that passage's context to see that similar injunctions about private prayer and almsgiving are made, yet these were still *de facto* community actions. The Lord's Prayer (Matt 6:9-13) is addressed to *our* Father, not merely to *my* Father, and the rest of its referents are in the plural. Additionally, most of the fasts described in Scripture were actually corporate in nature.[115] In OT history narratives, Israel frequently was called to corporate fasts, and these are generally held out as positive examples.[116] The ringing cry of the prophet Joel to consecrate a fast in a time of distress reminds us of how the community responded to threats of disaster (Joel 1:14, 2:12-15), and the classic story of the Ninevites' repentant response to Jonah's preaching was demonstrated with a city-wide fast (Jonah 3:5). It was this kind of corporate fast that John Calvin and John Knox saw as so valuable for their Reformed communities, and they set about finding practical ways to implement fast days whenever their communities faced serious difficulties.

The corporate fasts of the Bible most generally appear to receive divine commendation in their scriptural narratives. Yet one is also reminded by certain texts to go even further. Isaiah 58 criticizes the corporate fasts of Israel, but the reason is that their fasting was not accompanied by, or producing, a truly corporate spirit of social justice. The people were urged to fast truly by remembering the oppressed and loosening their burdens, feeding the hungry and clothing the naked (Isa 58:6-8). Similarly, Zechariah criticized the post-exilic community's mournful fasts because they did not reflect a just social situation (Zech 7:8-14). The prophet held out the eschatological ideal of fasting turned to feasting when the nation would reflect a true spirit of community justice that would even extend to the nations (Zech 8:16-23). As previously discussed, Calvin, Knox and the Puritans urged and practiced this kind of fasting in their communities.

Additionally, some of the NT references to fasting assume corporate contexts. Jesus' response to the synoptic fasting query uses plural references to describe the disciples in a time when "they will fast" (Matt 9:15; Mark 2:20; Luke 5:35).[117] The apostles were doing exactly that when they were fasting and praying together, in a corporate context, when the Spirit spoke to them (Acts 13:2-3). The early church seemed to see fasting and prayer as an appropriate way to solemnize the ordination of new leaders for their communities (Acts 14:23). When Paul lists "fastings" as part of his trials, he emphasizes that he went through these things for the sake of the ministry, on behalf of the churches (2 Cor 6:3-5, 11:27-28).[118] In light of these references, it would be difficult to maintain the idea that fasting is merely an individualistic concern without a potential corporate dimension.

A regular risk of the spiritual disciplines movement, as so often typified by ascetic movements, is to emphasize individual spirituality at the expense of the community. Richard Foster makes room for "corporate disciplines" like confession, worship, guidance and celebration, but fasting is grouped with prayer, meditation and study as "inward disciplines." His other category is "outward disciplines" of simplicity, solitude, submission and service.[119] While perhaps these distinctions may be helpful on a practical level, they tend to obscure the communitarian nature of all sanctification.

The Roman Catholic emphasis since Vatican II on fasting as solidarity demonstrates a move toward emphasizing community. While Protestants will want to understand Christian solidarity through a more spiritual and less strictly ecclesiastical bond than Catholics, the ultimate unity of all true believers is a biblical ideal toward which to strive.[120] This is especially valuable and relevant since the onset of the modern age of the individual.

Since the beginnings of the Christian era, as in the *Shepherd of Hermas*, St. Basil, and others, Isaiah 58 has stood as a model, if not the very definition, of proper fasting. When one voluntarily experiences hunger in fasting, perhaps one will think also of those who experience hunger and need involuntarily because of their social situations. When one learns by fasting to live with less, perhaps one will have more to share with those in need—not only from the relatively minor effects of the actual savings, but even more because of the increased capacity for sharing that could come from learning to live with less. Scripture, tradition, theology, and ethics unite in calling Christians to associate fasting with concern for others.

- ## Christian Fasting Encourages Discipline Without Mandating Methods

When the church considers the subject of spiritual disciplines, and fasting in particular, the inherent danger of legalism always lurks nearby. The reasoning could move fairly easily from the idea that if fasting is a useful tool for spirituality, then all Christians should practice it, and a sense of obligation could begin to dominate the practice. One might reasonably argue, as the 17th century Anglo-Catholic Peter Gunning did, that the church's members have chosen to submit to the church's authority, and this submission entails willing obedience.[121] But even modern Catholicism has moved more toward seeing fasting as a voluntary act, and has gone to great pains to try and rescue fasting from the grip of empty ritual. Too much historical baggage has associated with this practice, and the NT seems to regard the use of foods in religion as a matter generally left to the conscience of believers (Rom 14:17; 1 Cor 10:31; Col 3:16-17). So, it would be preferable for the church to hold out fasting as a useful discipline, encouraging people to practice it, perhaps even suggesting times and purposes, but to stop short of requiring fasting as an obligatory Christian duty.

Depending on one's view of the value of tradition, this may take differing forms. For instance, the Church of England has historically taken this approach in a liturgical context, urging traditional Catholic fasting practices without mandating them. In less liturgical environments, it may take effort to promote the positive virtues of fasting without laying burdens on people, and creativity will be in order. Perhaps the evangelical emphasis on spiritual disciplines will become a doorway to further renewal of the positive effects of fasting. The great traditions of the church could help to guide us toward more unity in this. Would there be anything wrong with suggesting that Christians might initiate fasting with relatively mild half-day fasts (like the traditional Christian fasts known as "stations" on Wednesdays or Fridays), as practiced by that evangelical here, John Wesley? Would it be all right to suggest that Christians might fast in anticipation of the Lord's Supper on a given Sunday in order to set apart the observance as special, as Augustine urged? This could remind Christians of Jesus' words at the Last Supper that he would not eat it or drink from the fruit of the vine "until it is fulfilled in the kingdom of God" (Luke 22:16, 18), and our people could receive sound eschatological teaching about the nature of the age. Maybe teaching concerning Lent could be considered, as a way of understanding what is of value in the Christian tradition and of memorializing Christ's passion. At least there would be benefit in understanding Christians who worship in liturgical environments as a sign of our solidarity with them. Protestants, and especially evangelicals, need to seriously consider the possibility that our tradition rejected these practices simply because they were too closely associated with a Catholicism whose doctrinal system could not be accepted. In this wholesale rejection, we may have made ourselves poorer by not considering the possible positive effects of such simple fasting practices.

And yet, in line with the Protestant Reformers' emphasis on the liberty of the believer's conscience in matters not commanded by Scripture, the Christian should be left free to follow the Spirit in individual calling, or vocation, within the body of Christ. Some Christians may be called to more extensive fasting, and these Christians may have lessons to teach the body as a whole. Some Christians may not be called to these practices, and they need not be coerced or cajoled into them. In these matters, "each of us will give an account of himself to God" (Rom 14:12).

Conclusion

Contemporary evangelical Christians have reawakened to the possibilities of fasting after long years of relative neglect. We may learn from the Orthodox about the value of fasting in tradition, and about rediscovering something of the importance of the body in spirituality. We may learn from post-Vatican II Roman Catholicism about the need for a theological orientation toward the community and a willingness to reform practices to honor the movements of the Spirit. And contemporary evangelical Protestants are already teaching a renewed form of spirituality in the application of the spiritual disciplines. In this climate, an integrated theology of fasting is needed that holds scriptural teachings in authority in conversation with tradition. Fasting has therefore been set within the context of God's work in Christ, and Christian practice is understood within the context of the eschatological nature of the age in which we find ourselves.

Any Christian fasting must be centered on Christ. An understanding of our place in redemptive history should prompt Christians to remember Christ, imitate him, and anticipate his presence and blessing. The bridegroom has been taken away, and in these days we will fast. In our fasting we are reminded of the body's basic goodness and the enjoyment that life in Christ can bring. We are reminded that Christ moves through his Spirit in and through us to others, and we see our bodies as part of a larger body that is his church. In Christian fasting we follow our Lord, who instructed us not to live "on bread alone" (Matt 4:4; Luke 4:4).

APPENDIX 1
Basil's Sermons *About Fasting*

As noted in chapter three, there are two authentic, extant Greek fasting homilies written by St. Basil the Great for Lent, Περὶ Νηστείας, also known by the Latin *De jejunio*. The text used here is from J. P. Migne's *Patrologia graeca*, which is available electronically.[1] They have been newly translated here as *About Fasting*, Sermons 1 and 2. (A third homily on fasting in the Basilian corpus is universally regarded as inauthentic.)[2] The only available English translation that the author has found, and that of only the first homily, is by Reginald Cardinal Pole, who appended a translation of it to his *Treatie of Iustification* in 1569.[3] That English is of good quality, but now antiquated in style.

It is hoped that this translation can make something of a modest contribution to the field of patristic studies, and studies of Basil in particular. So many works remain unavailable to the English reader, and so it is hoped that this effort will be a welcome addition to our literature from the great treasury of Christian antiquity. For a discussion of the themes in the content of the sermons, the reader is referred to chapter three.

Our Holy Father Basil, Archbishop of Caesarea, Cappadocia. *About Fasting* (*De jejunio*), Sermon 1.

[31.164] 1. "Sound the trumpet," he declares, "in the new moon, on the high day of your feast."[4] This command is from the prophets. But it's for us, too. The reading indicates the beginning of the feast days, and to us every trumpet is louder, and every musical instrument clearer.[5]

For we have come to know the gift of the fasts of Isaiah. While the Jewish manner of fasting has been set aside, a true fast has been handed down to us. Don't "fast unto judgment and strife," but "loose every chain of injustice."[6] And the Lord says: "Don't be like the gloomy-faced, but wash your face and anoint your head."[7] Therefore let's agree, as it has been taught, that we won't be looking gloomy on the days that are approaching. Rather, we will cheerfully, agreeably look forward to them, as is fitting for saints.

No one is passionless when he is receiving a victory crown! No one is gloomy when a victory monument is being erected for him. Don't make being healed gloomy! It's outrageous that you don't rejoice over the health of your soul, but grieve over changing foods. You appear to be giving more favors to the pleasure of your stomach than to the care of your soul.

While getting filled up does a favor for the stomach, fasting returns [31.165] benefits to the soul. Be encouraged, because the doctor has given you a powerful remedy for sin. Strong, powerful medicines can get rid of annoying worms that are living in the bowels of children. Fasting is like that, as it cuts down to the depths, venturing into the soul to kill sin. It is truly fitting to call it by this honorable name of medicine.

2. "Anoint your head, and wash your face."[8] The word calls to you in a mystery. What is anointed is christened; what is washed is cleansed.[9] Transfer this divine law to your inner life. Thoroughly wash the soul of sins. Anoint your head with a holy oil, so that you may be a partaker of Christ, and then go forth to the fast.

"Don't darken your face like the hypocrites."[10] A face is darkened when the inner disposition is feigned, arranged to obscure it to the outside, like a curtain conceals what is false.

An actor[11] in the theater puts on the face of another. Often one who is a slave puts on the face of a master, and a subject puts on royalty.[12] This also happens in life. Just as in the production cast of one's own life many act on the stage. Some things are borne in the heart, but others are shown to men for the sake of appearances. Therefore don't darken your face. Whatever kind it is, let it show.

Don't disfigure yourself toward gloominess, or be chasing after the glory of appearing temperate. Not even almsgiving[13] is of any profit when it is trumpeted, and neither is fasting that is done for publicity of any value. Ostentatious things don't bear fruit that lasts through the coming ages, but return back in the praises of men.

So run to greet the cheerful gift of the fast. Fasting is an ancient gift, but it is not worn out and antiquated. Rather, it is continually made new, and still is coming into bloom.

3. Do you think I am finding the ancient origin of fasting from the law? Fasting is even older than the law. If you will tolerate me a little while, you will find the truth from the word. Don't think that the Day of Atonement, commanded to Israel in the seventh month, the tenth day of the month,[14] was the beginning of fasting.

Indeed, come on and walk through the history, investigating its ancient origins. For the invention isn't new. It's an heirloom from the fathers. Everything of such great antiquity deserves respect for its importance. Show some respect for the gray head of fasting!

[31.168] Fasting is as old as mankind itself. It was given as a law in paradise. The first commandment Adam received was: "From the tree of the knowledge of good and evil do not eat."[15] Now this command, "do not eat," is the divine law of fasting and temperance. If Eve had fasted from the tree, we would not have to keep this fast now.

The strong don't need a doctor, but the sick do.[16] We were made sick through sin; let's be healed through repentance. But repentance[17] without fasting is ineffective. "For the earth is cursed, thorns and briars rise up to you."[18] You see, enduring pain has been prescribed for you, not delicate living.

Through fasting satisfaction is made to God. But the way of life of fasting in paradise is also an image, as people were sharing the life of angels. Even more than that, through contentment with little, humanity's likeness to the angels would have been established. But also because whatever kinds of diet human inventiveness later discovered, those in paradise had not yet come to understand. There wasn't the drinking of wine yet, nor the eating of meat,[19] nor anything clouding the human mind.

4. Since we did not fast, we fell from paradise. Well, now let's fast, so that we may go back again. Remember Lazarus, how through fasting he entered into paradise?[20] Don't imitate Eve's disobedience; don't again receive counsel from the serpent. That's how we were made subject to fleshly food. Don't make weakness of the body and illness a pretext. You aren't pretending to me, but you are talking to the One who knows.

Tell me, aren't you able to fast? But you're able to be filled up with this life, and to afflict the body with the weight of the things being eaten? Indeed, I know that doctors have ordered even sick people to abstain and go hungry, rather than eat all kinds of foods. How come somebody like that is able to do these things, but you pretend you aren't able to do that?

What's easier to the stomach? A plain diet that carries you through the night, or rich foods that weigh you down like a rock when you lie down? But even more than troubling you when you lie down, doesn't it frequently turn on you like an enemy, tearing through and causing you stomach contractions?

You would surely agree that the pilot of a merchant ship is better able to safely guide it to port if it is not fully loaded, when it is in excellent condition and light. The ship completely loaded down is sunk by a minor swell in the waters. But the boat that has a captain smart enough to toss overboard the extra weight will ride high above even surging waves.

That's like people in burdened down bodies. A person gets absorbed with filling up, getting weighed down until finally falling into ill health. But those who are well-equipped, light, and truly nourished, avoid the prospect of serious disease. [31.169] They are like the boat in stormy weather that goes right over a dangerous rock.

Contrast that with how relaxation from running, or taking a break from aging, actually makes you more miserable. But, you say, it is more fitting that those who are sick eat well, rather than a plain diet. However, the ability that governs the animal takes care of it through a plain diet and produces contentedness, and it learns to like being nourished. But if an animal is given expensive, exotic foods, it won't be satisfied in the end, and may even get all kinds of diseases.

5. But let the word walk you through history, passing through the antiquity of fasting. All the saints have protected it, like an inheritance passed down from the fathers. They in turn passed it down, like a father passing something down to a child. So we are the successors of this long line, and this possession has been entrusted to us.

Wine wasn't in paradise; there was not yet any slaughtering of animals, not yet any eating of meat. After the flood there was wine. After the flood, "you will eat all kinds of things, like you eat vegetables that grow from the ground."[21] When perfection was despaired, then the enjoyment of those things was allowed.

Now the wine is an example of inexperience, as Noah was ignorant of the use of wine. For it had not yet come into use in life, neither been known in human custom. Since he had neither seen another do it, nor tried it himself, he was unguardedly hurt by it. "For Noah planted a vineyard, and he drank from the fruit, and he got drunk."[22] He wasn't out-of-control drunk, he just wasn't aware of the potent thing he was consuming.

So the invention of wine drinking is younger than paradise, and the dignity of fasting is established as being even more ancient. But we have also been taught about the fasting of Moses when he came onto the mountain. He wouldn't have boldly faced the smoking summit, neither would he have had the courage to enter into the thick cloud, if he hadn't been completely armed with fasting.[23] Through fasting he received the commandments from the finger of God written on the tablets.

And while up above the divine law was being received with fasting, down below gluttony was disgorging itself into idolatry. "For the people sat down to eat and drink, and they got up to play."[24] Forty days devoted to fasting and waiting were made useless by one bout of drunkenness.

Fasting received the tablets written by finger of God, but drunkenness shattered them. The drunken crowd was judged unworthy to receive the divine law from the prophet of God. In one moment of time those people, who had been taught by the greatest miracle of God, were dragged off into Egyptian idolatry by their gluttonous inclination. Both of the arrangements are parallel— how fasting brings near to God, [31.172] and how luxury betrays salvation.

Come walk on down to later times.

6. What did Esau throw away, and so was made a slave of his brother? Didn't he sell his rights as first-born for a single meal?[25] By contrast, wasn't it with fasting and prayer that Hannah was favored to become the mother of Samuel?[26]

What great meal brought into being the invincible Samson? Wasn't it fasting, with which he was conceived in the womb of his mother?[27] Fasting conceived him, fasting nursed him, fasting made a man of him. The angel commanded his mother, "He must certainly not eat anything that comes from the vineyard, and he must certainly not drink wine or liquor."[28]

Fasting gives birth to prophets, shestrengthens the powerful.[29] Fasting makes lawmakers wise. She is a safeguard of a soul, a stabilizing companion to the body, a weapon for the brave, a discipline for champions. Fasting knocks over temptations, anoints for godliness. She is a companion of sobriety, the crafter of a sound mind. In wars she fights bravely, in peace she teaches tranquility. She sanctifies the Nazirite, and she perfects the priest.

How the law was introduced is figurative for true, mystical worship. One is not able to boldly face the divine presence without fasting. It made Elijah an observer of that marvelous vision. His soul was purified by fasting forty days, so that in the cave on Mt. Horeb he was considered worthy to see the Lord like one sees a man.[30]

By fasting he returned the widow's child to her—he became stronger than death through fasting![31] While fasting, a cry went out from his mouth that closed up the heavens for three years and six months from the lawbreaking people.[32] In order that the unbroken heart of the stubborn might be softened, he himself also took on the suffering of being condemned.

On account of this he said, "As the Lord lives, there will not be water on the land, except through my mouth."[33] And he laid on all the people a fast through the famine, so that the evil effects from their self-indulgence and unrestrained life might be corrected.

And what about the life of Elisha? How from the lodging place of the Shunemite he was driven away?[34] And how he himself entertained the prophets?[35] Wasn't he completely hospitable with wild vegetables and a little flour? When the poisonous gourd was added, those who had come in contact with it were about to be in danger. But the poison was neutralized by the prayer of fasting.

[31.173] Once fasting was discovered, all the saints were led by the hand into the divine way of life. There is a certain kind of substance, that the Greeks call *amianton*,[36] that is impervious to fire. When it is placed in the flame, it seems to be made of coal, but when it comes up out of the fire, it is cleaner than if it had been washed in water. That's what the bodies of those three children were like; they had bodies of *amianton* from fasting in Babylonia.[37] For in the great fiery furnace, their nature being like gold, was then demonstrated to be superior when they were drawn from the fire unhurt.

Here's how their nature was demonstrated to be stronger than gold: the fire did not refine them, but simply preserved their sincerity. When they had not yet even been cast into the fire, the flames were being fed naphtha and pitch and branches, and they streamed out above the furnace forty-nine cubits, so that many of the Chaldeans standing near it were destroyed.[38] Then, with fasting, when they were cast into the conflagration, they were able to walk around on their own feet, and they were breathing a little moistened air in the torrent of fire. And the fire didn't even damage their hair, because they had been strengthened by fasting.

7. Now Daniel (fasted) from desire,[39] and went without eating bread or drinking water for three weeks.[40] And when he was thrown down in their den, he taught the lions to fast![41] When one material strikes another, one is harder than the other, like bronze is harder than stone. Just so, the lions weren't able to sink their teeth into him. Fasting is like sharpening the edges of a man by dipping his body in iron—it makes him tougher than lions! They couldn't open their mouths against the saint.

Fasting quenches the power of fire; it closes the mouths of lions. Fasting sends prayer up into heaven, becoming like wings for its upward journey. Fasting is the increase of houses, the mother of health. It's an instructor of youth, an adornment to the old. It's a good companion for traveling, a secure living companion to those dwelling together.

A husband doesn't suspect a plot against his marriage, and lives in harmony with his wife when he sees her fasting. A wife doesn't fall apart in jealousy, and happily accepts the husband she sees fasting.

Who makes his own house decline by fasting? [31.176] Count the domestic benefits by considering the following things. No one has been deserted by those in the house on account of fasting.[42] There's no crying over the death of an animal, certainly no blood. Certainly nothing is missed by not bringing an unmerciful stomach out against the creatures.

The knives of the cooks have stopped; the table is full enough with things growing naturally. The Sabbath was given to the Jews, so that "you will rest," it says, "your animal and your child."[43] Fasting should become a rest for the household servants who slave away continually, all year long.

Give rest to your cook, give freedom to the table keeper, stay the hand of the cupbearer. For once put an end to all those manufactured meals! Let the house be still for once from the myriad disturbances, and from the smoke, and from the odor of burning fat, and from the running around up and down, and from serving the stomach as if it were an unmerciful mistress!

Even those who exact tribute sometimes give a little liberty to their subjects. The stomach should also give a vacation to the mouth! It should make a truce, a peace offering with us for five days.[44] That stomach never stops demanding, and what it takes in today is forgotten tomorrow. Whenever it is filled, it philosophizes about abstinence; whenever it is emptied, it forgets those opinions.

8. Fasting doesn't know the nature of usury. The one who fasts doesn't smell of interest tables.[45] The interest rates of fasting don't choke an orphan child's inheritance, like snakes curled around a neck. Quite otherwise, fasting is an occasion for gladness.

As thirst makes the water sweet,[46] and coming to the table hungry makes what's on it seem pleasant, so also fasting heightens the enjoyment of foods. For once fasting has entered deep into your being, and the continuous delight of it has broken through, it will give you a desire that makes you feel like a traveler who wants to come home for fellowship again. Therefore, if you would like to find yourself prepared to enjoy the pleasures of the table, receive renewal from fasting.

But, if you are overcome by the excess of delights, without knowing yourself the unseen delights, by the love of pleasure the real pleasure is ruined.

That's not really desirable, because if the enjoyment doesn't last, it comes to be despised. But possessions that are rare are much sought after for their enjoyment. So, too, this possession of fasting intends to bring about an exchange in our life, so that the grace of what has been given to us might remain with us.

Don't you see, that also the sun shines more brightly after the night? [31.177] And being awake is more pleasant after sleep? And health is more desirable after the experience of the opposite? A table is for that very reason more gratifying after fasting. It's like that both for the rich who live graciously, and for those with a simple and subsistence lifestyle.

9. You should be afraid of the example of the rich man.[47] That which is delightful throughout life cast him into the fire. It wasn't unrighteousness, but delicate living that accused him, roasted him in the flames of the furnace. So for that reason, it is necessary that we have water to extinguish that fire.

We ought not fast only because of what is going to happen, but in this flesh it is even more profitable. Those at the peak of health can have a turnaround and change, their natures get bent down, and they are no longer able to carry the burden of full health.

See to it that you don't go spitting on the water you're drinking now, and like the rich man,[48] afterward you desire a single drop.[49] No one ever got a hangover from water. No head ever ached because it was burdened with water. No one's feet were ever bound by living with another who was a water drinker.[50] No feet were bound, no hands ruined, because they were sprinkled with water.

It necessarily happens that those living luxuriously are working toward excessive diseases in their bodies, and their dissonance ripens for destruction.

One fasting has a healthy complexion, not breaking out in a shameless, blushing redness, but moderation is adorned with paleness. One fasting has a gentle eye, a calm gait, and a thoughtful face. There is no intemperate, arrogant laughter, but rather fitting speech, and purity of heart.

Remember the saints of old, "Of whom the world was not worthy, who went around in sheepskins, in goatskins, destitute, persecuted, mistreated."[51] Remember their mode of life, if indeed you are seeking after the same inheritance as them.

What was it that caused Lazarus to wake up in the bosom of Abraham? Wasn't it fasting?[52] John's life was one of fasting. He had no bed, no table, no fruitful piece of land, no plowing ox, no grain, no grinding and baking, nothing from the normal course of life.[53] Because of this, "No one born of women has arisen greater than John the Baptist."[54]

Like the others, fasting also marked Paul, who considered severe trials something to boast about, and he was caught up into the third heaven.[55]

But above all that has been said, our Lord took flesh and fortified it with fasting on behalf of us. Then in that condition he welcomed the assault of the devil,[56] teaching us to anoint and to train ourselves with fastings before struggling with temptations. So when he was wrestling in a state of need, an opportunity was given. The devil was not able to approach the Lord on account of the supernatural nature of his divinity, unless he came down to humanity through the state of need. However, when he had gone back into the heavens,[57] he partook of the food of the nature of the resurrected body of the believer.

[31.180] Doesn't it grieve you, that you are overgrown and fattened up? While the mind is wasting away of atrophy, not even a single word is spoken about the life-giving teaching of salvation? Don't you know, that just like when one army defeats the other, the flesh is handed over to the conquering spirit, and the spirit is changing the rank of the flesh to slavery? "These things are adversaries of each other."[58] So if you want to make the mind strong, tame the flesh through fasting!

This is what the apostle said, that "however much the outer man is wasting away, so much the inner man is being renewed."[59] And this: "Whenever I am weak, then I am strong."[60]

Won't you despise destructive foods? Wouldn't you rather receive a desire for the table in the kingdom, that fasting here prepares beforehand? Don't you know that by excessive filling you are preparing for yourself a fat worm to torture you?

Who has received anything of the fellowship of the spiritual gifts by abundant food and continual luxury? Moses, when receiving the law a second time, needed to fast a second time, too.[61] If the animals hadn't fasted together with the Ninevites, they wouldn't have escaped the threatened destruction.[62]

Whose bodies fell in the desert?[63] Wasn't it those who desired to eat flesh?[64] While those same people were satisfied with manna and water from the rock, they were defeating Egyptians, they were traveling through the sea, and "sickness could not be found in their tribes."[65] But when they remembered the pots of meat, they also turned back in their lusts to Egypt, and they did not see the Promised Land.[66] Don't you fear this example? Don't you shudder at gluttony, lest you be shut out from the good things you are hoping for?

Neither would the wise Daniel have seen visions, if he had not illuminated his soul with fasting. From fatty foods what sooty vapors rise up, like a frequent, punishing cloud! The rays from the presence of the Holy Spirit can barely penetrate it to shine on the mind.

Now if there is even a certain kind of food for angels, it is bread, as the prophet says: "Man ate the bread of angels."[67] It's neither flesh, nor wine, nor whatever those who are slaves to the stomach anxiously seek out.

Fasting is a weapon against the armies of demons: "For this kind doesn't go out [31.181] except by prayer and fasting."[68]

From fasting come so many good things, but fullness is the beginning of insolence. Immediately it rushes in together with the delicacy, and with drunkenness, and with all kinds of rich sauces. All kinds of licentious rs start grazing. After that, behaviomen become "lusty horses"[69] toward women, because the luxury makes a maddening itch enter into the soul. Those who are drunks pervert themselves against nature, using a male like a female, or vice-versa.[70]

But fasting even makes known how the proper boundaries of marriage work. The excesses of even things permitted by law are curtailed, introduced by agreement for an appropriate time, in order that the couple might be devoted to prayer.[71]

10. But don't limit the goodness of fasting by abstaining only from foods. For true fasting is the enemy of evil. "Loose the chains of injustice!"[72] Forgive your neighbor's offense, and forgive his debts. Don't "fast unto judgment and strife."[73] You don't eat meat, but you eat your brother. You abstain from wine, but stubbornly hold on to insolence. You patiently wait until evening to partake, but you spend the day in court.

"Woe to those who are drunk, but not from wine!"[74] Wrath is a drunkenness of the soul, making it senseless, like wine. Grief itself is also drunkenness, sinking down the mind. Fear is another drunkenness, whenever it fears things that don't need to be feared. For he says, "from fear of my enemy, deliver my soul."[75] Together, each of these passions, allowing the mind to be taken over and out of control, is rightly termed drunkenness.

Consider with me the one who is angry, how he is drunk with passion.

He isn't master of himself, he doesn't know himself, and he doesn't know who is standing around. He tries to hit everything, flailing all over, like somebody fighting in the dark. He declares that he is in control, he is hard to hold in, he reviles, he strikes, he threatens, he swears, he shouts, he curses.[76]

Guard against this kind of drunkenness, but don't be given over to the kind that comes from wine, either. Don't start being a water-drinker just because you've been drinking too much. Don't let drunkenness initiate you into fasting. The entryway into fasting doesn't come through drunkenness. Neither is greed the entryway into justice, nor is intemperance the way to sound judgment. To sum it up, evil never leads to virtue. There is another door into fasting. Drunkenness leads to intemperance, but contentment opens the door to fasting.

The athlete practices before the contest. The one who fasts is practicing self-control ahead of time. Don't approach these five days like you are coming to rescue them as if they need you, or like somebody who is trying to get around the intent of the law, by just laying aside intoxication. [31.184] If you do that, you are suffering in vain. You are mistreating the body, but not relieving its need.

This safe where you keep your valuables isn't secure; there are holes in the bottom of your wine-bottles.[77] The wine at least leaks out, and runs down its own path; but sin remains inside.

A servant runs away from a master who beats him. So you keep staying with wine, even though it beats your head every day? The best measure of the use of wine is whether the body needs it. But if you happen to go outside of the bounds, tomorrow you will feel overloaded, gaping, dizzy, smelling rotten from the wine. To you, everything will be spinning around; everything will seem to be shaking. Drunkenness brings a sleep that's a brother of death, but even being awake seems like being in a dream.

11. So, do you know whom you are about to receive? He who promised us, that "I myself, and the Father, we will come and make our home with him."[78] Why, then, would you get caught being drunk, and close the door against the Master? Why would you encourage the enemy to occupy your stronghold? Drunkenness doesn't make the Lord feel welcome; drunkenness chases away the Holy Spirit. For as smoke drives away bees, intoxication drives away the spiritual gifts.

Fasting is the proper decorum of a city, stability of the marketplace, peace of homes, saving of possessions. Do you want to see its dignity?

Compare with me today's evening to tomorrow, and you will see the city changed from its raging, surging sea into a deep tranquility.[79] But I pray, that both today might be like tomorrow in dignity, and tomorrow might leave none of today's joyousness behind.

Now, may the Lord who brought us through to the coming around of the season, grant to us, as competitors in these preliminary contests, that we may display enduring firmness and vigor, to attain also the crowns on the decisive day; now, in memory of the saving passions, but in the coming ages, by the recompense to us of the things done in life, by the righteous judgment of his Christ; because the glory belongs to him forever! Amen.

31.185 *About Fasting*, Sermon 2.

"Exhort the people, priests," it says; "speak into the ears of Jerusalem."[1] The nature of that word "exhort" is enough to intensify the desires of the earnest, but also to stir to readiness those who are idle and careless.

That's how commanders operate. They marshal the army into place, and give a speech before the battle is engaged. The exhortation has so much power that it often produces a disdain for death in many. Similarly, coaches and athlete trainers use exhortation. Before the games in the stadiums the athletes are brought forward, and they are given speeches that are full of how they have to exert themselves so they can win the crown. So by persuasion, many can be joined together in ambition for victory, even to the disregard of their own bodies.

And so it is now with me. The soldiers of Christ have been ordered to war against invisible enemies, and the athletes of godliness are preparing themselves for crowns of righteousness through self-control. So the word of exhortation is indispensable.

So, what am I saying, brethren? I'm saying it makes sense that those who practice battle tactics, and those who work out in wrestling school, take in more food for their bodies the more strenuous the exertions are that they participate in. But, to those for whom "the struggle is not against blood and flesh, but against rulers, against authorities, against cosmic powers of this darkness, against spiritual forces of wickedness,"[2] to these, it is absolutely necessary to be disciplined for struggle through self-control and fasting.

While oil bulks up the athlete, fasting is the strength-training of the godly. So whatever robs the flesh, of that you will make the soul shine[3] with spiritual health. Power to overcome invisible enemies doesn't come by bodily exertion, but by endurance of the soul. By patience trials are overcome.

2. Fasting is, therefore, useful all the time to those who take it up. (The abuse of demons can't challenge the one who fasts, and the angels who guard our lives love working more when they stay beside those who have made the soul clean through fasting.)

But now how much more, when all around the world the proclamation is being announced.[4] There isn't any island, land, city, nation, or remotest border where they haven't heard of the proclamation. Even armies and travelers, all alike hear the announcement, and they are receiving it joyfully.

So no one should leave himself off the list! People of every race, of all ages, and all different ranks are counted among those who fast. The angels are writing down the names of those who fast in each church. [31.188] See to it that you don't forfeit the angelic register through a little pleasurable food, and make yourself liable as a deserter, since you have been enlisted as a soldier by the scriptures.

The danger of the inexperienced soldier is that he will put down his shield when the battle is engaged. That's something that must be thoroughly warned against. Don't appear to be putting down the great weapon of fasting.

Are you rich? Don't insult the fast by refusing to eat at her[5] table, as if she were unworthy of you. Don't send her away from your house, when you have been happily living in pleasure, and never denying yourself in accord with the divine principle of fasting. If you do, your judgment will come many times over in times of want, or bodily sickness, or some other gloomy[6] circumstances. The poor should not pretend to ignore fasting, because in the past she lived together with you, and you had things in common.

Now women, fasting is as natural for your household as breathing. Children are nourished by fasting, just like thriving plants are sprinkled with water. From old times people have taken on the practice of it for themselves, and for the old it has made work light. Habitually practiced labors become less painful for those who have been trained.

To those who are traveling, fasting is a favorable traveling partner. While luxury forces them to bear burdens by carrying their enjoyments around, fasting prepares them to be light and unencumbered.

When a foreign war has been proclaimed and soldiers have been conscripted, they aren't furnished with luxuries. We have been sent out to war against invisible enemies. But after these victories we anticipate going to our home country up above. So isn't it appropriate that we be fed like an army, content with the conscription?

3. "Endure suffering as a good soldier,"[7] and contend lawfully, in order that you may be crowned. You know that "everyone who struggles is temperate in all things."[8]

But someone will undermine me perfectly by saying something that shouldn't be overlooked: that to those who are soldiers of the world, their provisions increase in proportion to their efforts. But on the contrary, to those who are heavily-armed spiritually, the less they have of food, the greater honor they have.

Our helmet contrasts with the perishable kind; theirs is made of bronze, but ours consists of the hope of salvation. Their shield is made of wood and leather, but we hold out the shield of faith.[9] [31.189] We wear the breastplate of righteousness, but they have coats of chain-mail around them.[10] We defend ourselves with the sword of the Spirit, but they carry iron.

So it's clear that foods don't produce the same kind of strength for both armies. The teachings of godliness strengthen us, even while they are enslaved by the fullness of their stomachs.

Now time has brought these much longed-for days around to us again. So let's welcome them into our homes like old nursemaids, who have been placed in the church for helping us to godliness.

Therefore, when you are going to fast don't be gloomy-faced like the Jews.[11] Rather, like gospel believers, adorn yourselves with rejoicing in the soul from spiritual enjoyment, not mourning your empty stomach.

You know that "The flesh desires what is opposed to the Spirit, and the Spirit is opposed to the flesh."[12] Therefore since "these things are adversaries to one another,"[13] let's rob the flesh of its comforts, and let's increase the soul's strength. Fasting will help us work through suffering until the victory feast is thrown for us, when we may be crowned with wreaths wrought by self-control.[14]

4. Now you should already be preparing yourselves to be worthy of the honorable fast. Don't be getting drunk today and ruin tomorrow's self-control.[15]

This kind of rationalizing is evil, a wicked notion: "Since five days of fasting have been proclaimed for us, let's drown ourselves in drunkenness today."

No man who is about to celebrate lawfully marrying a wife goes and cohabits with concubines and prostitutes beforehand. The lawful wife won't put up with those corrupted companions. So don't expect fasting to put up with it, if you begin with drunkenness—that public prostitute, that mother of shamelessness, that lover of laughter, that madman-maker, that friend of everything shameful.

Fasting and prayer will certainly not enter into the soul defiled by drunkenness. The Lord admits the one who is fasting inside the walls of holy places, but he doesn't approve of extravagance, he regards that as profane and unholy.

If you come tomorrow smelling of wine, and of this rotten stuff, how will I regard your extravagence as fasting? Consider this: I don't regard what's going on lately as being pure, because you aren't purified by wine. How will I categorize you? With the drunks, or with those who fast?

When drunkenness has passed it drags its victim around.[16] The presence of want corroborates the need for fasting.

It could be argued that drinking takes you into slavery, because it doesn't pay you fairly. The evidence exhibited that you were working as a slave is the odor of the wine that remains behind in the bottle.

Then the first of the fast days becomes unfavorable to you, on account of the remains of the drinking that have been stored up in you. [31.192] But if the beginning is unfavorable, then the whole time is also plainly rejected. "Drunkards will not inherit the kingdom of God."[17] If you come to the fast drinking, what do you think is the point? If drunkenness closes the kingdom of God from you, what's the use of you fasting?

Don't you see, that even those who are experienced in the breaking of racehorses expect a struggle, since they haven't been won over beforehand? But with malice toward yourself you gulp down your fill. You rush to gluttony like so many animals.

A full belly not only makes running a race difficult, it even makes sleep tough. When you are weighed down completely and can't find a way to rest, you are forced instead to continually turn from side to side.

5. Fasting guards infants, chastens the young, dignifies the old—for gray hair is more venerable when it's adorned with fasting.

It is an attractive ornament to women, a preventative for aging, a castle for couples, a nurse of virginity. There are people like this in each house who diligently pursue it.

But how is our public life in this society? The entire city has come together, and the entire region adopts good conduct, puts to sleep the shouting, gets rid of quarrels, and silences insults. What teacher can control the clamor of children when they have assembled like fasting, as it shows how it makes a throbbing city orderly?

What kind of revelry begins with fasting? What sort of sensual performance comes from fasting? Seductive laughter, songs of harlots, and passionate dances are suddenly withdrawn from the city, having been banished by the austere judge that is fasting.

If only everyone who needs a counselor would take her in, there would be nothing preventing a deep peace from abiding in each house. Nations wouldn't be attacking each other, and armies wouldn't be engaging in battle. Neither would weapons be forged, if fasting ruled. There would be no point in holding court, prisons would be unpopulated, and evildoers wouldn't have a place to hide. If slanderers were found in the cities, they would be thrown into the sea.

If all were disciples of fasting, to echo the words of Job, there wouldn't be heard any "voice of the taskmaster."[18] If fasting ruled our life, it wouldn't be full of groaning and sorrow.

It's clear that fasting would not only teach self-control in relation to all kinds of foods, but also how to entirely escape and get rid of covetousness, greed, and all kinds of evil. Having been set free, nothing [31.193] would hinder deep peace and calmness of soul from accompanying our lives.

6. But now those who have dismissed fasting and pursued after indulgence to make life happy, have instead found that swarms of evils have been introduced, and their own bodies are perishing anyway.

Pay attention with me to the difference in how the faces will appear to you this evening and tomorrow. Observing them today, they are somewhat reddish, wet with a little sweat, their eyes are watery and drooping, and a kind of mistiness seems to have taken over the clarity of their inward senses. But tomorrow they will have become quiet and solemn, the skin natural-looking, filled with meditation. The inner senses will be keen, since they have not had occasion to be darkened by physical exertions.

Fasting is the likeness of the angels, the tent-companion of the righteous, the moderation of life. It made the divine Mosaic Law.[19] Samuel is the fruit of fasting. Hannah was fasting when she prayed to God: "O sovereign Lord, God of hosts, if you will look upon your servant, and give me a male child, I will give him to you as a dedicated gift. Wine and liquor he will surely not drink, until the day he dies."[20]

Fasting brought about the great Samson, and brought him up until the time when he appeared publicly before men. Enemies were falling by the thousands, and many of their cities were being torn up, and lions were yielding to the strength of his hands. But when he came under the power of drinking and took up with harlots, he was easy prey for his enemies. He was bereaved of his eyes, and he was set out as a plaything for the children of foreigners.[21]

After Elijah fasted he closed up the heavens three years and six months.[22] After he saw how much wantonness had been born from the people's fullness, he thought it necessary to bring an involuntary fast upon them by means of famine. Through that he stood, while their excessive sins were already poured out, and fasting created such a burning, and cutting down of their evil leaders in pieces.[23]

7. Receive her,[24] poor common laborers, as your living companion and table partner. Slaves, you who hold the household together, receive her as a rest from your toils. You rich, receive her because she is curing you from the damage of excess. When she has worked her change in you, your daily life will be more pleasant, lived by the way of wisdom. You who are sick, receive her as the mother of health. You who are in good health, receive her as your prescribed good medicine.

Ask the doctors and they'll report it to you, that it's the most dangerous of all to be at the peak of health.[25] So even the most experienced should deprive themselves of overindulgence, so as not to start secretly weeping for the power of the burden of fleshiness. For when they have purged the excess [31.196] by firm purpose and through austerity, they prepare some open space for education, and a second beginning for promoting the power of growth. So it will have all kinds of bodily benefits for every activity, and it will go along well in houses and fields, by night and by day, in cities and wilderness.

So now, at such a time as this, let's receive her graciously and joyously into our homes for our own good. Let's obey the word of the Lord and not be like the gloomy-faced hypocrites,[26] but rather just letting the simple brightness of the soul show clearly.

And I suppose it's not really necessary for me to preach about the challenge of fasting, about how today should not be given over to the evils of drunkenness. Most of you receive fasting into your homes again as a habit, showing respect to yourself and one another. But I fear that the wine-lovers will try to rescue drunkenness, like an inheritance from their fathers.

It's as foolish to buy wine before five days of fasting, as it would be for those who are setting off on a long journey abroad. Who is so stupid that before even beginning to drink, he irrationally thinks about the things of drunkenness? Don't you know that a stomach won't safely care for what is entrusted to it? The stomach is a very unfaithful partner. It leaves the treasury unguarded. However many things you put away there, hoping to preserve them, it of course doesn't take care of them.

See to it that tomorrow, when you have come away from being drunk, the Lord doesn't have to say, "I haven't chosen this kind of fast."[27] Why do you dilute pure things? What communion has fasting with drinking? What fellowship does self-control have with drunkenness? "What concord has the temple of God with idols?"[28]

Those whom the Spirit of God indwells are God's temple.[29] But those who let drunkenness bring the refuse of intemperance into their lives are a temple of idols. Today is the gateway of the fast days. But surely the one who has profaned the front doors is not worthy to enter into the holy places.

No household slave who wants to win the favor of his master becomes friends with the champion of his enemy. Drunkenness is an enemy of God, but fasting is the beginning of repentance. So if you want to come near to God through confession, flee drunkenness, so that the loss will not be made more difficult for you.

So let's not be selfish as we begin the abstinence from foods that is the noble fast. Let's fast in an acceptable manner, one that's pleasing to God. A true fast is one that is set against evil, it's self-control of the tongue. It's the checking of anger, separation from things like lusts, evil-speaking, lies, and false oaths. Self-denial from these things is a true fast, so fasting from these negative things is good. But on the positive side, let's delight in the Lord, being in pursuit of the words of the Spirit. And let's delight in taking up the laws of salvation, and in all the doctrines that restore our souls.

Therefore let's guard the fast from these things in secret.[30] The prophet also rejects these things, saying, "The Lord will not let the soul of the righteous go hungry,"[31] and, "I have not seen the righteous forsaken, or his descendants looking for bread."[32] Now this isn't speaking about literal bread, such as what the children of our patriarch Jacob went down into Egypt for.[33] Rather, it's talking about spiritual food, the kind that goes inside us and perfects a person.

May the fasting threatened against the Jews not also come upon us: "For behold, days are coming, says the Lord, and I will bring upon this land a famine, not a famine of bread, neither thirst for water, but a famine of hearing the word of the Lord."[34] The righteous judge brought this upon them because their minds were suffering from hunger and in a state of atrophy without true teaching, and their bodies were growing fat and weighed down with flesh. So you should entertain the Holy Spirit joyfully every day without exception, both in the mornings and evenings.

No one should be left behind willingly from the spiritual feasting. Let's all share from this wineless bowl together. Wisdom has set it before us equally, and a special place for it has been set aside. "She has mixed her own bowl, and has slaughtered her own sacrifices."[35] This refers to the food of the mature, "Who because of practice have their senses trained to discern good and evil."[36] Once we have thoroughly taken our fill, may we also be found worthy of the exhilaration that comes in the bridal chamber of Christ Jesus our Lord![37] To him be the glory and the power forever! Amen.

APPENDIX 2
Fasting In Scripture

The following charts have been presented before in similar form, though minor changes have been made here.[1] They have been assembled by searching the Bible for texts that include the words in the "fasting" families,[2] as well as other narrative references to fasts which do not contain "fasting" words.

Scriptural References to Fasting

What follows is a comprehensive list of references to fasting in Scripture, with a brief summary of the contents of each passage (synoptic passages have been treated together). Notation is made of the extent of the fast (whether the fast is strictly individual or of a corporate nature), for the purpose of highlighting the corporate nature of biblical fasting in contrast to the frequent misconception that fasting was intended to be a strictly private, individualistic matter. Some text critical notes related to questionable NT passages are made here, but a fuller discussion may be found above in the discussion in the second chapter.

Reference	Extent	Summary
Exod 24:18, 34:28; Deut 9:9, 18, 10:10	individual	Moses twice spends forty days on Mount Sinai without eating or drinking, and in mourning over Israel's sin.
Judg 20:26	corporate	Israel fasts until evening to inquire of YHWH after loss to Benjamin.
1 Sam 1:7-8	individual	Hannah weeps and refuses to eat when her husband's other wife provokes her, and she prays for a son.
1 Sam 7:6	corporate	Israel fasts for a day to repent, Samuel prays, YHWH delivers them from the Philistines.
1 Sam 14:24-46	corporate	Saul places the army under oath not to eat until evening on the day of battle with the Philistines.
1 Sam 20:34	individual	Jonathan refuses to eat because of his grief over his father's mistreatment of David.
1 Sam 28:20	individual	Saul eats nothing all day and night when he consults with the witch of En-dor.
1 Sam 31:13; 1 Chr 10:12	corporate	Men of Jabesh fast seven days after recovering the bodies of Saul and Jonathan from the Philistines.
2 Sam 1:12	corporate	David's men fast until evening upon hearing the news of the death of Saul and Jonathan.
2 Sam 3:35	individual(?)	David refuses to eat food until evening when he heard of the death of Abner.
2 Sam 12:16-23	individual	David fasts and weeps seven days during the terminal illness of his son by Bathsheba.
1 Kgs 13:1-22	individual	An unnamed prophet is instructed by God not to eat or drink while on a mission to prophesy against Jeroboam's idolatry.
1 Kgs 19:8	individual	Elijah goes forty days on the strength of the food provided to him by an angel.
1 Kgs 21:4	individual	Ahab eats no food because he is sullen after Naboth refused to sell his vineyard.

1 Kgs 21:9-12	corporate	Jezebel calls a false day of fasting to accuse Naboth of cursing God.
1 Kgs 21:27-29	individual	Ahab fasts and puts on sackcloth in repentance after Elijah rebuked him, and God recognized Ahab's humility.
2 Chr 20:3	corporate	Jehoshaphat proclaims a fast throughout Judah to seek YHWH for fear of the armies of Ammon and Moab.
Ezra 8:21-23	corporate	Ezra calls a fast to seek God's protection for those leaving Babylon for Israel.
Ezra 10:6	individual	Ezra eats and drinks nothing because of his mourning over the unfaithfulness of the exiles.
Neh 1:4	individual	Nehemiah mourns and fasts for days over the news of the state of Jerusalem, confessing national sin.
Neh 9:1	corporate	The people of Israel assemble with fasting to confess their sin after Ezra reads from the law.
Esth 4:3	corporate	The Jews weep and fast when they hear of the king's decree for their destruction.
Esth 4:16	corporate	Esther, her maidens, and the Jews of Susa fast from food and drink for three days before she goes to the king.
Esth 9:31	corporate	Purim is established for the Jews with instructions for fasting and lamentations.
Job 3:24	individual	Job groans at the sight of food, and experiences great affliction and pain.
Job 33:19-20	individual	Elihu suggests that man (specifically, Job) is afflicted by God and unable to eat because God is chastening him.
Ps 35:13	individual	David defends his honor by saying that he fasted and prayed when his enemies were sick.
Ps 42:3	individual	The psalmist (Sons of Korah) says that tears are his food day and night.

Ps 69:10	individual	David's fasting, weeping and prayer was an object of scorn by his enemies.
Ps 102:4	individual	The afflicted psalmist forgets to eat bread because of his great grief.
Ps 107:17-18	individual	People in distress are pictured as near death, unable to eat, but YHWH saves them.
Ps 109:24	individual	David says his knees are weak from fasting, and his flesh has grown lean during his affliction from his enemies.
Isa 58:3-6	corporate	Israel's fasts are not heard by God because of their oppression and hypocrisy; He desires righteousness first.
Jer 14:12	corporate	Israel's fasts are not heard by God because of their oppression and hypocrisy.
Jer 36:6-9	corporate	The people of Judah assemble in Jerusalem for a fast, and Baruch reads Jeremiah's prophecy to them.
Ezek 24:18	individual	Ezekiel is instructed in special mourning rites, that include fasting, for the death of his wife.
Dan 6:18	individual	Darius fasts from food, entertainment, and sleep through the night while worrying for Daniel in the lion's den.
Dan 9:3	individual	Daniel fasts, confessing Israel's sin, upon reading Jeremiah's prophecy of the seventy weeks.
Dan 10:2-3	individual	Daniel mourns for three weeks, abstaining from tasty food, meat, wine, and ointment.
Joel 1:14	corporate	Joel calls for a nation-wide fast because of famine that is destroying the land.
Joel 2:12-15	corporate	YHWH calls the people to return to Him with fasting, rending their hearts, not garments; Joel again calls for a fast.

Jonah 3:5	corporate	All of Nineveh fasts, repenting at the preaching of Jonah of the destruction of the city.
Zech 7:5	corporate	YHWH rebukes the priests for their ritual fasts that were done more for themselves than for Him.
Zech 8:19	corporate	YHWH will transform the ritual fasts into feasts of joy when God's people have repented of sin and He grants them favor.
Matt 4:2; Luke 4:2	individual	Jesus fasts forty days in the wilderness, being tempted by the devil.
Matt 6:16-18	individual	Jesus teaches that fasting should be done privately for God, not for the purpose of being seen to be fasting, like the hypocrites.
Matt 9:14-15; Mark 2:18-20; Luke 5:33-35	corporate	Jesus tells John's disciples that his do not fast because the bridegroom is present, but when He is taken away they will.
Matt 15:32; Mark 8:3	corporate	Jesus did not wish to send the crowd away fasting,[3] since they had been with Him three days and have nothing (more?) to eat.
Matt 17:21;[4] Mark 9:29[5]	individual?	Jesus says that this kind of demon goes out only by means of prayer and fasting.[6]
Luke 2:37	individual	Anna serves in the temple night and day with fastings and prayers.
Luke 18:12	individual´	The Pharisee in Jesus' parable shows his self-righteousness by boasting that he fasts twice a week and tithes.
Acts 9:9	individual	Saul fasted from food and water three days after the Damascus Road experience.
Acts 10:30[7]	individual	Cornelius was fasting and praying when an angel instructed him to go to Peter.
Acts 13:2-3	corporate	Prophets and teachers in Antioch were ministering to the Lord and fasting before and after the Holy Spirit set apart Saul and Barnabas.

Acts 14:23	corporate	Paul and Barnabas appoint elders in the churches, having prayed with fasting.
Acts 23:12	corporate	Certain Jews bind themselves by oath not to eat or drink until they kill Paul.
Acts 27:9	corporate	Paul's voyage to Rome takes place after "the fast" was over, a reference to the Day of Atonement.
Acts 27:33	corporate	Paul encourages the ship's crew to eat, since they had gone 14 days fasting.[8]
1 Cor 7:5[9]	couples	Paul tells couples not to deprive one another sexually, except for brief periods devoted to prayer and fasting.
2 Cor 6:5; 2 Cor 11:27	individual	Paul lists "fastings"[10] among the hardships he suffered as a mark of his apostleship.

Summary of Biblical Purposes for Fasting

I. As a Sign of Sorrow
   A. For tragic events (Judg 20:26; 1 Sam 31:13/1 Chr 10:12; 2 Sam 1:12, 3:35; Esth 4:3; Jer 14:1-12; Joel 1:14, 2:12-15).
   B. For personal sorrow (1 Sam 1:7-8, 20:34; Job 3:24; Pss 42:3, 102:4, 107:17-18).
II. As a Sign of Repentance and Seeking Forgiveness
   A. National or corporate sins (Exod 34:28/Deut 9:9, 18, 10:10; 1 Sam 7:6; Ezra 9:1- 10:17; Neh 1:4-7, 9:1; Dan 9:3-14; Jonah 3:5-9; Zech 8:16-19).
   B. Personal sins (2 Sam 12:16-23; 1 Kgs 21:27-29; Ps 69:10; Acts 9:9?).
   C. As an opportunity for public exposure of sin (1 Kgs 21:9-12; Isa 58:1-5; Jer 36:6-9).
III. As an Aid in Prayer to God
   A. For others (2 Sam 12:16-23; Neh 1:8-10; Ps 35:13; Dan 6:18, 9:15-19).
   B. For self (1 Sam 1:7-11; Neh 1:11; Ps 109:21-24; Dan 9:3, 10:1-3).
   C. For success in battle (Judg 20:26; 1 Sam 7:6; 2 Chr 20:3) and in other endeavors (Ezra 8:21-23; Esth 4:16).
   D. For relief from famine (Jer 14:1-12; Joel 1:14, 2:12-15).
   E. As a means of personal or group devotion (Matt 6:16-18; Luke 2:37; Acts 10:30, 13:2-3; 1 Cor 7:5).

IV. As a Part of Experiencing God's Presence

    A. Supernatural sustaining by God (Exod 34:28/Deut 9:9, 18, 10:10; 1 Kgs 19:8).

    B. Reliance on God in times of temptation or spiritual warfare (Matt 4:2/Luke 4:2; Matt 17:21/Mark 9:29).

    C. Reflecting the reality of the absence of Christ's immediate presence with his followers (Matt 9:14-15/Mark 2:18-20/Luke 5:33-35).

    D. Going without food to remain longer under Jesus' teaching (Matt 15:32/Mark 8:3).

V. *As an Act of Ceremonial Public Worship* (Neh 9:1; Esth 9:31; Isa 58:3; Jer 36:6-9; Zech 7:3-5, 8:19; Acts 27:9).

VI. As Related to Ministry

    A. Preparation for significant ministry (Matt 4:2/Luke 4:2; Acts 9:9, 13:2-3, 14:23).

    B. Specific command of God while prophesying (1 Kgs 13:1-22).

    C. Suffering for the sake of the gospel (2 Cor 6:5/11:27).

VII. Negative Associations or Corrections of Fasting

    A. Fasting while engaging in hypocritical actions or attitudes (1 Sam 28:20; 1 Kgs 21:9-12; Isa 58; Jer 14:10-12; Jer 36:6-26; Zech 7:3-14; Matt 6:16-18; Luke 18:12).

    B. Fasting as a solemn binding for a foolish or sinful oath (1 Sam 14; Acts 23:12-21).

    C. Breaking a fast when God has commanded it (1 Kgs 13:8-24).

    D. A sulking refusal to eat (1 Kgs 21:4).

    E. Wrongly attributing the inability to eat as God's chastening (Job 33:19-20).

Bibliography

Abbo, John A. and Jerome D. Hannan. The Sacred Canons: A Concise Presentation of the Current Disciplinary Norms of the Church. St. Louis: Herder, 1952.

Achelis, H. "Fasting." The New Schaff-Herzog Encyclopedia of Religious Knowledge, ed. Samuel Macauley Jackson. Vol. 4: 281-84. Grand Rapids: Baker, 1950.

Ackroyd, Peter R. Exile and Restoration: A Study of Hebrew Thought of the Sixth Century B.C. Philadelphia: Westminster, 1968.

Akakios, Archimandrite. Fasting in the Orthodox Church: Its Theological, Pastoral, and Social Implications. Etna, Calif.: Center for Traditionalist Orthodox Studies, 1990.

Aland, Kurt, and Barbara Aland. The Text of the New Testament: An Introduction to the Critical Editions and to the Theory and Practice of Modern Textual Criticism, trans. Erroll F. Rhodes. Second ed. Grand Rapids: Eerdmans, 1989.

Albright, W. F., and C. S. Mann. Matthew. AB 26. Garden City, N.Y.: Doubleday, 1971.

Anderson, Andy. Fasting Changed My Life. Nashville: Broadman, 1977.

Anderson, Gary A., and Michael E. Stone, eds. A Synopsis of the Books of Adam and Eve, 2d. rev. ed. SBL, Early Judaism and Its Literature 17. Atlanta: Scholars, 1999.

Anglin, Thomas Francis. The Eucharistic Fast: An Historical Synopsis and Commentary The Catholic University of America Canon Law Studies 124. Washington: Catholic University of America, 1941.

Aquinas, Thomas. Summa Theologiæ, trans. Thomas Gilby. Vol. 43. New York: Blackfriars, McGraw-Hill, 1968.

_____. Summa Theologiæ, trans. Samuel Parsons and Albert Pinheiro. Vol. 53. New York: Blackfriars, McGraw-Hill, 1971.

_____. Summa Theologiæ, trans. James J. Cunningham. Vol. 57. New York: Blackfriars, McGraw-Hill, 1975.

_____. Summa Theologiæ, trans. Thomas Gilby. Vol. 59. New York: Blackfriars, McGraw-Hill, 1975.

Arbesmann, Rudolf. "Das Fasten bei den Greichen und Römern." Religionsgeschichtliche Versuche und Vorarbeiten 21, no. 1 (1929): 1-131.

_____. "Fasting and Prophecy in Pagan and Christian Antiquity." Traditio 7 (1949-51): 1-72.

Arndt, Herman. Why Did Jesus Fast? Cincinnati: By the author, 1922.

Augustine. Treatises on Various Subjects. The Fathers of the Church: A New Translation, ed. Roy J. Deferrari. New York: Fathers of the Church, 1952.

_____. The Works of Saint Augustine: A Translation for the 21st Century, ed. John E. Rotelle, trans. Edmund Hill. Hyde Park, N.Y.: New City, 1995.

Aumann, Jordan. "Origins of Monasticism." Monasticism: a Historical Overview. Word and Spirit 6. Still River, Mass.: St. Bede's, 1984.

Aune, David E., and John McCarthy, eds. The Whole and Divided Self: The Bible and Theological Anthropology. New York: Crossroad Herder, 1997.

Baird, John E., and Don DeWelt. What the Bible Says About Fasting. What the Bible Says Series. Joplin, Mo.: College Press, 1984.

Barbaric, Slavko. Fasting. Steubenville, Ohio: Franciscan University, 1988.

Barnes, Timothy David. Tertullian: A Historical and Literary Study. Oxford: Clarendon, 1985.

Barrett, C. K. A Commentary on the Second Epistle to the Corinthians. London: Adam and Charles Black, 1973.

Barré, Michael L. "Fasting in Isaiah 58:1-2: A Reexamination." Biblical Theology Bulletin 15 (July 1985): 94-97.

Barth, Markus, and Helmut Blanke. Colossians: A New Translation with Introduction and Commentary, trans. Astrid B. Beck. Vol. 34b The Anchor Bible. New York: Doubleday, 1994.

Barton, Wayne. "Toward an Understanding of Fasting in the New Testament." Th. D. diss., New Orleans Baptist Theological Seminary, 1954.

Basil. The Ascetic Works of Saint Basil, trans. W. K. L. Clarke. Translations of Christian Literature Series 1, Greek Texts. New York: MacMillan, 1925.

_____. Saint Basil: Ascetical Works, trans. M. Monica Wagner. Vol. 9 The Fathers of the Church: A New Translation, ed. Joseph Deferrari. New York: Fathers of the Church, 1950.

Bauer, W., F. W. Danker, W. F. Arndt, and F. W. Gingrich. A Greek-English Lexicon of the New Tetament and Other Early Christian Literature. 3rd ed. Chicago: University of Chicago, 2000.

Beatrice, Pier Franco. "Ascetical Fasting and Original Sin in the Early Christian Writers." In Prayer and Spirituality in the Early Church, ed. Pauline Allen, Raymond Canning, Lawrence Cross, Vol. 1. Everton Park, Queensland, Australia: Centre for Early Christian Studies, 1998.

Becon, Thomas. The Catechism of Thomas Becon, with Other Pieces The Parker Society for the Publication of the Works of the Fathers and Early Writers of the Reformed English Church, ed. John Ayre. Cambridge: University Press, 1844. Johnson Reprint, 1968.

Behm, Johannes. "νῆστις, νηστεύω, νηστεία." TDNT 4:924-35. Grand Rapids: Eerdmans, 1967.

Benedict. The Holy Rule of Our Most Holy Father Saint Benedict, ed. Benedictine Monks of St. Meinrad Archabbey. St. Meinrad, Ind.: Grail, 1956.

_____. The Rule of St. Benedict, trans. Anthony C. Meisel and M. L. del Mastro. New York: Image/Doubleday, 1975.

Benson, Bob, and Michael W. Benson. Disciplines for the Inner Life. Waco, Tex.: Word, 1985.

Berghuis, Kent D. "Pitirim Sorokin as Cultural Physician: His Diagnosis, Prognosis and Prescription." Paper presented at the 1997 ETS meeting, Santa Clara, Calif., 1997.

_____. "Teaching and Biblical Fasting." Paper presented at the ETS annual meeting, Orlando, Fla., 1998.

_____. "Fasting and the Nature of the Age." Paper presented at the ETS annual meeting, Boston, 1999.

_____. "A Biblical Perspective on Fasting" BSac 158 (2001) 86-103.

Bertholet, E. Le retour à la santé et la vie saine par le jeûne. 5th ed. Lausanne: P. Genillard, 1970.

Betz, Hans Dieter. The Sermon on the Mount: A Commentary on the Sermon on the Mount, Including the Sermon on the Plain (Matthew 5:3-7:27 and Luke 6:20-49). Hermeneia. Minneapolis: Augsburg Fortress, 1995.

Blass, F., and A. Debrunner. A Greek Grammar of the New Testament and Other Early Christian Literature, trans. Robert W. Funk. Chicago: University of Chicago, 1961.

Blomberg, Craig L. "Midrash, Chiasmus, and the Outline of Luke's Central Section." Gospel Perspectives: Studies in Midrash and Historiography, vol. 3, ed. R. T. France and David Wenham. Sheffield: JSOT Press, 1983.

Bock, Darrell L. Luke: Vol 1: 1:1-9:50. Baker Exegetical Commentary on the New Testament. Grand Rapids: Baker, 1994.

_____. Luke: Vol. 2: 9:51-24:53. Baker Exegetical Commentary on the NT. Grand Rapids: Baker, 1996.

Bockmuehl, Markus. The Epistle to the Philippians. BNTC. Peabody, Mass.: 1998.

Booij, T. "Negation in Isaiah 43:22-24." ZAW 94 (1982): 390-400.

Böhl, Felix. "Das Fasten an Mantagen und Donnerstagen: zur Geschichte einer pharisäischen Praxis (Lk 18,12)." Biblische Zeitschrift 31, no. 2 (1987): 247-50.

Bray, Gerald Lewis. Holiness and the Will of God: Perspectives on the Theology of Tertullian. Atlanta: John Knox, 1979.

Briggs, David Eddle. "Biblical Teaching on Fasting." Th.M. thesis, Dallas Theological Seminary, 1953.

Bright, Bill. The Coming Revival: America's Call to Fast, Pray, and 'Seek God's Face.' Orlando, Fla.: NewLife Publications, 1995.

Broadus, John. Commentary on the Gospel of Matthew. Valley Forge, Pa.: American Baptist Publication Society, 1886.

Brodie, Thomas L. The Crucial Bridge: The Elijah-Elisha Narrative as an Interpretive Synthesis of Genesis-Kings and a Literary Model for the Gospels. Collegeville, Minn.: Liturgical, 2000.

_____. Genesis as Dialogue: A Literary, Historical, and Theological Commentary. Oxford: Oxford University Press, 2001.

Brongers, H. A. "Fasting in Israel in Biblical and Post-Biblical Times." Instruction and Interpretation: Studies in Hebrew Language, Palestinian Archaeology and Biblical Exegesis. OTS, 20. Leiden: Brill, 1977.

Brooks, Phillips. The Candle of the Lord and Other Sermons. New York: Macmillan, 1905.

Brown, Harold O. J. The Sensate Culture: Western Civilization between Chaos and Transformation. Dallas: Word, 1996.

Brown, Peter. Augustine of Hippo: A Biography. Berkeley, Calif.: University of California, 2000.

Brown, Raymond E. The Birth of the Messiah: A Commentary on the Infancy Narratives in Matthew and Luke. Garden City, N.Y.: Doubleday, 1979.

Brox, Norbert. Der Hirt des Hermas. Kommentar zu den Apostolischen Vätern. Göttingen: Vandenhoeck & Ruprecht, 1991.

Bruce, F. F. The Acts of the Apostles: The Greek Text with Introduction and Commentary. Third rev. and enlarged ed. Grand Rapids: Eerdmans, 1990.

Bryan, David. Cosmos, Chaos and the Kosher Mentality. JSPSup 12. Sheffield: Sheffield Academic Press, 1995.

Bynum, Caroline Walker. Holy Feast and Holy Fast: The Religious Significance of Food to Medieval Women. Berkely, Calif.: University of California, 1987.

Callam, Daniel. "Fasting, Christian." In Dictionary of the Middle Ages, ed. Joseph R. Strayer, Vol. 5: 18-19. New York: Charles Scribner's Sons, 1985.

Calvin, John. Calvin: Institutes of the Christian Religion, trans. Ford Lewis Battles. The Library of Christian Classics 20, ed. John T. McNeill. Philadelphia: Westminster, 1960.

_____. A Harmony of the Gospels Matthew, Mark and Luke, trans. A. W. Morrison. Vol. 1, Calvin's Commentaries, ed. David W. Torrance and Thomas F. Torrance. Grand Rapids: Eerdmans, 1972.

_____. Isaiah The Crossway Classic Commentaries, ed. Alister McGrath and J. I. Packer. Wheaton, Ill.: Crossway, 2000.

_____. The Epistles of Paul the Apostle to the Galatians, Ephesians, Philippians and Colossians, trans. T. H. L. Parker. Calvin's Commentaries, vol. 11, ed. David W. Torrance and Thomas F. Torrance. Grand Rapids: Eerdmans, 1972.

Canon Law Society of America. Code of Canon Law: Latin-English Edition Washington: Canon Law Society of America, 1983.

Carroll, R. P. "The Elijah-Elisha Sagas: Some Remarks on Prophetic Succession in Ancient Israel." Prophecy in the Hebrew Bible: Selected Studies from Vetus Testamentum," ed. David E. Orton. Brill's Readers in Biblical Studies, vol. 5. Leiden: Brill, 2000. First published in VT 19 (1969): 400-415.

Carson, D. A. Jesus' Sermon on the Mount and His Confrontation with the World: An Exposition of Matthew 5-10. Toronto: Global Christian Publishers, 1999.

_____. Matthew. The Expositor's Bible Commentary. Vol. 8, ed. Frank E. Gaebelein. Grand Rapids: Zondervan, 1984.

Casey, Maurice. "Where Wright is Wrong: A Critical Review of N. T. Wright's Jesus and the Victory of God." JSNT 69 (1998): 95-103.

Casey, Robert Pierce ed. The Excerpta Ex Theodoto of Clement of Alexandria. In Studies and Documents, ed. Kirsopp Lake and Silva Lake, vol. 1. London: Christophers, 1934.

Cassian, John. John Cassian: The Conferences. Trans. Boniface Ramsey. ACW 57. New York: Paulist, 1997.

_____. John Cassian: The Institutes. Trans. Boniface Ramsey. ACW 58. New York: Paulist, 1997.

Cassuto, Umberto. A Commentary on the Book of Exodus, trans. Israel Abrahams. Jerusalem: Magnes, 1983.

Catechism of the Catholic Church. Mahwah, N.J.: Paulist, 1994.

Cavarnos, Constantine. Fasting and Science: A Study of the Scientific Support and Patristic Foundation for Fasting in the Orthodox Church, trans. Bishop Chrysostomos and Hieromonk Auxentios. Monographic Supplement Series 3. Etna, Calif.: Center for Traditionalist Orthodox Studies, 1988.

Chadwick, Owen. ed. and trans. Western Asceticism Library of Christian Classics 12. Philadelphia: Westminster, 1943.

Charles, J. Daryl. "Assessing Recent Pronouncements on Justification: Evidence from 'The Gift of Salvation' and the Catholic Catechism." Pro Ecclesia 8 (1999): 461.

Charles, Jerry. God's Guide to Fasting: A Complete and Exhaustive Biblical Encyclopedia. Madison, N.C.: Power Press, 1977.

Charles, R. H., ed. The Apocraypha and Pseudepigrapha of the Old Testament in English. Vol. 2. Oxford: Clarendon, 1963.

Chatham, R. D. Fasting: A Biblical Historical Study. South Plainfield, N.J.: Bridge Publishing, 1987.

Clancy, P. M. J. "Fast and Abstinence." New Catholic Encyclopedia. Vol. 5: 847-50. New York: McGraw-Hill, 1967.

Clark, Elizabeth A. "New Perspectives on the Origenist Controversy: Human Embodiment and Ascetic Strategies." In Forms of Devotion: Conversion, Worship, Spirituality, and Asceticism, ed. Everett Ferguson. Recent Studies in Early Christianity: A Collection of Scholarly Essays. New York: Garland, 1999.

Clarke, Kent D. Textual Optimism: A Critique of the United Bible Societies' Greek New Testament. JSNTSup 138. Sheffield: Sheffield Academic, 1997.

Clarke, K[ent] D., and K. Bales. "The Construction of Biblical Certainty: Textual Optimism and the United Bible Societies' Greek New Testament." Studies in the Early Text of the Gospels and Acts: Papers of the First Birmingham Colloquium on the Textual Criticism of the New Testament, ed. D. G. K. Taylor. TS Third Series 1. Birmingham: University of Birmingham, 1999.

Conrad, Edgar W. Zechariah. Readings: A New Biblical Commentary, ed. John Jarick. Sheffield: Sheffield Academic, 1999.

Constable, Giles. Attitudes Toward Self-Inflicted Suffering in the Middle Ages. Stephen J. Brademas, Sr., Lecture 9. Brookline, Mass.: Hellenic College, 1982.

Cooper, John W. Body, Soul and Life Everlasting: Biblical Anthropology and the Monism-Dualism Debate. Updated ed. Grand Rapids: Eerdmans, 2000.

Corrington, Gail Paterson. "The Defense of the Body and the Discourse of Appetite: Continence and Control in the Greco-Roman World." Semeia 57 (1992): 65-74.

Cremer, Franz Gerhard. Der Beitrag Augustins zur Auslegung des Fastenstreitsgesprächs: (Mk 2, 18-22 parr) und der Einfluss seiner Exegese auf die Mittelalterliche Theologie. Paris: Études Augustiniennes, 1971.

Davies, W. D. The Setting of the Sermon on the Mount. Cambridge: Cambridge University Press, 1964.

Davis, Kenneth Ronald. Anabaptism and Asceticism: A Study in Intellectual Origins. Studies in Anabaptist and Mennonite History 16. Kitchener. Ontario: Herald, 1974.

de Vogüé, Adalbert. To Love Fasting: The Monastic Experience, trans. Jean Baptist Hasbrouck. Petersham, Mass.: Saint Bede's, 1989.

de Ward, E. F. "Mourning Customs in 1,2 Sam II." JJS 23 (1972): 1-27, 145-66.

Dehnke, Gary D. "Fasting: Practice and Function in the New Testament and in the Early Church." M. Div. thesis, Concordia Theological Seminary, 1993.

Demetri, Bishop. His Grace Bishop Demetri's Message for Great Lent 2002, [article online] Antiochian Orthodox Christian Archdiocese of North America, accessed June 28 2002. Available from www.antiochian.org/midwest/Bishop/GreatLent_2002.htm; Internet.

Denis, A. M. "Ascèse et vie chrétienne." RSPT 47 (1963): 606-18.

Dieckhaus, Joseph C. "The Eucharistic Fast and Frequent Communion in the West: A Canonical and Liturgical Perspective." Licentiate in Canon Law Dissertation, Catholic University of America, 1991.

Dinkins, Frederic R. "The Biblical Practice and Doctrine of Fasting." Th. M. thesis, Columbia Theological Seminary, 1966.

Daniel M. Doriani. Putting the Truth to Work: The Theory and Practice of Biblical Application. Phillipsburg, N.J.: P&R, 2001.

Draper, Jonathan A. "Christian Self-Definition Against the 'Hypocrites' in Didache viii." The Didache in Modern Research, ed. Jonathan A. Draper. Leiden: Brill, 1996.

Duewel, Wesley L. Mighty Prevailing Prayer. Grand Rapids: Francis Asbury, 1990.

Dugan, Kathleen. "Fasting for Life: The Place of Fasting in the Christian Tradition." JAAR 63, no. 3 (1995): 539-48.

Dun, Angus. Not By Bread Alone. New York: Harper and Brothers, 1942.

Editorial. "Not a Fast Fix: It's Hard to Fast, and Even Harder to Do It for the Right Reasons." Christianity Today 43 (April 5, 1999): 30-31.

Elliott, J. K. The Apocryphal New Testament: A Collection of Apocryphal Christian Literature in an English Translation. Oxford: Clarendon, 1993.

Epstein, I. ed. The Babylonian Talmud. London: Soncino, 1938.

Estrada, Nelson P. "Praise for Promises Fulfilled: A Study on the Significance of the Anna the Prophetess Pericope." Asian Journal of Pentecostal Studies 2 (1999): 5-18.

Evans, C. F. "The Central Section of St Luke's Gospel." Studies in the Gospels, ed. D. E. Nineham. Oxford: Basil Blackwell, 1955.

Evans, Craig A. "The Pharisee and the Publican: Luke 18:9-14 and Deuteronomy 26." The Gospels and the Scriptures of Israel, ed. Craig A. Evans and W. Richard Stegner. JSNTSS 104, Studies in Scripture in Early Judaism and Christianity 3. Sheffield: Sheffield Academic, 1994.

_____. Mark 8:27-16:20. WBC 34B. Nashville: Thomas Nelson, 2001.

Falwell, Jerry. Fasting: What the Bible Teaches. Wheaton, Ill.: Tyndale, 1981.

Fee, Gordon D. Paul's Letter to the Philippians. NICNT. Grand Rapids: Eerdmans, 1995.

Felter, Thomas H. "The Relevance of the New Testament Treatment of Fasting to Modern Life." M. A. thesis, Wheaton College, 1960.

Feuillet, A. "Le récit lucanien de la tentation." Biblical Theology Bulletin 40 (1959):613-31.

Finch, Martha Lawrence. "Corporality and Orthodoxy in Early New England: Plymouth Colony, 1620-1692." Ph. D. diss., University of California, Santa Barbara, 2000.

_____. "Pinched with Hunger, Partaking of Plenty: Fasting and Thanksgiving in Early Puritan New England." Paper presented at the American Academy of Religion Annual Meeting. Nashville, Tenn., 2000.

Fink, Marion Michael, Jr. "The Responses in the New Testament to the Practice of Fasting." Ph. D. diss., The Southern Baptist Theological Seminary, 1974.

Fischer, Walter F. "Fasting and Bodily Preparation—A Fine Outward Training." Concordia Theological Journal 30 (December, 1959): 887-901.

Fitzmyer, Joseph A. The Acts of the Apostles. The Anchor Bible Vol. 31b. New York: Doubleday, 1998.

Flannery, Austin, ed. Vatican Council II: Volume 1, The Conciliar and Post Conciliar Documents. Northport, N.Y.: Costello, 1996.

Floyd, Ronnie W. The Power of Prayer and Fasting: 10 Secrets of Spiritual Strength. Nashville: Broadman & Holman, 1997.

Foster, Richard J. Celebration of Discipline: The Path to Spiritual Growth. Rev. ed. San Francisco: HarperSanFrancisco, 1988.

Fox, Samuel J. "An Investigation of Fasting in the Old Testament Literature." M. A. Thesis, Butler University, 1994.

Francis, Fred O. "Humility and Angelic Worship in Col 2:18." In Conflict at Colossae: A Problem in the Interpretation of Early Christianity Illustrated by Selected Modern Studies, ed. Fred O. Francis, and Wayne A. Meeks. Sources for Biblical Study 4. Missoula, Mont.: Scholars, 1975.

Frei, Hans. Theology and Narrative: Selected Essays, ed. George Hunsinger and William C. Placher. New York: Oxford University Press, 1993.

_____. The Eclipse of Biblical Narrative: A Study in Eighteenth and Nineteenth Century Hermeneutics. New Haven: Yale University, 1974.

Friedlander, Gerald, ed. and trans. Pirkê de Rabbi Eliezer. Fourth ed. New York: Sepher-Hermon, 1981.

Furnish, Victor Paul. II Corinthians. The Anchor Bible. Garden City, N.Y.: Doubleday, 1984.

Gadamer, Hans-Georg. Truth and Method. New York: Continuum, 1975.

Gamberoni, Johann. "Fasting." Encyclopedia of Biblical Theology, ed. Johannes B. Bauer, 257-60. New York: Crossroad, 1981.

Gardner, Christine J. "Hungry for God: Why More and More Christians Are Fasting for Revival." Christianity Today 43 (April 5, 1999): 32-38.

Gaster, Theodor H. The Dead Sea Scriptures in English Translation With Introduction and Notes. New York: Doubleday, 1956.

George, Timothy. "Evanngelicals and Catholics Together: A New Initiative." Christianity Today 41 (Dec. 8, 1997): 34-38.

George, Timothy, Thomas C. Oden, and J. I. Packer. "An Open Letter About 'The Gift of Salvation.'" Christianity Today 42 (April 27, 1998): 9.

Gerlitz, P. "Fasten als Reinigungsritus." ZRGG 20 (1968): 33-45.

Glare, P. G. W., ed. Oxford Latin Dictionary. Oxford: Clarendon, 1982.

Goodier, Alban. An Introduction to the Study of Ascetical and Mystical Theology. London: Burns Oates & Washbourne, 1938.

Green, Daniel D. The Use of Classical Spiritual Disciplines in Evangelical Devotional Life. D.Min. project, Trinity Evangelical Divinity School, 1994.

Greenstone, Julius H. "Fasting and Fast-Days." The Jewish Encyclopedia, ed. Isidore Singer, 5: 347-49. New York: Ktav, 1964.

Gregg, Robert C., trans. and ed. Athanasius: The Life of Antony and the Letter to Marcellinus. Classics of Western Spirituality. New York: Paulist, 1980.

Grimm, Veronika E. From Feasting to Fasting, the Evolution of a Sin: Attitudes to Food in Late Antiquity. London: Routledge, 1996.

Grudem, Wayne. Systematic Theology: An Introduction to Bible Doctrine. Grand Rapids: Zondervan, 1994.

Guillaume, Alexandre. Jeûne et charité: dans l'eglise latine, des origines au xiie siècle en particulier chez saint Léon le Grand. Rome: Pontificia Universitate Gregoriana, 1954.

_____. "Jeûne, prière, aumône dans le monde moderne." Assemblées du Seigneur 25 (1966): 71-83.

_____. Prière, jeûne et charité: des perspectives chrétiennes et une espérance pour notre temps. Paris: S. O. S., 1985.

_____. Prière, jeûne et charité: des perspectives chrétiennes et une espérance pour notre temps, abridged ed. Paris: S. O. S., 1988.

Gundry, Robert H. "Reconstructing Jesus." Christianity Today 42 (April 27, 1998): 76-79.

_____. Matthew: A Commentary on His Handbook for a Mixed Church under Persecution. Second ed. Grand Rapids: Eerdmans, 1994.

_____. Mark: A Commentary on His Apology for the Cross. Grand Rapids: Eerdmans, 1993).

Gunning, Peter. The Paschal or Lent Fast: Apostolical and Perpetual, new ed. Oxford: John Henry Parker, 1845.

Guthrie, H. H., Jr. "Fast, Fasting." IDB. Vol. 2: 241-44.

Hagner, Donald A. Matthew 1-13. WBC 33A. Dallas: Word, 1993.

_____. Matthew 14-28. WBC 33B. Dallas: Word, 1995.

Hall, Stuart George, and Joseph H. Crehan. "Fasten/Fasttage." TRE. Vol. 11: 41-59.

Hamilton, Victor P. The Book of Genesis Chapters 1-17. NICOT. Grand Rapids: Eerdmans, 1990.

Hargrave, William Loftin. "Fasting in the Early Church: Being a Study of Fasting Based Upon References to the Subject in the Old and New Testaments, and Upon the Writings of Some of the Ante-Nicene Fathers." S. T. M. thesis, University of the South, 1952.

Hauser, Alan J., and Russell Gregory. From Carmel to Horeb: Elijah in Crisis. JSOTSS 85. Bible and Literature Series 19. Sheffield: Almond, 1990.

Hawthorne, Gerald. Philippians. WBC 43. Waco, Tex.: Word, 1983.

Hellwig, Monika K. "Penance and Reconciliation." Commentary on the Catechism of the Catholic Church, ed. Michael J. Walsh. Collegeville, Minn.: Liturgical, 1994.

Hendriksen, William. New Testament Commentary: Exposition on the Gospel of Luke. Grand Rapids: Baker, 1978.

_____. New Testament Commentary: Exposition of Philippians. Grand Rapids: Baker, 1962.

Henning, Michael. "Man: 'a God by Grace?'" In On Fasting: The Scriptural and Spiritual Meaning of the Orthodox Christian Fasts. Dewdney, B. C.: Synaxis, 1997.

Hindringer, R. "Fasten." LTK. Vol. 2: 963-68.

Hoffeditz, David M. "A Prophet, a Kingdom, and a Messiah: The Portrayal of Elijah in the Gospels in Light of First-Century Judaism." Ph.D. diss., University of Aberdeen, 2000.

Holmes, Augustine. A Life Pleasing to God: The Spirituality of the Rules of St. Basil. London: Darton, Longman and Todd, 2000.

Holmes, Michael W., ed. The Apostolic Fathers: Greek Texts and English Translations of Their Writings, 2nd rev. ed. Grand Rapids: Baker, 1992.

Holmgren, Fredrick C. "The Pharisee and the Tax Collector: Luke 18:9-14 and Deuteronomy 26." Interpretation 48: 252-61.

Hoppe, Leslie J. "Isaiah 58:1-12, Fasting and Idolatry." Biblical Theology Bulletin 13 (April 1983): 44-47.

Horton, Michael S. Covenant and Eschatology: The Divine Drama. Louisville: Westminster John Knox, 2002.

_____, ed. "Spiritual Disciplines and Means of Grace: Contrast or Continuum? An Interview with Dallas Willard." Modern Reformation, July/Aug 2002, 41-43.

Houston, Walter. Purity and Monotheism: Clean and Unclean Animals in Biblical Law. JSOTSup 140. Sheffield: JSOT, 1993.

Hughes, Philip Edgcumbe. Paul's Second Epistle to the Corinthians: The English Text with Introduction, Exposition and Notes. NICNT. Grand Rapids: Eerdmans, 1962.

Isley, William. "Fasting: The Discipline for the In-between Time." Paper presented at the National Spiritual Formation Conference, Dallas, 2001.

Jacob, Thomas Wilson. "The Meaning and Importance of Fasting in the Teaching of Jesus." M. A. thesis, Wheaton College, 1976.

Janet, Richard J. "The Decline of General Fasts in Victorian England, 1832-1857." Ph.D. diss., University of Notre Dame, 1984.

Jayne, Francis John, ed. Anglican Pronouncements Upon Auricular Confession, Fasting Communion. London: Simpkin, Marshall and Co., 1907[?].

Jenks, Alan W. "Eating and Drinking in the Old Testament." In ABD, 2: 250-54. New York: Doubleday, 1992.

Jeremias, Joachim. The Parables of Jesus. Rev.ed. Trans. S. H. Hooke New York: Scribner's, 1963.

Jewett, Robert. Paul's Anthropological Terms: A Study of Their Use in Conflict Settings. Arbeiten zur Geschichte des antiken Judentums und des Urchristentums 10, ed. Otto Michel and Martin Hengel. Leiden: Brill, 1971.

Johnson, Charles W., Jr. "The Mysteries of Fasting." Spiritual Frontiers 5, no. 1 (1973): 44-51.

_____. Fasting, Longevity, and Immortality. Turkey Hills, Pa.: Survival Publishing, 1978.

Johnson, William Lee. "Motivations for Fasting in Early Christianity." Th. M. thesis, Southern Baptist Theological Seminary, 1978.

Johnson, Luke Timothy. The Acts of the Apostles. Sacra Pagina 5, ed. Daniel J. Harrington. Collegeville, Minn.: Liturgical, 1992.

Jones, Rhidian. The Canon Law of the Roman Catholic Church and the Church of England: A Handbook. Edinburgh: T&T Clark, 2000.

Josephus. Josephus, trans. Ralph Marcus H. St. J. Thackeray, Allen Wikgren and L. H. Feldman. 10 vols. LCL, ed. G. P. Goold. Cambridge, Mass.: Harvard University, 1986.

Justin Martyr. Writings of Saint Justin Martyr, trans. Thomas B. Falls. FC 6. New York: Christian Heritage, 1948.

_____. The First and Second Apologies, trans. Leslie William Barnard. ACW 56. New York: Paulist, 1997.

Kaiser, Walter C. Exodus. The Expositor's Bible Commentary, ed. Frank E. Gaebelein, vol. 2. Grand Rapids: Zondervan, 1990.

Keener, Craig S. A Commentary on the Gospel of Matthew. Grand Rapids: Eerdmans, 1999.

Kennedy, Robert P. "Fasting." Augustine through the Ages: An Encyclopedia, ed. Allan D. Fitzgerald. Grand Rapids: Eerdmans, 1999.

Kent, Homer A., Jr. Philippians. The Expositor's Bible Commentary, vol. 11. Grand Rapids: Zondervan, 1978.

Knox, John. The Works of John Knox, ed. David Laing. New York: Ames, 1966.

Koehler, Ludwig, and Walter Baumgartner. "צום." The Hebrew and Aramaic Lexicon of the Old Testament, ed. Rev. Baumgartner and Johann Jakob Stamm, trans. M. E. J. Richardson. 3: 1012. Leiden: Brill, 1996.

Koet, Bart J. "Holy Place and Hannah's Prayer: A Comparison of LAB 50-51 and Luke 2:22-39 À Propos 1 Samuel 1-2." Sanctity of Time and Space in Tradition and Modernity, ed. A. Houtman, M. J. H. M. Poorthuis and J. Schwarz. Jewish and Christian Perspectives Series 1. Leiden: Brill, 1998.

Lake, Kirsopp, ed. and trans. The Apostolic Fathers with an English Translation. 2 vols. LCL. Cambridge.: Harvard University, 1959.

Largement, R. "L'Ascétisme dans la Civilisation Suméro-Sémitique." ASSR 9 (1964): 27-34.

Lawless, George. Augustine of Hippo and his Monastic Rule. Oxford: Clarendon, 1987.

Leo the Great. The Letters and Sermons of Leo the Great, trans. Charles Lett Feltoe. Vol. 12 NPNF² 12, ed. Philip Schaff and Henry Wace. New York: Christian Literature Co., 1895.

_____. St. Leo the Great: Sermons, trans. Jane Patricia Freeland and Agnes Josephine Conway. FC 93, ed. Thomas P. Halton. Washington: Catholic University of America, 1996.

Leonard, F. "Shared Fasting." Clergy Review 57 (1972): 210-13.

Lewis, J. P. "Fast, Fasting." The Zondervan Pictorial Encyclopedia of the Bible, ed. Merrill C. Tenney 2: 501-4. Grand Rapids: Zondervan, 1976.

Leyser, Conrad. Authority and Asceticism from Augustine to Gregory the Great. Oxford Historical Monographs. Oxford: Clarendon, 2000.

Liddell, H. G., R. Scott, and H. S. Jones. A Greek-English Lexicon. 9th ed. Oxford: Clarendon, 1996.

Lindsay, Gordon. Prayer and Fasting: The Master Key to the Impossible. Dallas: Christ for the Nations, 1977.

Loisy, Alfred. Les Actes des Apotres. Paris: Nourry, 1920.

Louw, Johannes P., and Eugene A. Nida. Greek-English Lexicon of the New Testament based on Semantic Domains. New York: United Bible Societies, 1989.

Lowy, S. "The Motivation of Fasting in Talmudic Literature." JJS 9 (1958): 19-38.

Lunde, Martin J. "Understanding the Preeminence of Fasting in Tertullian's Practical Theology." M.A. thesis, Gordon-Conwell Theological Seminary, 2000.

Luther, Martin. Luther's Works, ed. Jaroslav Pelikan, et. al. Philadelphia: Fortress, 1958-74.

Macho, Alejandro Díez, ed. Neophyti 1: Targum Palestinense Ms de la Biblioteca Vaticana, vol. 3, trans. Martin McNamara and Michael Maher. Madrid: Consejo Superior de Investigacioned Científias, 1971.

Main, Keith. Prayer and Fasting: A Study in the Devotional Life of the Early Church. New York: Carlton, 1971.

Maloney, George A. A Return to Fasting. Pecos, N. Mex.: Dove Publications, 1974.

Malter, Henry, ed. and trans. The Treatise Ta'anith of the Babylonian Talmud. Philadelphia: Jewish Publication Society of America, 1978.

Mancantelli, John. "Fasting: A Christian View Based on The New Testament and Old Testament Jewish Antecedents." M. Div. thesis, St. Vladimir's Orthodox Theological Seminary, 1974. Micropublished, Portland, Ore.: TREN, 1990.

Mann, C. S. Mark. AB 27. Garden City, N.Y.: Doubleday, 1986.

Marjanen, Antti. "Thomas and Jewish Religious Practices." In Thomas at the Crossroads: Essays on the Gospel of Thomas, ed. Risto Uro. Edinburgh: T & T Clark, 1998.

Marsh, Clive. "Theological History? N. T. Wright's Jesus and the Victory of God." JSNT 69 (1998): 77-94.

Marshall, I. Howard. The Gospel of Luke: A Commentary on the Greek Text. Grand Rapids: Eerdmans, 1978.

_____. "Jesus—Example and Teacher of Prayer in the Synoptic Gospels." Into God's Presence: Prayer in the New Testament, ed. Richard N. Longenecker. McMaster New Testament Studies. Grand Rapids: Eerdmans, 2001.

Marti, Heinrich, ed. and trans. Rufin von Aquileia, De ieiunio I, II: zwei Predigten über das Fasten nach Basileios von Kaisareia. Sup. to VC 6. Leiden: Brill, 1989.

Martin, Ralph P. 2 Corinthians. WBC. Waco, Tex.: Word, 1986.

Mary, Agatha. The Rule of Saint Augustine: An Essay in Understanding. Villanova, Pa.: Augustinian, 1991.

Mason, Rex. "Some Echoes of the Preaching in the Second Temple?: Tradition Elements in Zechariah 1-8." ZAW 96 (1984): 221-35.

Mastrantonis, George. Fasting. [article online] Greek Orthodox Website www.goarch.org, accessed June 28 2002. Available from www.st-anthony.org/fasting.htm; Internet.

Mathewes-Green, Frederica. "To Hell on a Cream Puff." Christianity Today 39 (1995): 44-48.

Mathews, Susan. "The Biblical Evidence on Fasting." Diakonia 24 (1991): 93-108.

Maximus the Confessor. St. Maximus the Confessor: The Ascetic Life, and The Four Centuries on Charity, trans. Polycarp Sherwood. ACW 21. London: Longmans, Green and Co., 1955.

McAfee, James W. "The Practice of Fasting." Th. M. thesis, Dallas Theological Seminary, 1973.

McGowan, Andrew. Ascetic Eucharists: Food and Drink in Early Christian Ritual Meals. Oxford Early Christian Studies. Oxford: Clarendon, 1999.

M'Clintock, John, and James Strong, eds. "Fasting in the Christian Church." Cyclopaedia of Biblical, Theological, and Ecclesiastical Literature. Vol. III: 490-94. New York: Harper, 1891.

Meredith, A. "Asceticism—Christian and Greek." JTS 27 (1976): 313-32.

Merrill, Eugene H. Haggai, Zechariah, Malachi: An Exegetical Commentary. Chicago: Moody, 1994.

_____. Deuteronomy. NAC 4. Nashville: Broadman and Holman, 1994.

Metzger, Bruce M. A Textual Commentary on the Greek New Testament, Second Edition: A Companion Volume to the United Bible Societies' Greek New Testament (Fourth Revised Edition). New York: American Bible Society, 1994.

_____. The Text of the New Testament: Its Transmission, Corruption, and Restoration. Second ed. New York: Oxford University Press, 1968.

Meyers, Carol L., and Eric M. Meyers. Haggai, Zechariah 1-8: A New Translation with Introduction and Commentary. The Anchor Bible. Garden City, N.Y.: Doubleday, 1987.

Miles, Margaret R. Fullness of Life: Historical Foundations for a New Asceticism. Philadelphia: Westminster, 1981.

Miller, James. Systematic Fasting. Apollo, Pa.: West Publishing, 1951.

Mitchell, Curtis C. "The Practice of Fasting in the New Testament." BSac 147, no. 588 (Oct.-Dec., 1990): 455-69.

Mohrmann, Christine. "Statio." VC 7 (1953): 221-45.

Moiser, Jeremy. "The Meaning of koilia in Philippians 3:19." ExpTim 108 (1997): 365-66.

Moore, Art. "Does 'The Gift of Salvation' Sell Out the Reformation?" Christianity Today 42 (April 27, 1998): 17, 21.

Moore, Frederick Gordon. "The New Testament Concept, Practice, and Significance of Fasting: Its Historical Background and Present Implications." B. D. thesis, Western Conservative Baptist Theological Seminary, 1955.

Moulin, Léo. "Monks Fasted but Were Plump." In On Fasting and Feasting: A Personal Collection of Favourite Writings on Food and Eating, ed. Alan Davidson. London: Macdonald Orbis, 1988.

Muddiman, J. B. "Jesus and Fasting." In Jésus aux origines de la christologie, ed. J. Dupont, 2d ed. BETL 40. Louvain: Louvain University, 1989.

_____. "Fast, Fasting." In ABD, 2: 773-776. New York: Doubleday, 1992.

Musurillo, Herbert. "The Problem of Ascetical Fasting in the Greek Patristic Writers." Traditio 12 (1956): 1-64.

Nagosky, Basil. "The Purpose and Meaning of the Fast in the Orthodox Church." [M.A. thesis?], Saint Vladimir's Seminary, 1959.

Nairn, Stanley D. "Identification and Purposes of Fasting." M. Div. thesis, Grace Theological Seminary, 1976.

National Conference of Catholic Bishops. On Penance and Abstinence: Pastoral Statement of the National Conference of Catholic Bishops. 1966.

Neuhaus, Richard John, ed. "The Gift of Salvation." First Things, no. 79 (Jan. 1998): 20-23.

Neusner, Jacob. The Idea of Purity in Ancient Judaism. SJLA 1. Leiden: Brill, 1973.

_____. ed. The Two Talmuds Compared. Atlanta: Scholars, 1996.

Newberry, Ian. Available for God: A Study of the Biblical Teaching and the Practice of Fasting. Trans. Peter Coleman. Carlisle: OM/Paternoster, 1996.

Newman, Carey C., ed. Jesus and the Restoration of Israel: A Critical Assessment of N. T. Wright's Jesus and the Victory of God. Downers Grove, Ill.: InterVarsity, 1999.

Niederwimmer, Kurt. The Didache: A Commentary, trans. Linda M. Maloney. Hermeneia. Minneapolis: Fortress, 1998.

Nikodimos of the Holy Mountain, St., and St. Makarios of Corinth, compilers. The Philokalia, trans. and ed. G. E. H. Palmer, Philip Sherrard, and Kallistos Ware, 3 vols. London: Faber and Faber, 1979.

O'Brien, Peter. The Epistle to the Philippians: A Commentary on the Greek Text. NIGCT. Grand Rapids: Eerdmans, 1991.

O'Collins, Gerald, and Daniel Kendall. The Bible for Theology: Ten Principles for the Theological Use of Scripture. New York: Paulist, 1997.

O'Hara, J. "Christian Fasting (Mt 6:16-18)." Scripture 19 (1967): 3-18.

_____. "Christian Fasting (Mk 2:18-22)." Scripture 19 (1967): 82-95.

O'Leary, De Lacy. The Apostolical Constitutions and Cognate Documents, with Special Reference to Their Liturgical Elements. Early Church Classics. London: Society for Promoting Christian Knowledge, 1906.

O'Loughlin, Thomas. "Fasting: Western Christian." Encycopedia of Monasticism, ed., William M. Johnston. Chicago: Fitzroy Dearborn, 2000.

Okholm, Dennis L. "Being Stuffed and Being Filled." In Limning the Psyche: Explorations in Christian Psychology, ed. Robert C. Roberts and Mark R. Talbot. Grand Rapids: Eerdmans, 1997.

Osiek, Carolyn. Shepherd of Hermas: A Commentary. Hermeneia. Minneapolis: Fortress, 1999.

Paul VI. "Paentemini (Apostolic Constitution)." AAS 58 (1956): 177-98.

Paul VI and John Paul II. Fasting and Solidarity: Pontifical Messages for Lent. Vatican City: Pontifical Council Cor Unum, 1991.

Paul, Shalom M. "Gleanings from the Biblical and Talmudic Lexica in Light of Akkadian." Minhah le-Nahum: Biblical and Other Studies Presented to Nahum M. Sarna in Honour of his 70th Birthday, ed. Marc Brettler and Michael Fishbane. JSOTSup 154. Sheffield: JSOT, 1993.

Peterson, Michael D.. "Fasting: Eastern Christian." Encyclopedia of Monasticism, ed. William M. Johnston. Chicago: Fitzroy Dearborn, 2000.

Philo. Philo, trans. F. H. Colson. 10 vols. LCL. New York: Putnam, 1930.

_____. The Works of Philo: Complete and Unabridged, trans. C. D. Yonge. New Updated ed. Peabody, Mass.: Hendrickson, 1993.

Piper, John. A Hunger for God: Desiring God Through Prayer and Fasting. Wheaton, Ill.: Crossway, 1997.

Pokorny, P. "The Temptation Stories and Their Intention." NTS 20 (1974): 115-27.

Pole, Reginald. A Treatie of Iustification. Lovanii: Ioannem Foulerum, 1569. Reprint, Farnborough: Gregg, 1967.

Powell, Samuel M, and Michael E. Lodahl, ed. Embodied Holiness: Toward a Corporate Theology of Spiritual Growth. Downers Grove, Ill.: InterVarsity, 1999.

Prince, Derek. Shaping History through Prayer and Fasting. Old Tappan, N. J.: Revell, 1973.

_____. How to Fast Successfully. Ft. Lauderdale, Fla.: CGM Publishing, 1976.

Prokes, Mary Timothy. Toward a Theology of the Body. Grand Rapids: Eerdmans, 1996.

Puhalo, Lazar. "The Spiritual and Scriptural Meaning of the Fasts." In On Fasting: The Spiritual and Scriptural Meaning of the Orthodox Christian Fasts. Dewdney, B. C.: Synaxis, 1997.

Quinley, Charles W. "Not By Bread Alone: A Study in the Christian Discipline of Fasting." D.Min. diss., Asbury Theological Seminary, 1989.

Rabbinowitz, J., ed. and trans. Ta'anith. In I. Epstein, ed., The Babylonian Talmud: Seder Mo'ed, vol. 4. London: Soncino, 1938.

Ranwez, C. "Le jeûne. Abandon ou réhabilitation?" La vie spirituelle 118 (1968): 271-91.

Régamey, P. R. Redécouverte du jeûne. Paris: Les Éditions du Cerf, 1959.

_____. ed. Wiederentdeckung des Fastens, trans. F. Kollmann et al. Wien: Herold, 1963.

Ricoeur, Paul. Time and Narrative, trans. Kathleen McLaughlin and David Pellauer. Chicago: University of Chicago, 1984.

Ridderbos, Herman. Paul: An Outline of His Theology, trans. John Richard De Witt. Grand Rapids: Eerdmans, 1975.

Roberts, Alexander, and James Donaldson, eds. Ante-Nicene Christian Library 17. Edinburgh: T. & T. Clark, 1870.

_____. The Ante-Nicene Fathers. Grand Rapids: Eerdmans, 1962.

Roberts, Richard Owen, ed. Sanctify the Congregation: A Call to the Solemn Assembly and to Corporate Repentance. Wheaton, Ill.: International Awakening, 1994.

Robinson, John A. T. The Body: A Study in Pauline Theology. Bristol, Ind.: Wyndham Hall, 1988.

Rogers, Eric N. [Pseudonym]. Fasting: The Phenomenon of Self-Denial. Nashville: Thomas Nelson, 1976.

Rordorf, Willy. "Baptism According to the Didache." The Didache in Modern Research, ed. Jonathan A. Draper. Leiden: Brill, 1996.

Rothenberg, F. S. "Fast." New Testament Theology, ed. Colin Brown. Vol. 1: 611-13. Grand Rapids: Zondervan, 1975.

Ru, G. De. "The Conception of Reward in the Teaching of Jesus." NovT 8 (1966): 202-22.

Rubenson, Samuel. "Antony, St." In Encyclopedia of Monasticism, ed. William M. Johnston. Chicago: Fitzroy Dearborn, 2000.

_____. "Asceticism: Christian Perspectives." Encycopedia of Monasticism, ed. William M. Johnston. Chicago: Fitzroy Dearborn, 2000.

Ruddy, James. The Apostolic Constitution Christus Dominus: Text, Translation and Commentary, with Short Annotations on the Motu Proprio Sacram Communionem The Catholic University of America

Canon Law Studies 390. Washington: Catholic University of America, 1957.

Rufe, Joan Brueggeman. "Early Christian Fasting: A Study of Creative Adaptation." Ph.D. diss., University of Virginia, 1994.

Ryan, Thomas. Fasting Rediscovered: A Guide to Health and Wholeness for Your Body-Spirit. New York: Paulist, 1981.

Sarna, Nahum M. Genesis. The JPS Torah Commentary. Philadelphia: Jewish Publication Society, 1989.

_____. Exodus. The JPS Torah Commentary. Philadelphia: Jewish Publication Society, 1991.

Schaff, Philip and Henry Wace, trans. and eds. Nicene and Post-Nicene Fathers of the Christian Church, 2nd Series. New York: Scribner's, 1900.

Schäfer, K. Th. "... Und dann werden sie fasten." Synoptische Studien: Festschrift für A. Wikenhauser, ed. J. Schmid and A. Vögtle. München: Karl Zink Verlag, 1953, pp. 124-47.

Scherman, Nosson and Meir Zlotowitz, eds. The Mishnah. Artscroll Mishnah Series. Brooklyn: Mesorah, 1969.

Schmidt-Clausing, F. "Fasten." RGG. Vol. 2: 881-85.

Schnackenburg, Rudolf. The Gospel According to St John, trans. Kevin Smyth. New York: Crossroad, 1982.

Schneemelcher, Wilhelm, ed. New Testament Apocrypha. Louisville: Wetminster/John Knox, 1992.

Schochet, Elijah Judah. Animal Life in Jewish Traditions: Attitudes and Relationships. New York: Ktav, 1984.

Schümmer, J. "Die altchristliche Fastenpraxis: mit besonderer Berücksichtigung der Schriften Tertullians." LQF 27: 164-78.

Schwartz, Oded. In Search of Plenty: A History of Jewish Food. London: Kyle Cathie, 1992.

Scotti, Paschal. "The Times of Fasting in the Early Church." Licentiate in Canon Law thesis, Catholic University of America, 1995.

Seifrid, Mark A. "The Gift of Salvation: Its Failure to Address the Crux of Justification." Paper presented at the 50th annual conference of the Evangelical Theological Society, Orland, Fla., 1998.

Shannon, Peter. "The Code of Canon Law: 1918-1967." Canon Law Postconciliar Thoughts: Renewal and Reform of Canon Law. Concilium 28. New York: Paulist, 1967.

Shaw, Teresa M. The Burden of the Flesh: Fasting and Sexuality in Early Christianity. Minneapolis, Minn.: Fortress, 1998.

Siebrunner, Barbara. Die Problematik der Kirchlichen Fasten- und Abstinenzgesetzgebung: Eine Untersuchung zu dem im Zuge des Zweiten Vatikanischen Konzils erfolgten Wandel European University Studies Series 23, Theology 736. Frankfurt am Main: Peter Lang, 2001.

Silva, Moisés. Philippians. The Wycliffe Exegetical Commentary. Chicago: Moody, 1988.

Smith, David R. Fasting: A Neglected Discipline. Fort Washington, Pa.: Christian Literature Crusade, 1954.

Sorokin, Pitirim. The Crisis of Our Age. Oxford: Oneworld, 1992.

Staley, Vernon. The Liturgical Year: An Explanation of the Origin, History and Significance of the Festival Days and Fasting Days of the English Church. London: A. R. Mowbray, 1907.

Stein, Robert H. "N. T. Wright's Jesus and the Victory of God: A Review Article." JETS 44 (2001): 207-18.

Steinsaltz, Adin, ed. The Talmud: The Steinsaltz Edition. New York: Random House, 1995.

Stewart, Columba. Cassian the Monk. Oxford Studies in Historical Theology. Oxford: Oxford University, 1998.

Stolz, F. "צום." In TLOT 2: 1066. Peabody, Mass.: Hendrickson, 1997.

Sullivan, Jordan Joseph. Fast and Abstinence in the First Order of Saint Francis: A Historical Synopsis and a Commentary. The Catholic University of America Canon Law Studies 374. Washington: The Catholic University of America, 1957.

Syrien, Ephrem le. Hymnes sur le jeûne, trans. Dominique Cerbelaud. Spiritualité 69. Maine-&-Loire: abbaye de Bellefontaine, 1997.

Tertullian. Apologetic and Practical Treatises, trans. C. Dodgson. A Library of Fathers of the Holy Catholic Church 1. Oxford: John Henry Parker, 1842.

_____. On Fasting. In ANF, ed. Alexander Roberts and James Donaldson, 4. Grand Rapids: Eerdmans, 1956.

_____. Disciplinary, Moral and Ascetical Works. FC 40. New York: Fathers of the Church, 1959.

Tigay, Jeffrey H. Deuteronomy. The JPS Torah Commentary (Philadelphia: Jewish Publication Society, 1996.

Towns, Elmer L. Fasting for Spiritual Breakthrough: A Guide to Nine Biblical Fasts. Ventura, Calif.: Regal, 1996.

Townsend, John T., trans. Midrash Tanhuma (S. Buber Recension): Translated into English with Introduction, Indices and Brief Notes. Hoboken, N. J.: KTAV, 1989.

Tyrrell, Bernard J. Christotherapy II: The Fasting and Feasting Heart. New York: Paulist, 1982.

Vall, Gregory. "Psalm 22 and the Vox Christi: A Hermeneutical Test Case." Paper presented at the Southwest Commision on Religious Studies Regional Meeting, Irving, Texas, 2000.

VanGemeren, Willem. The Progress of Redemption: The Story of Salvation from Creation to the New Jerusalem. Grand Rapids: Baker, 1988.

von Rad, Gerhard. Genesis: A Commentary. Rev. ed., trans. John H. Marks. Philadelphia: Westminster, 1972.

Vos, Geerhardus. Biblical Theology: Old and New Testaments. Grand Rapids: Eerdmans, 1948. Reprint, 1975.

Vööbus, Arthur. History of Asceticism in the Syrian Orient. CSCO 14. Louvain: CSCO, 1958.

Wallace, Daniel B. Greek Grammar Beyond the Basics: An Exegetical Syntax of the New Testament. Grand Rapids: Zondervan, 1996.

Wallis, Arthur. God's Chosen Fast. Fort Washington, Pa.: Christian Literature Crusade, 1968.

Ware, Kallistos (Timothy). The Orthodox Church. New ed. New York: Penguin, 1997.

Way, Robert J. "צום." NIDOTTE 3: 780-83. Grand Rapids: Zondervan, 1997.

Wennink, H. A. The Bible on Asceticism. Du Pere: St. Norbert Abbey, 1966.

Wesley, John. The Journal of the Rev. John Wesley, A.M. Standard ed., ed. Nehemiah Curnock. New York: Eaton & Mains, 1909.

_____. The Works of Wesley: Wesley's Standard Sermons. Vol. 1. 4th annotated ed., ed. Edward H. Sugden. Grand Rapids: Francis Asbury, 1955.

_____. The Works of John Wesley, Vol. 11: The Appeals to Men of Reason and Religion and Certain Related Open Letters, ed. Gerald R. Cragg. Oxford: Clarendon, 1975.

_____. The Works of John Wesley: Sermons. Vol. 4. Bicentennial ed., ed. Albert C. Outler. Nashville: Abingdon, 1987.

Wessel, Walter W. Mark. The Expositor's Bible Commentary, vol. 8. Grand Rapids: Zondervan, 1984.

Whitchurch, Irl Goldwin. The Philosophical Bases of Asceticism in the Platonic Writings and in Pre-Platonic Tradition. New York: Longmans, Green & Co., 1923.

Wickwire, Daniel Edward. "The Role of Prayer and Fasting in Binding and Loosing with Special Reference to the Problem of Reaching the Unreached People of the World Today." M.A. thesis, The Columbia Graduate School of Bible and Missions, Columbia, S.C., 1983.

Wilcox, Max. "Luke 2, 36-38: 'Anna Bat Phanuel, of the Tribe of Asher, a prophetess ...': A Study in Midrash in Material Special to Luke." In The Four Gospels 1992: Festschrift, Frans Neirynck, ed. F. Van Segbroeck, C. M. Tuckett, G. Van Belle and J. Verheyden, Leuven: Leuven University Press, 1992.

Willard, Dallas. The Spirit of the Disciplines: Understanding How God Changes Lives. San Francisco: Harper & Row, 1988.

_____. "Christ-Centered Piety." In Where Shall My Wond'ring Soul Begin? The Landscape of Evangelical Piety and Thought, ed. Mark A. Noll and Ronald F. Thiemann, 27-36. Grand Rapids: Eerdmans, 2000.

Williams, D. H. Retrieving the Tradition and Renewing Evangelicalism: A Primer for Suspicious Protestants. Grand Rapids: Eerdmans, 1999.

Wimbush, Vincent L., ed. Ascetic Behavior in Greco-Roman Antiquity: A Sourcebook. Studies in Antiquity and Christianity. Minneapolis: Fortress, 1990.

Wimmer, Joseph F. Fasting in the New Testament: A Study in Biblical Theology Theological Inquiries: Studies in Contemporary Biblical and Theological Problems, ed. Lawrence Boadt. New York: Paulist, 1982.

Winter, Naphtali, ed. Fasting and Fast Days, ed. Raphael Posner, Popular Judaica Library. Jerusalem: Keter, 1975.

Winter, Donald Vinson. "Fasting: A Biblical and Practical Approach." M.A. thesis, Columbia Bible College Graduate School of Bible and Missions, 1976.

Witherington, Ben, III. The Acts of the Apostles: A Socio-Rhetorical Commentary. Grand Rapids: Eerdmans, 1998.

Wright, N. T. The New Testament and the People of God. In Christian Origins and the Question of God, Vol. 1. Minneapolis: Fortress, 1992.

_____. Jesus and the Victory of God. In Christian Origins and the Question of God, Vol. 2. Minneapolis: Fortress, 1996.

Zalba, Marcellino. "Fasting." Sacramentum Mundi: An Encyclopedia of Theology, ed. Karl Rahner, 2: 334-35. New York: Herder and Herder, [n.d.].

Zijpp, N. van der. "Fasting." In The Mennonite Encyclopedia, ed. Harold S. Bender and C. Henry Smith, 2: 317. Scottdale, Pa.: Mennonite, 1956.

Zumkeller, Adolar. Augustine's Rule: A Commentary, trans. Matthew J. O'Connell, ed. John E. Rotelle. Villanova, Pa.: Augustinian, 1987.

Zwingli, Ulrich. The Latin Works and the Correspondencee of Huldreich Zwingli, Together with Selections from His German Works, trans. Walter Lichtenstein, Henry Preble, and Lawrence A. McLouth. Vol. 1, ed. Samuel Macauley Jackson. New York: G. P. Putnam's Sons/Knickerbocker, 1912.

_____. Commentary on True and False Religion, ed. Samuel Macauley Jackson and Clarence Nevin Heller. Durham, N. C.: Labyrinth, 1981.

_____. Huldrych Zwingli Writings, trans. E. J. Furcha. Vol. 1. 500th Anniversary Volume ed. Allison Park, Pa.: Pickwick, 1984.

Abstract

Abbreviations and technical terms used in this work are intended to conform to standards in *The SBL Handbook of Style for Ancient Near Eastern, Biblical, and Early Christian Studies*, Hendrickson Publishers, 1999.

Endnotes

Introduction: Contribution and Methodology

[1] For recent Roman Catholic works related to fasting, see Adalbert de Vogüé, *To Love Fasting: The Monastic Experience*, trans. Jean Baptist Hasbrouck (Petersham, Mass.: Saint Bede's, 1989). George A. Maloney, *A Return to Fasting* (Pecos, N.Mex.: Dove Publications, 1974); Thomas Ryan, *Fasting Rediscovered: A Guide to Health and Wholeness for Your Body-Spirit* (New York: Paulist, 1981); Slavko Barbaric, *Fasting* (Steubenville, Ohio: Franciscan University Press, 1988). P. R. Régamey, *Redécouverte du jeûne* (Paris: Les Éditions du Cerf, 1959), 386-436. Alexandre Guillaume, *Prière, jeûne et charité: des perspectives chrétiennes et une espérance pour notre temps* (Paris: S. O. S., 1985); Marcellino Zalba, "Fasting," *Sacramentum Mundi: An Encyclopedia of Theology*, ed. Karl Rahner (New York: Herder and Herder, 1968), 2: 334-35; P. M. J. Clancy, "Fast and Abstinence," *New Catholic Encyclopedia* (New York: McGraw-Hill, 1967), vol. 5: 847-50. Barbara Siebrunner, *Die Problematik der kirchlichen Fasten- und Abstinenzgesetzgebung: eine Untersuchung zu dem im Zuge des zweiten Vatikanischen Konzils erfolgten Wandel*, European University Studies Series 23, Theology 736 (Frankfurt am Main: Peter Lang, 2001); Canon Law Society of America, *Code of Canon Law: Latin-English Edition* (Washington: Canon Law Society of America, 1983), 446-47. Paul VI, "Paentemini (Apostolic Constitution)," *AAS* 58 (1956); National Conference of Catholic Bishops, *On Penance and Abstinence: Pastoral Statement of the National Conference of Catholic Bishops* (1966); Thomas Francis Anglin, *The Eucharistic Fast: An Historical Synopsis and Commentary*, The Catholic University of America Canon Law Studies 124 (Washington: Catholic University of America, 1941); James Ruddy, *The Apostolic Constitution Christus Dominus: Text, Translation and Commentary, with Short Annotations on the Motu Proprio Sacram Communionem*, The Catholic University of America Canon Law Studies 390 (Washington: Catholic University of America, 1957); Joseph C. Dieckhaus, "The Eucharistic Fast and Frequent Communion in the West: A Canonical and Liturgical Perspective" (Licentiate in Canon Law Dissertation, Catholic University of America, 1991); Paul VI and John Paul II, *Fasting and Solidarity: Pontifical Messages for Lent* (Vatican City: Pontifical Council Cor Unum, 1991).

[2] The most influential evangelical works on the spiritual disciplines are Richard J. Foster, *Celebration of Discipline: The Path to Spiritual Growth* (San Francisco:

HarperSanFrancisco, 1988), and Dallas Willard, *The Spirit of the Disciplines: Understanding How God Changes Lives* (San Francisco: Harper & Row, 1988). Popular works promoting fasting include Angus Dun, *Not By Bread Alone* (New York: Harper, 1942); James Miller, *Systematic Fasting* (Apollo, Pa.: West, 1951); David R. Smith, *Fasting: A Neglected Discipline* (Fort Washington, Pa.: Christian Literature Crusade, 1954); Arthur Wallis, *God's Chosen Fast: A Spiritual and Practical Guide to Fasting* (Fort Washington, Pa.: Christian Literature Crusade, 1968); Derek Prince, *Shaping History through Prayer and Fasting* (Old Tappan, N. J.: Revell, 1973); *How to Fast Successfully* (Ft. Lauderdale, Fla.: CGM Publishing, 1976); Charles W. Johnson, Jr. "The Mysteries of Fasting," *Spiritual Frontiers* 5, no. 1 (1973): 44-51; *Fasting, Longevity, and Immortality* (Turkey Hills, Pa.: Survival Publishing, 1978); Eric N. Rogers [Pseudonym], *Fasting: The Phenomenon of Self-Denial* (Nashville: Thomas Nelson, 1976); Andy Anderson, *Fasting Changed My Life* (Nashville: Broadman, 1977); Jerry Charles, *God's Guide to Fasting: A Complete and Exhaustive Biblical Encyclopedia* (Madison, N.C.: Power Press, 1977); Gordon Lindsay, *Prayer and Fasting: The Master Key to the Impossible* (Dallas: Christ for the Nations, 1977); Jerry Falwell, *Fasting: What the Bible Teaches* (Wheaton, Ill.: Tyndale, 1981); John E. Baird and Don DeWelt, *What the Bible Says About Fasting,* What the Bible Says Series (Joplin, Mo.: College Press, 1984); Bob and Michael W. Benson, *Disciplines for the Inner Life* (Waco, Tex.: Word, 1985); Wesley L. Duewel, *Mighty Prevailing Prayer* (Grand Rapids: Francis Asbury, 1990); Bill Bright, *The Coming Revival: America's Call to Fast, Pray, and 'Seek God's Face'* (Orlando: NewLife Publications, 1995); Ian Newberry, *Available for God: A Study of the Biblical Teaching and the Practice of Fasting,* trans. Peter Coleman (Carlisle: OM/Paternoster, 1996); Elmer L. Towns, *Fasting for Spiritual Breakthrough: A Guide to Nine Biblical Fasts* (Ventura, Calif.: Regal, 1996); John Piper, *A Hunger for God: Desiring God Through Fasting and Prayer* (Wheaton, Ill.: Crossway, 1997); Ronnie W. Floyd, *The Power of Prayer and Fasting: 10 Secrets of Spiritual Strength* (Nashville: Broadman & Holman, 1997).

[3] Samuel J. Fox, "An Investigation of Fasting in the Old Testament Literature" (M. A. thesis, Butler University, 1944); William Loftin Hargrave, "Fasting in the Early Church: Being a Study of Fasting Based Upon References to the Subject in the Old and New Testaments, and Upon the Writings of Some of the Ante-Nicene Fathers" (S. T. M. thesis, University of the South, 1952); David Eddle Briggs, "Biblical Teaching on Fasting" (Th. M. thesis, Dallas Theological Seminary, 1953); Wayne Barton, "Toward an Understanding of Fasting in the New Testament" (Th. D. diss., New Orleans Baptist Theological Seminary, 1954); Frederick Gordon Moore, "The New Testament Concept, Practice, and Significance of Fasting: Its Historical Background and Present Implications" (B.

D. thesis, Western Conservative Baptist Theological Seminary, 1955); Frederic R. Dinkins, "The Biblical Practice and Doctrine of Fasting" (Th. M. thesis, Columbia Theological Seminary, 1966); James W. McAfee, "The Practice of Fasting" (Th. M. thesis, Dallas Theological Seminary, 1973); Donald Vinson Winter, "Fasting: A Biblical and Practical Approach" (M. A. thesis, Columbia Bible College Graduate School of Bible and Missions, 1976); Thomas Wilson Jacob, "The Meaning and Importance of Fasting in the Teaching of Jesus" (M. A. thesis, Wheaton College, 1976); Stanley D. Nairn, "Identification and Purposes of Fasting" (M. Div. thesis, Grace Theological Seminary, 1976); William Lee Johnson, "Motivations for Fasting in Early Christianity" (Th. M. thesis, Southern Baptist Theological Seminary, 1978); Gary D. Dehnke, "Fasting: Practice and Function in the New Testament and in the Early Church" (M. Div. thesis, Concordia Theological Seminary, 1983); Daniel Edward Wickwire, "The Role of Prayer and Fasting in Binding and Loosing with Special Reference to the Problem of Reaching the Unreached People of the World Today" (Masters thesis, The Columbia Graduate School of Bible and Missions, Columbia, S. C., 1983); R. D. Chatham, *Fasting: A Biblical Historical Study* (South Plainfield, N.J.: Bridge Publishing, 1987); Charles W. Quinley, "Not By Bread Alone: A Study in the Christian Discipline of Fasting" (D. Min. diss., Asbury Theological Seminary, 1989); Thomas H. Felter, "The Relevance of the New Testament Treatment of Fasting to Modern Life" (M. A. thesis, Wheaton College, 1960); Keith Main, *Prayer and Fasting: A Study in the Devotional Life of the Early Church* (New York: Carlton, 1971); Marion Michael Fink, Jr., "The Responses in the New Testament to the Practice of Fasting" (Ph.D. diss, The Southern Baptist Theological Seminary, 1974).

[4] Joseph F. Wimmer, *Fasting in the New Testament: A Study in Biblical Theology* (New York: Paulist, 1982); Caroline Walker Bynum, *Holy Feast and Holy Fast: The Religious Significance of Food to Medieval Women* (Berkely, Calif.: University of California, 1987); Veronika E. Grimm, *From Feasting to Fasting, the Evolution of a Sin: Attitudes to Food in Late Antiquity* (London: Routledge, 1996); Teresa M. Shaw, *The Burden of the Flesh: Fasting and Sexuality in Early Christianity* (Minneapolis, Minn.: Fortress, 1998).

[5] Some of the more important that have been noted are R. Arbesmann, "Das Fasten bei den Greichen und Römern," *Religionsgeschichtliche Versuche und Vorarbeiten* 21, no. 1 (1929), H. A. Brongers, "Fasting in Israel in Biblical and Post-Biblical Times," in *Instruction and Interpretation: Studies in Hebrew Language, Palestinian Archaeology and Biblical Exegesis*, Ots (Leiden: Brill, 1977); Susan Mathews, "The Biblical Evidence on Fasting," *Diakonia* 24 (1991); J. B. Muddiman, "Jesus and Fasting," in *Jésus aux origines de la christologie*, ed. J. Dupont (Leuven (Belgium): Leuven University Press, 1989); Herbert Musurillo, "The Problem of Ascetical Fasting in the Greek Patristic Writers," *Traditio* 12

(1956); J. Schümmer, "Die altchristliche Fastenpraxis: mit besonderer Berücksichtigung der Schriften Tertullians," *LQF* 27.

[6] H. Achelis, "Fasting," in *The New Schaff-Herzog Encyclopedia of Religious Knowledge*, ed. Samuel Macauley Jackson (Grand Rapids: Baker, 1950); Johannes Behm, "Νηστί, Νηστεύω, Νηστεία," *TDNT* (Grand Rapids: Eerdmans, 1967); P. M. J. Clancy, "Fast and Abstinence," in *New Catholic Encyclopedia* (New York: McGraw-Hill, 1967); "Fasting in the Christian Church," in *Cyclopaedia of Biblical, Theological, and Ecclesiastical Literature*, ed. John M'Clintock and James Strong (New York: Harper, 1891); Johann Gamberoni, "Fasting," in *Encyclopedia of Biblical Theology*, ed. Johannes B. Bauer (New York: Crossroad, 1981); Julius H. Greenstone, "Fasting and Fast-Days," in *The Jewish Encyclopedia*, ed. Isidore Singer (New York: Ktav, 1964); Stuart George Hall and Joseph H. Crehan, "Fasten/Fasttage," *TRE* 11, R. Hindringer, "Fasten," *LTK* 2; Robert P. Kennedy, "Fasting," in *Augustine through the Ages: An Encyclopedia*, ed. Allan D. Fitzgerald (Grand Rapids: Eerdmans, 1999); Ludwig Koehler and Walter Baumgartner, "צוֹם," in *The Hebrew and Aramaic Lexicon of the Old Testament*, ed. Rev. Baumgartner and Johann Jakob Stamm (Leiden: Brill, 1996); J. P. Lewis, "Fast, Fasting," in *The Zondervan Pictorial Encyclopedia of the Bible*, ed. Merrill C. Tenney (Grand Rapids: Zondervan, 1976); J. B. Muddiman, "Fast, Fasting," in *The Anchor Bible Dictionary*, ed. David Noel Freedman (New York: Doubleday, 1992); Thomas O'Loughlin, "Fasting: Western Christian," in *Encyclopedia of Monasticism*, ed. William M. Johnston (Chicago: Fitzroy Dearborn, 2000); Michael D. Peterson, "Fasting: Eastern Christian," in *Encyclopedia of Monasticism*, ed. William M. Johnston (Chicago: Fitzroy Dearborn, 2000); F. S. Rothenberg, "Fast," in *New Testament Theology*, ed. Colin Brown (Grand Rapids: Zondervan, 1975); F. Schmidt-Clausing, "Fasten," *RGG* 2, F. Stolz, "צוֹם," in *Theological Lexicon of the Old Testament*, ed. Ernst Jenni and Claus Westermann (Peabody, Mass.: Hendrickson, 1997); Robert J. Way "צוֹם," in *New International Dictionary of Old Testament Theology & Exegesis*, ed. Willem VanGemeren (Grand Rapids: Zondervan, 1997); Naphtali Winter, ed., *Fasting and Fast Days*, ed. Raphael Posner, Popular Judaica Library (Jerusalem: Keter, 1975); Marcellino Zalba, "Fasting," in *Sacramentum Mundi: An Encyclopedia of Theology*, ed. Karl Rahner (New York: Herder and Herder); N. van der Zijpp, "Fasting," in *The Mennonite Encyclopedia*, ed. Harold S. Bender and C. Henry Smith (Scottdale, Pa.: Mennonite, 1956).

[7] Perhaps the closest work in this regard is R. D. Chatham's *Fasting: A Biblical-Historical Study* (South Plainfield, N. J.: Bridge, 1987). But her work, while reasonably good in surveying biblical and historical references to fasting, falls short of integrating fasting into a theological framework.

[8] As used here, an integrated theology might be defined as one that examines and develops ideas first from Scripture and then from various historical and contemporary Christian communities, then contextualizes a synthetic statement of its conclusions to its particular setting (and here that is the general community of Protestant evangelicalism at the beginning of the twenty-first century). Cf. Gordon R. Lewis and Bruce A. Demarest, *Integrative Theology* (Grand Rapids: Zondervan, 1996), 25-26.

[9] These sermons are commonly known by their Latin title, *De jejunio* (occasionally *De ieiunio*), and are found in PG 31:164-97.

[10] Sermon 1 was actually published in English translation as an appendix to Reginald Pole, *A Treatie of Iustification* (Lovanii: Ioannem Foulerum, 1569; reprint, Farnborough: Gregg, 1967). Although this translation was certainly excellent for its day, its dated nature and rather obscure publication clearly does not preclude a contemporary version. No English translation of Sermon 2 has been located.

Chapter 1: In the Old Testament and Ancient Judiasm

[1] Gerald O'Collins and Daniel Kendall, *The Bible for Theology: Ten Principles for the Theological Use of Scripture* (New York: Paulist, 1997), 24. The authors go on to explain: "Obviously the principle of convergence emphasizes the unity of the canonical scriptures more than their diversity, that unity effected by the Holy Spirit over against the diversity due to the human authors and the complex differences between the OT and NT. To expect convergent biblical testimony presupposes that one takes the Bible to exhibit, in and through its diverse witnesses and the tension between their perspectives, much more unity than a mere anthology of ancient, religious writings held together by the covers of one book. Ultimately it is the divine authorship by the one Holy Spirit that forges the christological unity of the Bible in the convergence of its many witnesses."

[2] Ibid., 27-28. An important qualification follows: "This sixth principle does not aim to repeat the naive appeals to 'authoritative' biblical concepts that James Barr, Brevard Childs, and others rightly criticized years ago. It simply aims at noting the existence of patterns of divine activity and promise that recur in the Bible, yield an overall picture, evoke varying human responses, and throw light, above all, on Jesus' activity and identity. Any adequate theology will be sustained by the biblical metathemes and metanarratives."

[3] Daniel M. Doriani, *Putting the Truth to Work: The Theory and Practice of Biblical Application* (Phillipsburg, N.J.: P&R, 2001), 81-91.

[4] Doriani, 86-87.

[5] Ibid., 195-96, 207-10. Hans Frei (*Theology and Narrative: Selected Essays*, ed. George Hunsinger and William C. Placher [New York: Oxford University Press, 1993], 113-14), following Karl Barth, describes the three stages of hermeneutics of narrative: "(1) *Explicatio*, the sheer retelling of the story or other texts, together with the philological and other aids that go into that activity for the more technically trained; (2) *meditatio*, the conceptual redescription or (more generally) refraction of the text through the structures of our minds—whether we think of this as taking place by virtue of a unified phenomenon, an internal process, or through the discovery of deep structures shared by synchronically ordered texts into which the interpreter himself becomes intercalated, or other forms of what this autonomous intellectual activity might best be described to be; and finally (3) *applicatio*, or use, which is in its own way as inclusive as the second stage. It is the skill to relate the story (or other texts) to the context, the judgment that we do or do not share a world with the text and with the community in which it has functioned since its first telling. The text is meaningful by appropriation, its meaning is performatively or existentially realized."

[6] A more thorough discussion of narrative, hermeneutics, and theology would need to interact with several more philosophical and methodological questions, such as those raised and discussed in the following primary sources and the many secondary sources surrounding them: Hans W. Frei, *The Eclipse of Biblical Narrative: A Study in Eighteenth and Nineteenth Century Hermeneutics* (New Haven: Yale University, 1974); Hans-Georg Gadamer, *Truth and Method* (New York: Continuum, 1975); and Paul Ricoeur, *Time and Narrative*, trans. Kathleen McLaughlin and David Pellauer (Chicago: University of Chicago, 1984). It is beyond the scope of this dissertation to explicitly critique and/or bring these works to bear on the material presented below.

[7] H. A. Brongers, "Fasting in Israel in Biblical and Post-Biblical Times," in *Instruction and Interpretation: Studies in Hebrew Language, Palestinian Archaeology and Biblical Exegesis*, OtSt 20 (Leiden: Brill, 1977), 1.

[8] H. H. Guthrie, Jr., "Fast, Fasting," *IDB* 2: 241-42; John Muddiman, "Fast, Fasting," *The Anchor Bible Dictionary* 2: 773; Julius H. Greenstone, "Fasting and Fast-Days," *The Jewish Encyclopedia* 5: 347-49.

[9] Brongers, 2.

[10] R. Largement, "L'ascétisme dans la civilisation Suméro-Sémitique," *ASSR* 9 (1964): 22-34. Largement also draws connections between the related practices of virgins dedicated by celibacy to the gods and the psalms with superscriptions to virgins (*'alamoth*). From this he surmises a celibate virgin cult ritual in

Jerusalem, which he also speculates as forming a background for later Christian celibacy practices. He also compares Pss 89:39 and 51:3-6 to a ceremony on the fifth day of the Babylonian New Year festival, in which the king of Israel humbly confesses sin in contrast to the Babylonian king who professed perfect innocence. These highly speculative ideas cannot really be substantiated, but there is clearly the likelihood that Israelite religious asceticism and fasting (and perhaps the early Christian forms that grew from it) reflect wider cultural traditions of their day.

[11] F. Stolz, "צום," *Theological Lexicon of the Old Testament*," ed. Ernst Jenni and Claus Westermann, trans. Mark E. Biddle (Peabody, Mass.: Hendrickson, 1997), 2: 1066.

[12] See Appendix I for a complete listing of biblical passages that first appeared in Kent D. Berghuis, "A Biblical Perspective on Fasting," *BSac* 158 (2001): 97-101.

[13] Stolz, 1066.

[14] BDB, 847.

[15] Ludwig Koehler and Walter Baumgartner, *The Hebrew and Aramaic Lexicon of the Old Testament*, rev. Baumgartner and Johann Jakob Stamm, trans. M. E. J. Richardson (Leiden: Brill, 1996), 3: 1012.

[16] Robert J. Way, "צום," *New International Dictionary of Old Testament Theology & Exegesis*, ed. Willem VanGemeren (Grand Rapids: Zondervan, 1997), 3: 780.

[17] Ibid., 781.

[18] Brongers, 3.

[19] For a full list of references and sub-categories, see the Appendix, "Master Summary of Biblical Purposes for Fasting," that first appeared in Berghuis: 102-3. A sixth category that appeared there, that of fasting as an accompaniment of ministry, has been subsumed under the category here of experiencing the sustaining presence of God.

[20] Brongers, 2, comments that fasting is more properly categorized with "customs and manners" rather than with legal prescriptions.

[21] Nahum M. Sarna, *Genesis*, The JPS Torah Commentary (Philadelphia: Jewish Publication Society, 1989), 21.

[22] הָאָדָם, primarily referred to generically in the context as the "man," and probably not as the proper name "Adam."

[23] The context moves from Adam's creation in the garden (2:1-15), the prohibition (2:16-17), Eve's creation (2:18-25), the questioning of the prohibition (3:1-5).

[24] Interestingly, the man is presented as alone in the giving of the command by God, while the woman is presented as alone in the questioning of the command by the serpent. This may already be suggestive of a subverting of the exclamation of the man in Gen 2:23, emphasizing separateness that is being brought into the creation. But as in Gen 3:5, וִהְיִיתֶם and other verbs in the passage are plural, so the serpent is including the man and woman together in the speech.

[25] This assertion by the serpent suggests that Elohim knew evil experientially, which would be contrary to sound faith in later biblical theology.

[26] The reference in this verse is singular.

[27] Sarna, Genesis, 27.

[28] The reference to "offspring" is in the singular, which could function collectively, but is grammatically used here as being personified in the singular, as the pronoun הוּא (3:15) would suggest.

[29] אִישֵׁךְ, recalling the created relationship of Gen 2:23.

[30] Sarna, Genesis, 28.

[31] Thomas L. Brodie, Genesis as Dialogue: A Literary, Historical, and Theological Commentary (Oxford: Oxford University Press, 2001), 151.

[32] John Mancantelli, "Fasting: A Christian View Based on The New Testament and Old Testament Jewish Antecedents" (M. Div. thesis, St. Vladimir's Orthodox Theological Seminary, 1974; Micropublished, Portland, Oreg.: TREN, 1990), 8.

[33] The versions may be compared in Gary A. Anderson and Michael E. Stone, eds., A Synopsis of the Books of Adam and Eve, 2d. rev. ed., SBL Early Judaism and Its Literature 17 (Atlanta: Scholars Press, 1999).

[34] As in the words of comfort in Isa 6:13, 41:8, 43:5, 44:3, 45:19, 25, 48:19, 53:10, 54:3, 59:21, 61:9, 65:9, 23, and 66:22. Jeremiah also views the people collectively as the seed of Abraham, though often in more judgmental tones (cf. 36:31), yet he provides similar themes of assurance to the chosen seed in Jer 31:27, 36-37, and 33:22-26 (which additionally reasserts the Abrahamic promise of innumerable multiplied seed to the Davidic line).

[35] Victor P. Hamilton, The Book of Genesis Chapters 1-17, NICOT (Grand Rapids: Eerdmans, 1990), 190, citing J. T. Walsh, "Genesis 2:4b-3:24: A Synchronic Approach," JBL 96 (1977): 166.

[36] The LXX version of Gen 3:6b reads, καὶ λαβοῦσα τοῦ καρποῦ αὐτοῦ ἔφαγεν, καὶ ἔδωκεν καὶ τῷ ἀνδρὶ αὐτῆς μετ᾽ αὐτῆς, καὶ ἔφαγον. In the NT passages, the Greek uses the same verbs consistently.

[37] Cf. Matt 22:1-14, 25:1-13; Rev 19:7-9.

[38] Gen 2:7b reads: וַיִּפַּח בְּאַפָּיו נִשְׁמַת חַיִּים וַיְהִי הָאָדָם לְנֶפֶשׁ חַיָּה.

[39] Gerhard von Rad, *Genesis: A Commentary*, rev. ed, trans. John H. Marks (Philadelphia: Westminster, 1972), 77.

[40] Jeffrey H. Tigay, *Deuteronomy*, The JPS Torah Commentary (Philadelphia: Jewish Publication Society, 1996), 100-01, discusses the possibility of Deuteronomy referring to the three instances in Exodus or whether Deuteronomy has references to three partial reports of one prayer condensing the three into a single instance: "In either case, Deuteronomy is not interested in a chronological report but in presenting information about Moses' prayer(s) at the points where it is most effective in illustrating Moses' theme. In the present section (vv. 7-21), the contents of the narrative are determined by its focus on Israel's sin and God's anger, and Moses' prayer(s) is mentioned only briefly."

[41] Walter C. Kaiser, *Exodus*, The Expositor's Bible Commentary, ed. Frank E. Gaebelein, vol. 2 (Grand Rapids: Zondervan, 1990), 487.

[42] Nahum M. Sarna, *Exodus*, The JPS Torah Commentary (Philadelphia: Jewish Publication Society, 1991), 220. Cf. Tigay, 99: "Moses' ability to survive for so long a time without food or drink can only be due to divine support"; Umberto Cassuto, *A Commentary on the Book of Exodus*, trans. Israel Abrahams (Jerusalem: Magnes, 1983), 447: "Hence it is further recorded here: *he neither ate bread nor drank water*, indicating that he was uplifted above the everyday plane of life and tangibly approached the Divine sphere. In the light of this development, we can understand the statement in the next paragraph that the skin of Moses' face shone."

[43] Tigay, 99-100.

[44] Eugene H. Merrill, *Deuteronomy*, NAC 4 (Nashville: Broadman and Holman, 1994), 192.

[45] E.g., Johann Gamberoni, "Fasting," *Encyclopedia of Biblical Theology: The Complete Sacramentum Verbi*, ed. Johannes B. Bauer (New York: Crossroad, 1981), 257; Muddiman, "Fast, Fasting," 773; Greenstone, 347.

[46] Note the expansion on the HB text in *Tg. Neof.* Lev 23:27-32 [ca. second century AD]: "But on the tenth day of this seventh month is the fast of atonement (צומה דכיפורייה). It shall be for you a feast day and a holy convocation. You shall fast (ותצומרן) on it, and you shall offer sacrifices before the Lord. 28 And you shall not do any work on that same day for it is the fast day (יום צומה) of the atonement, to make atonement for you before the Lord your God. 29 For whoever eats on a day of fast (למצום) and does not fast (ציימה) at

the time of the fast day (יום צומה) of the atonement shall be blotted out from the midst of the people. 30 And whoever does any work on that same day, I shall blot out that person from the midst of the people. 31 You shall do no work. It is an everlasting statute for your generations in every place where your dwellings are. 32 It shall be for you a sabbath of solemn rest, and on it you shall fast (ותציימר). On the ninth day of the month from evening until (the following) evening you shall make your fasts (צימי), you shall take your rest and you shall observe the times of your appointed feasts with joy" (Alejandro Díez Macho, ed., *Neophyti 1: Targum Palestinense Ms de la Biblioteca Vaticana*, vol. 3, trans. Martin McNamara and Michael Maher [Madrid: Consejo Superior de Investigacioned Científias, 1971], 398). Similar additions occur in *Tg. Ps.-J.* Lev 23:27 [date unknown; however, the additions to the text of Neofiti in these passages seem to suggest a later date]: "And you shall afflict your souls from food, drink, and the enjoyment of the bath and anointing, sexual intercourse and sandals. And you shall sacrifice sacrifices before the Lord" (Ibid., 508). Other passages, such as Lev 16:29, 31, 25:9; and Num 29:7 specifically refer to fasting in the Targums where the HB does not, some adding references to other forms of abstinence as above.

1QpHab 11.8 [ca. 1st century BC to 1st Century AD]: "*Woe unto him that plies his neighbor with drink, that pours out his flask* [hematho], *yea, makes him drunk, in order to gaze on their festivals! This refers to the wicked priest, who chased after the true exponent of the Law, right to the house where he was dwelling in exile, in order to confuse him by a display of violent temper [hamatho], and who then, on the occasion of the rest-day of Atonement, appeared to them in full splendor in order to confuse them and trip them up on the day of the fast, the day of their sabbatical rest*" (Theodor H. Gaster, *The Dead Sea Scriptures in English Translation With Introduction and Notes* [New York: Doubleday, 1956], 255). This refers to the Jewish tradition of changing the date of the day of Atonement by lengthening the previous month so as to avoid the holy day falling on a Sabbath, a practice the Qumran community rejected. Cf. also Acts 27:9.

[47] Cf. also Isa 58:5.

[48] BDB, 772-77, lists three other roots with the same radicals (ענה): I. "answer, respond"; II. "be occupied, busied with"; III. "be bowed down, afflicted" (the usage under discussion here); and IV. "sing."

[49] Another term, כָּנַע, "to be humble," functions similarly (note especially the reflexive uses in Lev 26:41; 2 Chr 7:14, 12:6, 7, 12, 30:11, 32:26, 33:12, 19, 23, 34:27, 36:12; 1 Kgs 21:29; 2 Kgs 22:19); also compare Isaiah's preferred term, שָׁפֵל, "to become low, be abased" (Isa 2:9, 11, 5:15, 10:33, 52:15; Jer 13:18; Dan 5:22).

[50] Cf. Pss 9:12[13], 37:11, 140:12[13], 147:6; Prov 3:34; 2 Sam 22:28, and many others.

[51] Gregory Vall, "Psalm 22 and the *Vox Christi*: A Hermeneutical Test Case" (paper presented at the Southwest Commission on Religious Studies Regional Meeting, Irving, Texas, 4-5 March 2000). In addition to the references to Psalm 22 at Christ's crucifixion, Isaiah 53 also uses עָנָה to present God's servant as one who will be afflicted with suffering (53:4, 7). Cf. Matt 18:4, 23:12; Jas 4:6-10; 1 Pet 5:5-6.

[52] Oded Schwartz, *In Search of Plenty: A History of Jewish Food* (London: Kyle Cathie, 1992) provides a fascinating look into the everyday nature of Jewish food through time. Writers occasionally note that apparently humanity in paradise enjoyed a vegetarian existence, and only after the flood was meat-eating permitted, with the proviso of the blood taboo (cf. Gen 1:29-30, 9:3-4; but also note that God covered Adam and Eve in animal skins [3:21], and Abel offered animal sacrifices to God [4:4-5], both of which seem to point away from the adequacy of vegetation after the fall). For a fuller discussion of the place of animals in Judaism, including a discussion of vegetarianism, see Elijah Judah Schochet, *Animal Life in Jewish Traditions: Attitudes and Relationships* (New York: Ktav, 1984).

[53] Jacob Neusner, *The Idea of Purity in Ancient Judaism*, SJLA 1 (Leiden: Brill, 1973), 18. Neusner cites biblical texts mentioning unclean animals and food: Gen 7:2,8, Deut 14:3-20; Judg 13:4, 7, 14; Ezek 4:14; and unclean people and food: Deut 12:15, 22; 1 Sam 20:26; 2 Chr 30:18-19.

[54] For a fuller discussion, see Walter Houston, *Purity and Monotheism: Clean and Unclean Animals in Biblical Law*, JSOTSup 140 (Sheffield: JSOT, 1993), and David Bryan, *Cosmos, Chaos and the Kosher Mentality*, JSPSup 12 (Sheffield: Sheffield Academic Press, 1995), 130-67.

[55] Bryan, 144-60. Bryan points out their respective weaknesses: the cultic explanation of Noth lacks real evidence, the hygienic approach does not seem to fit ancient mentalities as much as modern ones, and the ethical explanation does not get one far enough into the mind of priests drawing up the laws.

[56] For other instances of fasting for the death of a king or leader, see 1 Sam 31:13/1 Chr 10:12, and 2 Sam 1:12, 3:35.

[57] See also similar contexts in Ezra 9:1-10:17, Joel 2:12-15, and Zech 7:5, 8:16-19.

[58] This also occurs in the apocryphal 2 Esdras 5:15, 6:31, and 9:23.

[59] One might note Elijah's conversation with YHWH in 1 Kgs 19:9-18, which stresses Elijah's role as a prophet to whom the people apparently have not

listened, in contrast to the words of Deut 18:15. Alan J. Hauser and Russell Gregory (*From Carmel to Horeb: Elijah in Crisis*, JSOTSS 85, Bible and Literature Series 19 [Sheffield: Almond, 1990], 144-46) highlight the contrast between Moses and Elijah as prophetic figures.

[60] Thomas L. Brodie, *The Crucial Bridge: The Elijah-Elisha Narrative as an Interpretive Synthesis of Genesis-Kings and a Literary Model for the Gospels* (Collegeville, Minn.: Liturgical, 2000), 46. David M. Hoffeditz provides a thorough discussion of the later connections to Elijah in the Gospels, in "A Prophet, a Kingdom, and a Messiah: The Portrayal of Elijah in the Gospels in Light of First-Century Judaism," D. Phil. thesis, University of Aberdeen, 2000.

[61] R. P. Carroll, "The Elijah-Elisha Sagas: Some Remarks on Prophetic Succession in Ancient Israel," in *Prophecy in the Hebrew Bible: Selected Studies from Vetus Testamentum*, ed. David E. Orton, Brill's Readers in Biblical Studies 5 (Leiden: Brill, 2000), 56-71. First published in *VT* 19 (1969): 400-415.

[62] Similar words are also found in Jer 14:10-12 and 36:6-26.

[63] Because the same category of people that fasts is called to repentance and social justice, it would appear that the community at large is in view and not merely priests or religious leaders. This follows the reasoning of Michael L. Barré, "Fasting in Isaiah 58:1-2: A Reexamination," *Biblical Theology Bulletin* 15 (July 1985): 94-97, in response to Leslie J. Hoppe, "Isaiah 58:1-12, Fasting and Idolatry," *Biblical Theology Bulletin* 13 (April 1983): 44-47.

[64] Cf. also 58:13.

[65] Barré, 96, quoting Th. Booij, "Negation in Isaiah 43:22-24," *ZAW* 94 (1982): 397.

[66] Barré, 96-97.

[67] The unity of the entire chapter is assumed here, including the supposedly dissimilar verses 13-14, in agreement with Barré (who cites J. Muilenburg and N. E. A. Andraeson favorably), 95-96. This is based on the similar structure of the "if/then" clauses throughout and the similar thematic material from the beginning to the end of the chapter (again in contrast to Hoppe, "Isaiah 58:1-2," and the position that Barré cites as held by the majority of commentators, including J. L. McKenzie and C. Westermann).

[68] For a good discussion of the nature of sermonic material in Zechariah as a case study in the post-exilic prophets and second temple period, see Rex Mason, "Some Echoes of the Preaching in the Second Temple? Tradition Elements in Zechariah 1-8," *ZAW* 96 (1984): 221-35.

[69] This reference to the envoy being from Bethel is in line with the NASB, as well as Carol L. and Eric M. Meyers, *Haggai, Zechariah 1-8: A New Translation with Introduction and Commentary*, The Anchor Bible (Garden City, N.Y.: Doubleday, 1987), 382-83, and Eugene H. Merrill, *Haggai, Zechariah, Malachi: An Exegetical Commentary* (Chicago: Moody, 1994), 206-8. This somewhat difficult passage could be translated differently, as Ackroyd does: "Then Bethelsharezer the Rab-mag of the king and his men sent to seek the favour of Yahweh ..." (Peter R. Ackroyd, *Exile and Restoration: A Study of Hebrew Thought of the Sixth Century B.C.* [Philadelphia: Westminster, 1968], 206-07). This would clarify the use of the first person in Zech 7:3. But the readily recognizable town of Bethel should not be too easily dismissed in favor of a person nowhere else mentioned, bearing a title which is based on textual emendation (supported by the Syriac and Ethiopic versions) and which would perhaps more easily be a proper name, as in the NASB. It may be significant that "Bethel" means "House of God/El," and the messengers are being sent to the "House of YHWH" in Jerusalem, suggesting the prominence of Jerusalem as YHWH's dwelling place and the main centralizing factor in Israel and Judah's religion (Edgar W. Conrad, *Zechariah*, Readings: A New Biblical Commentary, ed. John Jarick [Sheffield: Sheffield Academic Press, 1999], 133). These men from Bethel come to "seek the favor of the Lord," anticipating something the peoples and inhabitants of many cities will one day do (8:20-21; Conrad, 135). However, it seems to go too far to suggest that at this point El is viewed as a rival deity to YHWH, as Conrad seems to suggest (137). The contrast in Zech 7:5-6 is not between YHWH and El, but rather between YHWH and the people's own selfishness, a connection Conrad mentions but appears to misunderstand, as he says the meaning "is not totally clear" (138).

[70] See discussion on *Ta'anit*, below.

[71] BDB, 634. Merrill cites J. Kühlewein, *TWAT* 2:50, as pointing out that the verb "in the niphal occurs four times (Lev 22:2; Ezek 14:7; Hos 9:10; Zech 7:3) in the sense of separation from unclean things, from YHWH Himself, or from food" (Merrill, 208).

[72] Merrill, 209. The fast of the seventh month, Tishri, was apparently in memorial of the murder of Gedaliah.

[73] Conrad suggests that "a question about mourning and practising abstinence for one month (the fifth month) has been answered with reference to 'seasons of joy' during four months of the year" (Conrad, 137). However, in light of the brief summary of the presumably longer conversation between the messengers and Zechariah, it would seem that this conclusion is unnecessary. Perhaps by mentioning the four fasts in Zech 8:19, Zechariah uses literary skill in avoiding redundancy while further elucidating the nature of the original conversation.

[74] Mason, 229-30, citing Ackroyd, 209.

[75] Ackroyd, 209.

[76] Naphtali Winter, ed., *Fasting and Fast Days*, Popular Judaica Library, ed. Raphael Posner (Jerusalem: Keter, 1975), 10, 17.

[77] Willem VanGemeren, *The Progress of Redemption: The Story of Salvation from Creation to the New Jerusalem* (Grand Rapids: Baker, 1988), 296.

[78] Shalom M. Paul, "Gleanings from the Biblical and Talmudic Lexica in Light of Akkadian," *Minhah le-Nahum: Biblical and Other Studies Presented to Nahum M. Sarna in Honour of his 70th Birthday*, ed. Marc Brettler and Michael Fishbane, JSOTSup 154 (Sheffield: JSOT, 1993), 244-48, provides a helpful explanation of Zech 8:23 in light of cultural backgrounds.

[79] 1 Esd 8:50: "There I proclaimed a fast for the young men before our Lord, to seek from him a prosperous journey ..."; 8:71-73: "As soon as I heard these things I tore my garments and my holy mantle, and pulled out hair from my head and beard, and sat down in anxiety and grief. And all who were ever moved at the word of the Lord of Israel gathered around me, as I mourned over this iniquity, and I sat grief-stricken until the evening sacrifice. Then I rose from my fast, with my garments and my holy mantle torn, and kneeling down and stretching out my hands to the Lord" (NRSV).

[80] Cf. also 2 Esd 20 and 6:31, 35.

[81] It should be noted, however, that Anna's fasting is associated with temple service and eschatological anticipation (as discussed in the following chapter), while Judith's fasting apparently was only for the purpose of a sign of mourning. Also, Judith's beauty and heroic deeds do not find any correspondence in Anna.

[82] References to the following pseudepigraphal materials are found in R. H. Charles, ed., *The Apocrypha and Pseudepigrapha of the Old Testament in English*, vol. 2 (Oxford: Clarendon, 1963). Joseph F. Wimmer, *Fasting in the New Testament: A Study in Biblical Theology*, ed. Lawrence Boadt, Theological Inquiries: Studies in Contemporary Biblical and Theological Problems (New York: Paulist, 1982), 10-17, contains a very nice summary of Jewish intertestamental sources.

[83] Charles, ed., 301.

[84] Ibid., 347. Cf. also *T. Jos.* 4:8; also reminiscent of Daniel 1.

[85] Ibid., 349. Cf. also *T. Jos.* 4:3.

[86] Ibid., 343.

[87] Wimmer, 11.

[88] Charles, ed., 635.

[89] Wimmer, 12.

[90] CD 4.18-20; 1QpHab 11.4-8; TS 25.10-17.10.

[91] See Wimmer, 17-22, for a thorough discussion of the broader implications of asceticism in the community as a possible link to fasting.

[92] *De Posteritate Caini*, 13.48, Philo, *The Works of Philo: Complete and Unabridged*, trans. C. D. Yonge, new updated ed. (Peabody, Mass.: Hendrickson, 1993), 136.

[93] *Mos.* 2.23.1. See also *Decal.* 159.5; *Spec.* 1.169.1, 1.186.3, 2.41.8, 2.193.1, *Legat.* 306.5.

[94] *Ebr.* 148, *Philo*, trans. F. H. Colson, LCL (New York: Putnam, 1930), 3: 397.

[95] *Migr.* 204, *Philo*, LCL, 4: 251-53; cf. *Migr.* 98.7.

[96] Wimmer, 27-30, provides a thorough discussion of this community.

[97] *De Agr.* (*On Husbandry*) 8.37-38, *Philo*, LCL 3: 127.

[98] See especially the discussion of John Cassian in the fourth chapter, below.

[99] Ibid., 22.

[100] For examples of references to OT narratives, see *Ant.* 5.159, 5.166, 8.358, 10.93, 11.134, 11.228. For references to the Day of Atonement as "the Fast," see *Ant.* 3.240, 14.487, 17.165, 17.166 (this interesting account tells of a high priest relieved from his duties for one day on the Day of Atonement because of a sexual dream defiling him for the day); 18.94; *Wars* 5.236. Note that he refers to the taking of Jerusalem by the Romans on "the Fast," apparently a reference to the Day of Atonement, in *Ant.* 14.66; this is probably a chronological error, due to Josephus following sources that mistakenly referred to the sabbath day as a fast, as in Strabo 16.763, who says Pompey took Jerusalem "on a fast day, they say, when the Jews refrain from all work," as noted in *Josephus*, trans. Ralph Marcus, LCL (Cambridge, Mass: Harvard University Press, 1986), 7: 480-81.

[101] *Life* 290.2.

[102] *Ant.* 20.89-91.

[103] Wimmer, 22, citing *Ap.* 2.282.

[104] Winter, ed., 23.

[105] Note the relationship to the Hebrew root ענה. The noun תַּעֲנִית from which the tractate derives its title occurs only once in the OT, in Ezra 9:5, "But at the

evening offering I arose from my *humiliation*, even with my garment and my robe torn, and I fell on my knees and stretched out my hands to the LORD my God" (NASB). Editions consulted here include Avrohom Yoseif Rosenberg, trans., "Tractate Taanis," *The Mishnah*, Seder Moed vol. 4, Artscroll Mishnah Series, ed. Nosson Scherman and Meir Zlotowitz (Brooklyn: Mesorah, 1969); J. Rabbinowitz, ed. and trans., *Ta'anith*, in I. Epstein, ed., *The Babylonian Talmud: Seder Mo'ed*, vol. 4 (London: Soncino, 1938), v-vi; Henry Malter, ed. and trans., *The Treatise Ta'anith of the Babylonian Talmud*, (Philadelphia: Jewish Publication Society of America, 1978), xi-xliii; Adin Steinsaltz, *The Talmud: The Steinsaltz Edition*, vols. 13-14, "Tractate Ta'anit," ed. and trans. Israel V. Berman (New York: Random House, 1995); Jacob Neusner, ed., *The Two Talmuds Compared*, vol. I. F (Atlanta: Scholars, 1996), 105-232.

[106] Steinsaltz, *Talmud*, vol. 14, 1.

[107] Preserved in these traditions here we see some of the very additions to fasting (restrictions from bathing and anointing in particular) that Jesus criticized in Matt 6:16-18. While it is unclear exactly when such practices emerged in Judaism, Jesus' words, along with the material in the Targums on the Day of Atonement already examined, can be taken as evidence that at least some of these practices were prevalent in the first century.

[108] R. Eliezer said that the king and the bride could wash their faces, and a new mother could wear shoes, things which the Mishnah says the other sages prohibited. However, the Talmud records the haggling over the possible exceptions to these regulations, and the halachah eventually allowed for a good deal of latitude.

[109] S. Lowy, "The Motivation of Fasting in Talmudic Literature," *JJS* 9 (1958): 19-38.

[110] Ibid., 21.

[111] Ibid., 29.

[112] Ibid., 22-23; also noted are *Bab. Mes.* 85a; *y. Ta'an.* 2.13, 66a; *y. Meg.* 1.6, 70d; *y. Ned.* 8.2, 40d.

[113] Lowy, 23-24.

[114] Lowy, 25-26, traces some of the early Christian conflict over fasting to its Jewish counterpart. Christians saw great value in fasting, but rejected Jewish fasting as insincere, and as Lowy points out, ignoring many of the rabbinic calls for caution. Perhaps early Christians were also repudiating what they perceived as Jewish disregard for Jesus, and fasting practices were used to highlight the

differences. See especially the discussion of the *Didache* below in the third chapter.

Chapter 2: Fasting in the New Testament

[1] On these methodological points, see the discussion of O'Collins and Kendall, *The Bible for Theology*, and Doriani, *Putting the Truth to Work*, at the beginning of the first chapter.

[2] Marion Michael Fink, Jr., "The Responses in the New Testament to the Practice of Fasting" (Ph.D. diss, The Southern Baptist Theological Seminary, 1974); Joseph F. Wimmer, *Fasting in the New Testament: A Study in Biblical Theology*, ed. Lawrence Boadt, Theological Inquiries: Studies in Contemporary Biblical and Theological Problems (New York: Paulist, 1982).

[3] Rudolf Arbesmann, "Das Fasten bei den Greichen und Römern," *Religionsgeschichtliche Versuche und Vorarbeiten* 21, no. 1 (1929): 1-131; and "Fasting and Prophecy in Pagan and Christian Antiquity," *Traditio* 7 (1949-51): 1-72.

[4] Fink, 288.

[5] Wimmer, 123-24.

[6] *TDNT* 4:924-25. BDAG, 672, defines νῆστις as "not eating, hungry," and the only biblical texts cited are Dan 6:19 (LXX, which certainly could be intererpreted as "fasting" where the king Darius "spent the night fasting and weeping for Daniel," καὶ ηὐλίσθη νῆστις καὶ ἦν λυπούμενος περὶ τοῦ Δανιηλ), Matt 15:32 (where Jesus refers to the crowd following and, and "does not want to send them away hungry," ἀπολῦσαι αὐτοὺς νήστεις οὐ θέλω), and Mark 8:3 (which is parallel). LSJ, 1175, lists the definitions as "not eating, fasting," or as a substantival "famine," "hunger," "the one fasting," "causing hunger, starving."

[7] BDAG, 671-71, cites only two NT verses for νηστεία as hunger or going without food by necessity, 2 Cor 6:5 and 11:27 (where Paul refers to himself as "in fastings often," ἐν νηστείαις πολλάκις), but these could refer to intentional fasts as well (see discussion of these texts below). LSJ, 1175, only uses the definition "fast."

[8] *TDNT* 4: 925. BDAG, 672, only defines νηστεύω as "to fast," then cites a variety of examples (as a devotional rite, as a sign of grief, with lamentation and prayer, and some miscellaneous references) without any distinct definitions. LSJ,

1175, defines νηστεύω as "fast," and also as "abstain from κακότητος," citing only the single example of Empedocles 144, where it is used metaphorically.

[9] L&N, 253 (23.31).

[10] Ibid., 541 (53.65).

[11] Ibid., 530 (51.11).

[12] Fink, 60-61, citing Onasander, *The General*, xii; Aeschylus, *Agamemnon*, 1616ff.; *Prometheus Bound*, 569ff., 599ff.; *Agamemnon*, 1014ff.; Homer, *The Iliad*, xix 155ff., 205ff.; Aristotle, *Parts of Animals*, III. xiv (675b-676a); Aeschylus, *The Libation Bearers*, 246ff.; and Athenaeus, *The Deipnosophists*, vii. 307d-f, which is an extended quotation that Fink includes in his text, describing numerous (usually derogatory) comparisons to people who engage in fasting to mullet fish. Mullets were described as fasters because they did not retain food in their stomachs.

[13] Wimmer, 23.

[14] Ibid., 24-25.

[15] *TDNT* 4:925. The minor exceptions inlcude Esth 4:16, in which צוּם appears twice and is translated the second time, perhaps only as a stylistic difference, by ἀσιτέω (a slightly broader word which might normally mean "to hunger," but could include fasting), and Esth 4:3 and 9:1 do not translate the word at all. The LXX also used forms of νηστεύω to translate צָבָא, a word describing female religious servants, perhaps suggesting a fasting role for these women, though the evidence is scanty, in Exod 38:8 (LXX 38:26; Fink, 44, mistakenly references these as Exod 28:8 and LXX 28:8); νηστείαν for עֲצָרָה, a word for a solemn assembly in Isa 1:13; and changed 1 Kgs 21:9 (LXX 3 Kgs 20:9) from קִרְאוּ־צוֹם to νηστεύσατε νηστείαν.

[16] John does not mention fasting explicitly in any context. The closest possible reference is John 4:32, in which Jesus tells his disciples who were urging him to eat, "I have food to eat that you do not know about" (NASB). Although this may possibly indicate that Jesus was intentionally fasting, it is more likely that the situation of needing food (especially kosher food in Samaria) prompted the disciples to go get some, and they returned expecting Jesus to eat. He then used the opportunity for a double-entendre lesson in his mission. This also provides an introduction to the more lengthy discussion of himself as the bread of life in John 6. See Rudolf Schnackenburg, *The Gospel According to St John*, trans. Kevin Smyth (New York: Crossroad, 1982), 1: 445-48.

[17] Hagner, Donald A., *Matthew 1-13*, WBC 33a (Dallas: Word, 1993), 64.

[18] The difficulties for a literalistic reading have prompted some biblical scholars to regard the story as a kind of Hellenistic Judeo-Christian "haggada, in which the teaching of Dt about Israel was used to present Jesus as the prototype of those who remain faithful to God in the course of temptation" (Wimmer, 33). Wimmer concludes that the evidence for calling the account this sort of genre is overwhelming, citing rabbinic parallels, the references to Moses and Israel in the desert as a textual commentary on Deuteronomy 6-8, the symbolic nature of the account, the use of Psalm 91 by the devil, the fact that Jesus is quoting the LXX, the private nature of the temptations, and the reflection on the meaning of the proclaimed title "Son of God" immediately preceding the context. Wimmer, 33-34, lists A. Meyer, R. Bultmann, H. A. Kelley, S. Schulz, B. Gerhardsson, B. Rigaux, X. Léon Dufour, and H. Schürmann in support.

[19] Geerhardus Vos, *Biblical Theology: Old and New Testaments* (Grand Rapids: Eerdmans, 1948; reprint, 1975), 331.

[20] Ibid., 332.

[21] Cf. the Pauline doctrine in Rom 5:12-21, with its emphasis on the relationship between Adam, Moses and Christ. Cf. also 1 Cor 15:45. See also Darrell L. Bock, *Luke: Vol 1: 1:1-9:50*, Baker Exegetical Commentary on the New Testament (Grand Rapids: Baker, 1994), 367-74.

[22] D. A. Carson, *Matthew*, ed. Frank E. Gaebelein, The Expositor's Bible Commentary, vol. 8 (Grand Rapids: Zondervan, 1984), 148. This is seen in the six verses that begin, "You have heard that it was said," and transition to "But I say …". Jesus cites Mosaic laws, as commonly misunderstood by the people of his day, concerning murder, adultery, divorce, false vows, talionic justice, and love of neighbor with the hatred of enemies. In contrast, he tells his disciples to obey these commandments at an attitudinal, or heart level: the command not to murder is kept by not being angry with another, not committing adultery and divorcing is prevented by not lusting, not breaking a vow is prevented by not making a vow at all, and talionic justice is replaced by loving one's enemies and doing them good. This, at least thematically, is consistent with the need for the law to be written not merely on tables of stone, but on the heart, as seen in the figure of the circumcised heart in the restoration in Deut 30:6, and the new covenant promise of Jer 31:33. This theme is picked up by Paul in 2 Cor 3:1-4, in which his new covenant ministry in the gospel of Christ is one of writing the law of Christ through the Spirit on the hearts of his converts, which stands in contrast to the letters written in stone.

[23] William Hendriksen, *New Testament Commentary: Exposition on the Gospel of Luke* (Grand Rapids: Baker, 1978), 233.

[24] Ibid., 233-34; Cf. also Bock, *Luke* 1: 371; A. Feuillet, "Le récit lucanien de la tentation," *Bib* 40 (1959): 613-631.

[25] Wimmer, 34.

[26] Much of the material for this section was first presented in Kent D. Berghuis, "Fasting and the Nature of the Age," (paper presented at the ETS annual meeting, Boston, 1999).

[27] Bock, *Luke* 1: 503.

[28] Cf. Matt 7:25-34 in which allegiance to Christ is the key to overcoming worry about these matters; Matt 22:1-14, 25:1-13, Luke 12:35-37, and Rev 19:7-10 all link the eating and drinking of wedding feasts to the appropriate attire for such occasions.

[29] N. T. Wright, *The New Testament and the People of God*, Christian Origins and the Question of God, vol. 1 (Minneapolis: Fortress, 1992), 234-35. See discussion below for further interaction with how this fasting question and answer qualifies Wright's eschatological thesis.

[30] Bock, *Luke* 1: 517.

[31] Alan W. Jenks, "Eating and Drinking in the Old Testament," *Anchor Bible Dictionary* 2: 250-54 (New York: Doubleday, 1992).

[32] I. Howard Marshall, *The Gospel of Luke: A Commentary on the Greek Text* (Grand Rapids: Eerdmans, 1978), 226. In "Jesus—Example and Teacher of Prayer in the Synoptic Gospels," *Into God's Presence: Prayer in the New Testament*, ed. Richard N. Longenecker, McMaster New Testament Studies (Grand Rapids: Eerdmans, 2001), 123-25, Marshall adds that other references to fasting by Jesus simply assume the current Jewish practice, and do not argue for continued practice of fasting after the joyous event of the resurrection. He does allow for fasting as a special accompaniment of prayer, though he sees it as relatively marginal to NT prayer on the whole.

[33] Examples include Basil's homily *About Fasting* 2.7, and Augustine's Sermon 210.4, mentioned in the following chapter below. There is no reason to suggest that there was any misunderstanding in any of the links between the words of Jesus, the writing of these passages, and their early church reception.

[34] John Piper, *A Hunger for God: Desiring God Through Fasting and Prayer* (Wheaton: Crossway, 1997), 84-85.

[35] Carson, *Matthew*, 228.

[36] Jenks, *ABD* 2: 254.

[37] For critiques of Wright's thesis about the restoration of Israel (especially as found in *Jesus and the Victory of God*), see Carey C. Newman, ed., *Jesus and the Restoration of Israel: A Critical Assessment of N. T. Wright's* Jesus and the Victory of God (Downers Grove, Ill.: InterVarsity, 1999); Clive Marsh, "Theological History? N. T. Wright's *Jesus and the Victory of God*," *JSNT* 69 (1998): 77-94; Maurice Casey, "Where Wright is Wrong: A Critical Review of N. T. Wright's *Jesus and the Victory of God*," *JSNT* 69 (1998): 95-103; Robert H. Stein, "N. T. Wright's *Jesus and the Victory of God*: A Review Article," *JETS* 44 (2001): 207-18; Robert H. Gundry, "Reconstructing Jesus," *Christianity Today* 42 (April 27, 1998): 76-79.

[38] N. T. Wright, *The NT and the People of God*, 234.

[39] N. T. Wright, *Jesus and the Victory of God*, Christian Origins and the Question of God, vol. 2 (Minneapolis: Fortress, 1996), 433-34.

[40] Wimmer, 93.

[41] Keith Main, *Prayer and Fasting: A Study in the Devotional Life of the Early Church* (New York: Carlton, 1971), 37.

[42] See especially his discussion of his understanding of Jesus' eschatology in his response in Carey C. Newman, ed., *Jesus and the Restoration of Israel*, 261-72. It is evident here that Wright is very hesitant to build on the idea of Jesus speaking to an ultimate future eschatology, even though he seems to acknowledge the possibility.

[43] Wright, *The NT and the People of God*, 459-64.

[44] W. D. Davies, *The Setting of the Sermon on the Mount* (Cambridge: Cambridge University Press, 1964), 93.

[45] Matt 6:1 reads, Προσέχετε [δὲ] τὴν δικαιοσύνην ὑμῶν μὴ ποιεῖν ἔμπροσθεν τῶν ἀνθρώπων πρὸς τὸ θεαθῆναι αὐτοῖς· εἰ δὲ μή γε, μισθὸν οὐκ ἔχετε παρὰ τῷ πατρὶ ὑμῶν τῷ ἐν τοῖς οὐρανοῖς. This is the structure maintained by each of the following three sections, and so almsgiving, prayer, and fasting are all considered τὴν δικαιοσύνην.

[46] See especially the discussion of Leo the Great in the following chapter.

[47] Hans Dieter Betz, *The Sermon on the Mount: A Commentary on the Sermon on the Mount, Including the Sermon on the Plain (Matthew 5:3-7:27 and Luke 6:20-49)*, Hermeneia (Minneapolis: Augsburg Fortress, 1995), 330-32, 337.

[48] D. A. Carson, *Jesus' Sermon on the Mount and His Confrontation with the World: An Exposition of Matthew 5-10* (Toronto: Global Christian Publishers, 1999), 60.

[49] B. Ta'an 15B-16A describes the practice of putting ashes on oneself during fasting; 12A-B describes refraining from wearing sandals, bathing, anointing, and marital relations. These may help illustrate the contrast here between the different approaches offered by the Pharisees and Jesus to hygiene during fasting.

[50] Betz, 420.

[51] Ibid., citing Horace *Sat.* 1.5.101-3.

[52] Ibid., citing Ps.-Plato *Alc. min.* 150ff., in *Plato*, LCL v. 12, 228-73.

[53] The phrase here is Ὅταν δὲ νηστεύητε, with the temporal particle plus the present subjunctive defined as: "Usually of (regularly) repeated action *whenever, as often as, every time that*" (BDAG, 730-31). The phrase implies that Jesus' disciples will fast, and when they do so, here is how it is to be done. It is to be taken in a general, rather than absolute, sense.

[54] Michael W. Holmes, ed., *The Apostolic Fathers: Greek Texts and English Translations of Their Writings*, ed. J. B. Lightfoot and J. R. Harmer, 2nd ed. (Grand Rapids: Baker, 1992), 259.

[55] Carson, *Matthew*, 164., citing John Broadus, *Commentary on the Gospel of Matthew* (Valley Forge, Penn.: American Baptist Publication Society, 1886).

[56] Jesus' fasting in the desert in Matt 4:1-4 and Luke 4:1-4, as well as the fasting query of Matt 9:14-17, Mark 2:18-22, and Luke 5:33-39.

[57] C. F. Evans, "The Central Section of St Luke's Gospel," *Studies in the Gospels*, ed. D. E. Nineham (Oxford: Basil Blackwell, 1955), 37-53.

[58] Craig A. Evans, "The Pharisee and the Publican: Luke 18:9-14 and Deuteronomy 26," *The Gospels and the Scriptures of Israel*, ed. Craig A. Evans and W. Richard Stegner, JSNTSS 104, Studies in Scripture in Early Judaism and Christianity 3 (Sheffield: Sheffield Academic Press, 1994), 342-55.

[59] *Ant.* 4.8.22 ← 242-43.

[60] Craig A. Evans, 354.

[61] Craig L. Blomberg, "Midrash, Chiasmus, and the Outline of Luke's Central Section," *Gospel Perspectives: Studies in Midrash and Historiography* 3, ed. R. T. France and David Wenham (Sheffield: JSOT Press, 1983), 217-61, criticizes the approach of C. F. Evans and his followers rather strongly. Blomberg thinks there is a lack of evidence for correspondence for a number of the pericopes, and that Luke does not fit the general category of Midrash well, since Midrashim normally are more explicit in their dependence on OT Scriptures and do not generally follow the kind of neat linear order proposed. Craig Evans is aware of

Blomberg's criticisms, and seeks to answer Blomberg's concerns and avoid falling into the errors Blomberg rightly points out.

[62] That is, hypothetically, if the Pharisee were to be truly considered righteous before God. Holmgren's words here do not make that completely clear, although that is the thrust of his point. Obviously the parable does not present the Pharisee here as justified (Luke 18:14 explicitly says that he was not).

[63] Fredrick C. Holmgren, "The Pharisee and the Tax Collector: Luke 18:9-14 and Deuteronomy 26," *Interpretation* 48 (1994): 259-60.

[64] Bock notes, "The Pharisee manages to refer to himself in the first person five times in two verses and describes himself in the prayer with the active voice. The tax collector has God as the subject and sees himself as a passive figure" (*Luke: Vol. 2: 9:51-24:53*, Baker Exegetical Commentary on the NT [Grand Rapids: Baker, 1996], 1458).

[65] Joachim Jeremias remarks, "Our passage is the only one in the Gospels in which the verb δικαιοῦν is used in a sense similar to that in which Paul generally uses it.... . Our passage shows, on the other hand, that the Pauline doctrine of justification has its roots in the teaching of Jesus" (*The Parables of Jesus*, rev. ed., trans. S. H. Hooke [New York: Scribner's, 1963], 141).

[66] B. *Ta'an* 12A says that individuals may take vows to fast on Monday and Thursday throughout the entire year, beyond the prescribed days.

[67] Felix Böhl, "Das Fasten an Montagen und Donnerstagen: Zur Geschichte einer pharisäischen Praxis (Lk 18,12), *Biblische Zeitschrift* 31 (1987): 247-50. Bock says the days reflected the traditional days that Moses went up and came down from Mount Sinai, "but the real reason may be simply that it divided the week nicely" (*Luke* 2: 1463).

[68] *Midrash Tanhuma (S. Buber Recension)* 4 (Wayyera): 16 (Genesis 19:24ff., Part I), trans. John T. Townsend (Hoboken, N. J.: KTAV, 1989), vol. 1: 102-3.

[69] Nelson P. Estrada ("Praise for Promises Fulfilled: A Study on the Significance of the Anna the Prophetess Pericope," *Asian Journal of Pentecostal Studies* 2 [1999]: 5-18) provides a summary of the promise-fulfillment-praise motif in the infancy narratives in general and the Anna story in particular.

[70] Bart J. Koet, "Holy Place and Hannah's Prayer: A Comparison of LAB 50-51 and Luke 2:22-39 À Propos 1 Samuel 1-2," *Sanctity of Time and Space in Tradition and Modernity*, ed. A. Houtman, M. J. H. M. Poorthuis and J. Schwarz, Jewish and Christian Perspectives Series 1 (Leiden: Brill, 1998). "LAB survived only in a Latin text from the 4th century. It is generally assumed that the Latin text is a translation of a Greek text, which in turn is a translation of a

Hebrew text from the 1st century." While there is debate about dating it before or after the fall of Jerusalem, "there seems to be nearly a *communis opinio* about dating LAB to the latter part of the 1st century" (45).

[71] Ibid., 46.

[72] Ibid., 60.

[73] Raymond E. Brown, *The Birth of the Messiah: A Commentary on the Infancy Narratives in Matthew and Luke* (Garden City, N. Y.: Doubleday, 1979), 451; also cited by Koet, "Holy Place," 60.

[74] Cf. Bock, *Luke* 1:251.

[75] Max Wilcox, "Luke 2, 36-38: 'Anna Bat Phanuel, of the Tribe of Asher, a prophetess ...': A Study in Midrash in Material Special to Luke," *The Four Gospels 1992: Festschrift, Frans Neirynck*, ed. F. Van Segbroeck, C. M. Tuckett, G. Van Belle and J. Verheyden, vol. 2, BETL 100 (Leuven: Leuven University Press, 1992).

[76] Cf. Gerald Friedlander, ed. and trans., *Pirkê de Rabbi Eliezer*, fourth ed. (New York: Sepher-Hermon, 1981), 384-85. In this translation, when Serah (or Serach, as here) hears about Moses, she says, "He is the man who will redeem Israel in the future from Egypt, for thus I did hear, 'I have surely visited you' (Ex. iii.16). Forthwith the people believed in their God and in His messenger, as it is said, 'And the people believed, and when they heard that the Lord *had visited* the children of Israel.'"

[77] The reference is actually to Sarah wife of Abraham, but Wilcox thinks this is due to a confusion of traditions (Wilcox, 1576).

[78] This recalls the discussion in the first chapter on deriving doctrine from narrative, and combines within a context that focuses on the narrative of the history of redemption elements of what Doriani, 86-91, refers to as "exemplary acts" and "biblical images or symbols."

[79] F. F. Bruce, *The Acts of the Apostles: The Greek Text with Introduction and Commentary*, third revised and enlarged ed. (Grand Rapids: Eerdmans, 1990), 236. See also the discussion by Alfred Loisy, *Les Actes des Apotres* (Paris: Nourry, 1920), 403. This text has historically been seen by some as an example of fasting before baptism. While Saul's experience was likely not understood by him to be a ritual for that purpose, it could certainly be seen as a historical experience that later believers imitated.

[80] Cf. Phil 3:3-6.

[81] Joseph A. Fitzmyer, *The Acts of the Apostles*, AB 31b (New York: Doubleday, 1998), 497.

[82] Luke Timothy Johnson, *The Acts of the Apostles*, ed. Daniel J. Harrington, Sacra Pagina 5 (Collegeville, Minn.: Liturgical, 1992), 254.

[83] These narrative passages would seem to fit the principles mentioned in the first chapter, offered by Doriani, 195, 207: "Where there is no direct teaching, narrative provides guidance," and "Biblical narratives guide readers in their proper use."

[84] Fitzmyer, 723.

[85] Ben Witherington, III, *The Acts of the Apostles: A Socio-Rhetorical Commentary* (Grand Rapids: Eerdmans, 1998), 694. He cites *m. Ned.* 3.3.

[86] For a good discussion, see Bruce, 515. He arrives at the date of October 5, A.D. 59.

[87] Witherington, 772.

[88] Ralph P. Martin, *2 Corinthians*, WBC (Waco, Tex.: Word, 1986), 174-75. Martin mistakenly cites Barrett in support of his view, when in actuality Barrett argues against it.

[89] Philip Edgcumbe Hughes, *Paul's Second Epistle to the Corinthians: The English Text with Introduction, Exposition and Notes*, NICNT (Grand Rapids: Eerdmans, 1962), 226; C. K. Barrett, *A Commentary on the Second Epistle to the Corinthians* (London: Adam and Charles Black, 1973), 186; Victor Paul Furnish, *II Corinthians*, AB (Garden City, N.Y.: Doubleday, 1984), 355.

[90] Ralph Martin, 175, however, uses this point to follow just the opposite line of reasoning.

[91] Fink, 283-85.

[92] Keith Main, *Prayer and Fasting: A Study in the Devotional Life of the Early Church* (New York: Carlton, 1971).

[93] For a discussion of deriving theological application from narrative literature, see Doriani, 161-212, and the more thorough interaction with these ideas at the beginning of the first chapter above.

[94] Ps 34 [35]:13; Isa 58:3; Ezra 8:21; the Day of Atonement passages in Lev 16:29, 31, 23:27, 29.

[95] Markus Barth, and Helmut Blanke, *Colossians: A New Translation with Introduction and Commentary*, trans. Astrid B. Beck, AB 34b (New York: Doubleday, 1994), 344.

[96] John Muddiman, "Fast, Fasting," *ABD* (New York: Doubleday, 1992), 2: 775. See also Fred O. Francis, "Humility and Angelic Worship in Col 2:18," in *Conflict at Colossae: A Problem in the Interpretation of Early Christianity Illustrated by Selected Modern Studies*, ed. Fred O. Francis, and Wayne A. Meeks, Sources for Biblical Study (Missoula, Mont.: Scholars Press, 1975), 167-71.

[97] Francis, 168.

[98] The phrase for "bodily discipline" in Greek here is σωματικὴ γυμνασία, not *askesis* as Muddiman writes ("Fast, Fasting," 775).

[99] L&N 88.53.

[100] Bruce M. Metzger, *The Text of the New Testament: Its Transmission, Corruption, and Restoration*, second ed. (New York: Oxford University Press, 1968), 203.

[101] Bruce M. Metzger, *A Textual Commentary on the Greek New Testament, Second Edition: A Companion Volume to the United Bible Societies' Greek New Testament*, fourth rev. ed. (New York: American Bible Society, 1994), 85.

[102] Cf. Robert H. Gundry, *Mark: A Commentary on His Apology for the Cross* (Grand Rapids: Eerdmans, 1993), 502; C. S. Mann, *Mark*, AB 27 (Garden City, N.Y.: Doubleday, 1986), 371; Craig A. Evans, *Mark 8:27-16:20*, WBC 34B (Nashville: Thomas Nelson, 2001), 47; Walter W. Wessel, *Mark*, The Expositor's Bible Commentary, vol. 8 (Grand Rapids: Zondervan, 1984), 704.

[103] Kurt Aland and Barbara Aland, *The Text of the New Testament: An Introduction to the Critical Editions and to the Theory and Practice of Modern Textual Criticism*, trans. Erroll F. Rhodes, second ed. (Grand Rapids: Eerdmans, 1989), 301. Their discussion goes on to cite several verbal changes in the manuscript tradition from Mark 9:29 to Matt 17:21, as "a further indication of the seondary character of Matt. 17:21 that the influence of the Marcan text occurred at various times and in various forms. ℵ* (the verse is added typically by the second hand) B θ 33.892* *pc* e ff¹ sy^s and sy^c as wekk as the preponderance of the Coptic tradition are more than adequate evidence for the originality of the omission of verse 21 from Matthew's text. On the other hand, no one would have deleted a text of such popular appeal, and the relatively great number of witnesses for the omission (particularly astonishing is the presence of the Old Syriac and the Coptic traditions, representing cultures where monasticism and fasting were especially esteemed) offers further confirmation of the hardy tenacity characteristic of the New Testament textual tradition."

[104] Carson, *Matthew*, 392.

[105] Craig S. Keener, *A Commentary on the Gospel of Matthew* (Grand Rapids: Eerdmans, 1999), 442, n. 128. Cf. also Robert H. Gundry, *Matthew: A Commentary on His Handbook for a Mixed Church under Persecution*, second ed. (Grand Rapids: Eerdmans, 1994), 353; Donald A. Hagner, *Matthew 14-28*, WBC 33B (Dallas: Word, 1995), 501; W. F. Albright and C. S. Mann, *Matthew*, AB 26 (Garden City, N.Y.: Doubleday, 1971), 209.

[106] Aland and Aland, 301, however, are confident that "א* B 0274 k and Clement of Alexandria are quite adequate support for the shorter form of Mark 9:29."

[107] Cf. Judg 20:26; 1 Sam 1:7-11, 7:6; 2 Sam 12:16-23; 2 Chr 20:3; Ezra 8:21-23; Neh 1:8-11; Esth 4:16; Pss 35:13, 109:21-24; Jer 14:1-12; Joel 1:14, 2:12-15; Dan 6:18, 9:3, 15-19; Matt 6:16-18; Luke 2:37; Acts 13:2-3.

[108] Metzger, *Textual Commentary*, 330.

[109] For critiques of the optimism about textual certainty evidenced in UBS[4], see Kent D. Clarke, *Textual Optimism: A Critique of the United Bible Societies' Greek New Testament*, JSNTSup 138 (Sheffield: Sheffield Academic, 1997), and K[ent] D. Clarke and K. Bales, "The Construction of Biblical Certainty: Textual Optimism and the United Bible Societies' *Greek New Testament*," *Studies in the Early Text of the Gospels and Acts: Papers of the First Birmingham Colloquium on the Textual Criticism of the New Testament*, ed. D. G. K. Taylor, TS Third Series 1 (Birmingham: University of Birmingham, 1999).

[110] Ibid., 331.

[111] Ibid., 488.

[112] O'Collins and Kendall, 6, 25-27.

[113] The situation seems to be analogous to the OT references to the Day of Atonement and their application in Judaism as discussed in the previous chapter. Although the Scriptural texts in Lev 16:29-30, 23:27-32, and Num 29:7 do not explicitly command fasting, the Targums frequently added fasting to the requirements, reflecting how fasting was universally practiced by the Jews by that time. The NT acknowledges the Day of Atonement as "the Fast" (Acts 27:9), and we have no reason to believe that the early Christians saw these practices as subversive of the meaning of the OT Scriptures, with the understanding that Jesus qualified how his disciples should fast in Matt 6:16-18, as discussed above.

Chapter 3: Fasting Through the Patristic Era

[1] Joan Brueggeman Rufe, "Early Christian Fasting: A Study of Creative Adaptation" (Ph.D. diss., University of Virginia, 1994), iii.

[2] Herbert Musurillo, "The Problem of Ascetical Fasting in the Greek Patristic Writers," *Traditio* 12 (1956): 2.

[3] Ibid.: 62.

[4] Ibid.: 63.

[5] Kirsopp Lake, ed. and trans., *The Apostolic Fathers with an English Translation*, vol. 1, LCL (Cambridge: Harvard University Press, 1959), 155.

[6] Ibid., 293.

[7] Ibid., 349.

[8] Michael W. Holmes, ed. and rev., *The Apostolic Fathers: Greek Texts and English Translations of Their Writings*, 2d ed., J. B. Lightfoot and J. R. Harmer, eds. and trans. (Grand Rapids: Baker, 1992), 541.

[9] Lake, *Apostolic Fathers*, 1: 308-09, 320-21.

[10] Ibid., 1: 309.

[11] The phrase referencing fasting is generally viewed as evidence of a later interpolation into the oral gospel tradition, as it does not appear in the Gospels. Kurt Niederwimmer, *The Didache: A Commentary*, trans. Linda M. Maloney, ed. Harold W. Attridge, Hermeneia (Minneapolis: Fortress, 1998), 74. Cf. also Luke 6:27-28.

[12] Considering the strong theme in the *Didache* to distinguish the Christian community from the Jews, it is likely that the enemies envisioned here come from Judaism (Niederwimmer, 74).

[13] Lake, *Apostolic Fathers*, 1: 321.

[14] Rufe, 161, LSJ and BAGD note that this verb appears elsewhere only in Herodotus II.40 and Hippocrates. *de nat mul.* 95; Niederwimmer, 129, mentions that Lampe also notes Ammonius of Alexandria, *Fragmenta in Acta apostolorum* 13.2 (PG 85:1541A), and that the Wengst edition of the *Didache* has νηστευσάτω in this passage like *Constitutions*.

[15] Rufe, 164, also notes possible parallels with mystery religions' initiation rites and the possibility of viewing baptism as an act of exorcism, which may have appealed to Gentile converts to Christianity. Probably the main influence is from the biblical and Jewish heritage, but over time accommodations for the Gentile culture were being made.

[16] *Did.* 9.5 makes it clear that only baptized converts were allowed to participate in the Eucharist, with the citation of Matt 7:6, "Give not that which is holy to the dogs."

[17] Willy Rordorf, "Baptism According to the Didache," *The Didache in Modern Research*, ed. Jonathan A. Draper (Leiden: Brill, 1996), 216; citing J. Schümmer, "Die altchristliche Fastenpraxis: mit besonderer Berücksichtigung der Schriften Tertullians" (*LQF* 27: 164-78), 169. Niederwimmer, 130, however, thinks that the group fasting practice rather declined and can scarcely be connected to the later Easter ritual.

[18] Lake, *Apostolic Fathers*, 1: 321.

[19] Whether or not the writer of the *Didache* had access to Matthew's written gospel, or was simply relying upon a similar oral tradition, is a debated point (Rufe, 152, n. 24).

[20] Jonathan A. Draper, "Christian Self-Definition Against the 'Hypocrites' in Didache VIII," *The Didache in Modern Research*, ed. Jonathan A. Draper (Leiden: Brill, 1996), 234. Niederwimmer,131, however, says that "these are freely chosen days of fasting imposed by individual Christians on themselves. (Nothing is said about the motives for such fasting.) Thus this section is not intended to introduce the custom of fasting but simply to fix the commonly accepted custom in a certain way and with more precision."

[21] Daniel B. Wallace, *Greek Grammar Beyond the Basics: An Exegetical Syntax of the New Testament* (Grand Rapids: Zondervan, 1996), 202. Wallace cites the example of Matt 4:2 in which Jesus fasted forty days and forty nights, and since the reference is in the accusative it means that he fasted not only on those days, but throughout the entire period. He suggests that *Did.* 8.1 makes a qualitative distinction between the fasting practices of the two groups. Rufe, 155, notes that Audet, Rordorf and Tuilier support this interpretation, but she notes that the temporal dative can also be used to answer the question of "how long," which suggests to her that "the Didachist might not have been as rigorous in his use of the forms as some scholars surmise." BDF 161.2 describes the use of the accusative of extent of time, 201.1 the temporal dative.

[22] Rufe, 154.

[23] For a caution on the parochial nature of the *Didache* and its use in comparison to the NT and early Christianity, see Wayne Grudem, *Systematic Theology: An Introduction to Bible Doctrine* (Grand Rapids: Zondervan, 1994), 67, n. 32.

[24] Carolyn Osiek, *Shepherd of Hermas: A Commentary*, ed. Helmut Koester, Hermeneia (Minneapolis: Fortress, 1999), 18-20.

[25] Ibid., 54.

[26] Lake, *Apostolic Fathers*, 2: 55.

[27] This is probably a loan word from Latin, having military associations. Tertullian would later say that Christians observed stations because they were God's militia (*De orat.* 19, *De jejun.* 10). Although the exact nature of the practices in this early period of the church's history is not clear, the witness to fasting twice a week in *Did.* 8.1, here, and to Tertullian may give some idea of the growth of customary station fasting. Christine Mohrmann, "Statio," *VC* 7 (1953): 221-45; Rufe, 202-07; Osiek, 169; Norbert Brox, *Der Hirt des Hermas,* Kommentar zu den Apostolischen Vätern (Göttingen: Vandenhoeck & Ruprecht, 1991), 308-9.

[28] Cf. vineyard imagery in Isa 5:1-11; Mark 12:1-12/Matt 21:33-46/Luke 20:9-19; Matt 24:45-51/Luke 12:41-46; Mark 13:34; Matt 25:14-30; Luke 12:27 (Osiek, 171).

[29] Parallels can be found in *Didasc.* 19 and *Ap. Const.* 5.1.3 (Osiek, 174).

[30] J. K. Elliott, *The Apocryphal New Testament: A Collection of Apocryphal Christian Literature in an English Translation* (Oxford: Clarendon, 1993), 5, 9-10.

[31] Ibid., 150, 156.

[32] Ibid., 136.

[33] Ibid., 137.

[34] Ibid., 139.

[35] Ibid., 146.

[36] For an extensive discussion of the problems, see Antti Marjanen, "*Thomas* and Jewish Religious Practices," in *Thomas at the Crossroads: Essays on the Gospel of Thomas,* ed. Risto Uro, Studies of the New Testament and Its World (Edinburgh: T & T Clark, 1998), 164-74.

[37] Ibid., 172.

[38] Elliott, 49, 57.

[39] Ibid., 48.

[40] Ibid., 334.

[41] Ibid., 364.

[42] Ibid., 368.

[43] Ibid., 379.

[44] Ibid., 382.

[45] Ibid., 383.

[46] Ibid., 383-84.

[47] Wilhelm Schneemelcher, ed., *New Testament Apocrypha*, rev. ed., 2 vols. (Louisville: Wetminster/John Knox, 1992), 2: 271-83.

[48] Ibid., 2: 287.

[49] Ibid., 2: 288.

[50] Ibid., 2: 300.

[51] Ibid., 2: 305.

[52] Ibid., 2: 323.

[53] Arthur Vööbus, *History of Asceticism in the Syrian Orient*, CSCO 184: 14 (Louvain: CSCO, 1958), 85-86.

[54] Schneemelcher, ed., 2: 340.

[55] Ibid., 2: 347. Cf. also *Acts Thom.* 9.96; 9.104; 12.145

[56] Ibid., 2: 351.

[57] Ibid., 2: 373.

[58] Ibid., 2: 485.

[59] PG 2:300-301; Schneemelcher, ed., 2: 488.

[60] PG 2:336-38; Alexander Roberts and James Donaldson, eds., *Ante-Nicene Christian Library* 17 (Edinburgh: T. & T. Clark, 1870), 216-18.

[61] *Ante-Nicene Christian Library* 17: 185-86. The *Apostolical Constitutions* are sometimes regarded as Pseudo-Clementine literature since the manuscripts bear Clement's name, but probably date from later centuries. Various Eastern Orthodox communities regard them as bearing apostolic authority, but they were largely unknown in the West until modern times. See De Lacy O'Leary, *The Apostolical Constitutions and Cognate Documents, with Special Reference to Their Liturgical Elements*, Early Church Classics (London: Society for Promoting Christian Knowledge, 1906), 11-13; *Ante-Nicene Christian Library* 17: 3-4.

[62] *Ps.-Clem. Rec.* 3.67, PG 1:1511; *Ps.-Clem. Rec.* 6.15, PG 1:1355-56; *Ps.-Clem. Rec.* 7.34-37, PG 1:1368-70.

[63] *Ante-Nicene Christian Library* 17: 186.

[64] *Ante-Nicene Christian Library* 17: 130, 134, 138-39.

[65] Limitations of time and space have prevented an exhaustive analysis of primary sources related to fasting in all the church fathers. In addition to the material

presented in the following sections, material in such important figures as Origen, Chrysostom and Jerome could prove useful for further study. However, these authors do not offer extended treatments of fasting but rather mention it in diverse and scattered contexts. Therefore, I have chosen to focus more on those authors who write directly about fasting, examining numerous other references to fasting that they also mention, in order to get a deeper understanding of those key individuals.

[66] Justin Martyr, *The First and Second Apologies*, trans. Leslie William Barnard, ACW 56 (New York: Paulist, 1997), 48-49.

[67] Ibid., 66

[68] Justin Martyr, *Writings of Saint Justin Martyr*, FC 6, trans. Thomas B. Falls (New York: Christian Heritage, 1948), 170-71.

[69] Cf. also *Dial. Tr.* 46.2.5; 111.1.3.

[70] FC 6: 209.

[71] *Stromata* 3 describes those who are eunuchs for the kingdom of God as performing a kind of fast to the world (which is not exactly fasting, but the connection to sexuality is here made explicit). This book remains untranslated from Latin in the *ANF* series due to its subject matter and the sensibilities of the populace. *ANF* 2: 381, 399-400.

[72] *Who Is the Rich Man that Shall Be Saved? ANF* 2, 603-4.

[73] Robert Pierce Casey, ed., *The Excerpta Ex Theodoto of Clement of Alexandria*, Studies and Documents 1, ed. Kirsopp Lake and Silva Lake (London: Christophers, 1934), 91.

[74] *Eclog. ex Scrip. Proph.* 14; PG 9:704-05.

[75] Tertullian, *On Baptism* 20, Tertullian, *Apologetic and Practical Treatises*, trans. C. Dodgson, A Library of Fathers of the Holy Catholic Church 1 (Oxford: John Henry Parker, 1842), 278.

[76] Tertullian, *On Repentance* 9, *Apologetic and Practical Treatises*, 365.

[77] Tertullian, *On Patience* 13, *Tertullian: Disciplinary, Moral and Ascetical Works*, Fathers of the Church, vol. 40 (New York: Fathers of the Church, 1959), 216.

[78] Tertullian, *On Prayer* 18, *Apologetic and Practical Treatises*, 310-11.

[79] Tertullian, *On Prayer* 23, *Apologetic and Practical Treatises*, 317.

[80] Tertullian, *To His Wife*, 2.4, *Apologetic and Practical Treatises*, 425-26.

[81] Tertullian, *On Fasting, ANF* 4 (Grand Rapids: Eerdmans, 1956).

[82] Tertullian, *On Fasting* 1, ANF 4: 102.

[83] Although Tertullian links eating and sexual pleasure frequently, Gerald Bray notes that in Tertullian's overall work, fasting occupies much less of his attention than continence in his approach to sanctification. This may be because fasting as a religious ritual would have little meaning to the larger Roman world in general, and also because total fasting is impossible, as food is necessary for life. Gerald Lewis Bray, *Holiness and the Will of God: Perspectives on the Theology of Tertullian* (Atlanta: John Knox, 1979), 134. This statement should qualify the title of the thesis by Martin J. Lunde, "Understanding the Preeminence of Fasting in Tertullian's Practical Theology" (M.A. thesis, Gordon-Conwell Theological Seminary, 2000).

[84] Timothy David Barnes, *Tertullian: A Historical and Literary Study* (Oxford: Clarendon, 1985), 83; Lunde, 6.

[85] Rufe, 284, n. 147.

[86] Tertullian, *On Fasting* 2, ANF 4: 103.

[87] Tertullian, *On Fasting* 3, ANF 4: 103-4.

[88] Tertullian, *On Fasting*, 3, ANF 4: 104.

[89] Lunde, 35, 38.

[90] Tertullian, *On Fasting* 4, ANF 4: 104-5.

[91] Tertullian, *On Fasting* 6, ANF 4: 105-6.

[92] Tertullian, *On Fasting* 8, ANF 4: 107. Also, references to the casting out of demons by fasting in Matt 17:21 and Mark 9:29, and Cornelius fasting in Acts 10:30, demonstrate that these NT textual variants were already established in the textual tradition and were viewed as authoritative by Tertullian.

[93] Tertullian, *On Fasting* 9, ANF 4: 108.

[94] Tertullian, *On Fasting* 10, ANF 4: 108-9. Mohrmann, 221-45, traces the use of the "station," both for fasting days of the week as well as eucharistic practice, from *The Didache*, *The Shepherd of Hermas* and Tertullian through later Catholic practice.

[95] Tertullian, *On Fasting* 12, ANF 4: 110.

[96] Tertullian, *On Fasting* 15, ANF 4: 112.

[97] Tertullian, *On Fasting* 16, ANF 4: 113.

[98] Tertullian, *On Fasting* 17, ANF 4: 114.

[99] These are generally known by the Latin title *De jejunio* (PG 31:163-98), and they have been newly translated here from Greek and included in the appendix.

[100] The *Longer Rules* may be found in English in Augustine Holmes, *A Life Pleasing to God: The Spirituality of the Rules of St. Basil* (London: Darton, Longman and Todd, 2000); *Saint Basil: Ascetical Works*, FC 9, 223-339; both the *Longer Rules* and *Shorter Rules* may be found in English in Basil, *The Ascetic Works of Saint Basil*, trans. W. K. L. Clarke, Translations of Christian Literature Series 1, Greek Texts (New York: MacMillan, 1925).

[101] Holmes, 241-43.

[102] Ibid., 244.

[103] Ibid., 246.

[104] Basil, *The Ascetic Works*, trans. Clarke, 277.

[105] *Shorter Rules* 128, Basil, *The Ascetic Works*, trans. Clarke, 277.

[106] *Shorter Rules* 223, Basil, *The Ascetic Works*, trans. Clarke, 311.

[107] PG 31:163-84 and PG 31:185-98, respectively.

[108] PG 31:1507-10.

[109] Reginald Pole, *A Treatie of Iustification* (Lovanii: Ioannem Foulerum, 1569; reprint, Farnborough: Gregg, 1967), 48-57.

[110] *About Fasting* 1.1.

[111] Ibid., 2.1.

[112] This can be seen when he says the stomach "should make a truce, a peace offering with us for five days" (*About Fasting* 1.7), and also when he rhetorically quotes the possible carnal reasoning of his parishioners, "'Since five days of fasting have been proclaimed for us, let's drown ourselves in drunkenness today'" (*About Fasting* 2.4).

[113] *About Fasting* 2.2.

[114] Ibid.

[115] Ibid., 1.3.

[116] Ibid.

[117] Pier Franco Beatrice, "Ascetical Fasting and Original Sin in the Early Christian Writers," in *Prayer and Spirituality in the Early Church*, ed. Pauline Allen, Raymond Canning, Lawrence Cross (Everton Park, Queensland, Australia: Centre for Early Christian Studies, 1998), 227-28.

[118] Ibid., 211-15. See also discussion below on Augustine.

[119] Musurillo: 5-11.

[120] *About Fasting* 1.5.

[121] Ibid., 1.6.

[122] Ibid., 1.7.

[123] Ibid., 1.9.

[124] Ibid.

[125] Ibid.

[126] Cf. also *About Fasting* 2.6 for similar lists.

[127] *About Fasting* 1.2.

[128] Ibid., 1.9; cf. 2.3.

[129] Ibid., 1.10.

[130] Ibid., 2.4.

[131] Ibid., 2.7.

[132] Ibid., 1.4.

[133] Ibid.

[134] Ibid., 1.9.

[135] Ibid., 1.8.

[136] Ibid., 1.9; cf. 2.6.

[137] Ibid., 1.7.

[138] Ibid., 1.9.

[139] Ibid., 1.10.

[140] Ibid., 2.5.

[141] Ibid.

[142] Ibid., 1.11.

[143] Ibid.

[144] Ibid.

[145] Ibid., 1.9.

[146] Ibid., 2.7.

[147] Robert P. Kennedy, "Fasting," *Augustine through the Ages: An Encyclopedia*, ed. Allan D. Fitzgerald (Grand Rapids: Eerdmans, 1999), 354-55.

[148] Ibid., 355.

[149] *Discourse of Augustine the Bishop Against the Pagans*, Sermon 198, *The Works of Saint Augustine: A Translation for the 21st Century*, pt. 3, vol. 11, ed. John E. Rotelle, trans. Edmund Hill (Hyde Park, NY: New City, 1995), 229, n. 1.

[150] *On The Three Ways of Understanding Christ in Scripture*, Sermon 341.26, *Works of St. Augustine* 3.11: 304-05: "Those of you here today who didn't fast yesterday should grieve that you spent the other festival days of the pagans in this way, while we were feeling so sad for you, and should please have the goodness, some time or other, to relieve us of our sadness and yourselves of your vile behavior."

[151] *Against the Pagans* 5, *The Works of St. Augustine* 3.11: 184.

[152] *Against the Pagans* 6, *The Works of St. Augustine* 3.11: 184-85.

[153] *Against the Pagans* 9, *The Works of St. Augustine* 3.11: 187.

[154] *Against the Pagans* 56, *The Works of St. Augustine* 3.11: 223.

[155] *On the Beginning of Lent*, Sermon 205.1, *The Works of St. Augustine* 3.6: 103.

[156] This must have been a personally vexing issue, as it creeps into every annual Lenten sermon with fairly strong and pertinent comments; cf. Sermons 207.2, 208.1, 209.3, 210.10-11.

[157] *On the Beginning of Lent*, Sermon 205.1-3, *The Works of St. Augustine* 3.6: 103-5. Cf. Sermon 209.1.

[158] *On the Beginning of Lent*, Sermon 206.2-3, *The Works of St. Augustine* 3.6: 107-08.

[159] *On Almsgiving* 1, Sermon 390, *The Works of St. Augustine* 3.10: 413.

[160] *On the Beginning of Lent*, Sermon 207.1, *The Works of St. Augustine* 3.6: 109-110.

[161] *On the Beginning of Lent*, Sermon 210, *The Works of St. Augustine* 3.6: 118-27.

[162] Ser. 210.7, *The Works of St. Augustine* 3.6: 122.

[163] Ser. 210.8, *The Works of St. Augustine* 3.6: 122-23.

[164] Ser. 210.9, *The Works of St. Augustine* 3.6: 123. One wonders whether Augustine's married hearers would agree with his entirely positive assessment of what married chastity did for them, as they would likely have found pleasure in returning to normalcy, just as with eating.

[165] *Answer to the Pelagians: The Punishment and Forgiveness of Sins and the Baptism of Little Ones* 3.6.12, *Works of St. Augustine* 1.23: 127-28.

[166] *Answer to the Pelagians: The Perfection of Human Righteousness* 8.18, *Works of St. Augustine* 1.23: 296.

[167] On the use of Basil's sermons by Augustine, translations available to him and a chart of relationships of various editions, see Heinrich Marti, ed. and trans., *Rufin von Aquileia, De ieiunio I, II: zwei Predigten über das Fasten nach Basileios von Kaisareia* (Leiden: Brill, 1989), xxviii-xxix.

[168] *Answer to the Pelagians, II: Answer to Julian* 1.17, 32, *Works of St. Augustine* 1.24: 279, 291.

[169] *Arianism and Other Heresies: Heresies 53, Works of St. Augustine* 1.18: 47.

[170] *Heresies 82, Works of St. Augustine* 1.18: 53.

[171] *Answer to Julian* 4.71, *Works of St. Augustine* 1.24: 420-21.

[172] Franz Gerhard Cremer, *Der Beitrag Augustins zur Auslegung des Fastenstreitsgesprächs: (Mk 2, 18-22 parr) und der Einfluss seiner Exegese auf die Mittelalterliche Theologie* (Paris: Études Augustiniennes, 1971), 45-49.

[173] *De utilitate jejunii*, PL 40; cf. Augustine, *The Usefulness of Fasting*, in *Treatises on Various Subjects*, The Fathers of the Church: A New Translation, ed. Roy J. Deferrari (New York: Fathers of the Church, 1952), 395-422; *On the Value of Fasting*, Sermon 400, *Works of St. Augustine* 3.10: 471-83.

[174] *Works of St. Augustine* 3.10: 482, n. 1.

[175] Ibid., 471.

[176] Ibid.

[177] Ibid., 473.

[178] *Value of Fasting* 3, *Works of St. Augustine* 3.10: 473.

[179] *Value of Fasting* 4, *Works of St. Augustine* 3.10: 474, referring to Eph 5:29.

[180] *Value of Fasting* 5, *Works of St. Augustine* 3.10: 474.

[181] *Value of Fasting* 6, *Works of St. Augustine* 3.10: 475.

[182] *Value of Fasting* 7, *Works of St. Augustine* 3.10: 476.

[183] *Value of Fasting* 8-11, *Works of St. Augustine* 3.10: 476-80.

[184] *Value of Fasting* 12-13, *Works of St. Augustine* 3.10: 480-81.

[185] George Lawless, *Augustine of Hippo and his Monastic Rule* (Oxford: Clarendon, 1987), 60. Cf. also Peter Brown, *Augustine of Hippo: A Biography* (Berkeley, Calif.: University of California, 2000), 125-30 for a description of his pre-monastic life in Thagaste, and 131-38, 193-95 for a description of monastic life in Hippo.

[186] Ibid., 85, 111.

[187] Adolar Zumkeller, *Augustine's Rule: A Commentary*, trans. Matthew J. O'Connell, ed. John E. Rotelle (Villanova, Penn.: Augustinian, 1987), 66-67.

[188] Also mentioned in *Value of Fasting* 3, *Works of St. Augustine* 3.10: 473.

[189] Agatha Mary, *The Rule of Saint Augustine: An Essay in Understanding* (Villanova, Penn.: Augustinian, 1991), 116; cf. P. G. W. Glare, ed., *Oxford Latin Dictionary* (Oxford: Clarendon, 1982), 1:571-72.

[190] Ibid., 117.

[191] Zumkeller, 66.

[192] *Rule* 3.2, Lawless, 85.

[193] *Rule* 3.5, Lawless, 87.

[194] Zumkeller, 68.

[195] A selection of sermons has been translated in *The Letters and Sermons of Leo the Great*, NPNF[2] 12; the full set of available sermons is translated in *St. Leo the Great: Sermons*, FC 93, in which see esp. Ser. 12-20, 39-50, and 86-94.

[196] NPNF[2] 12: 123.

[197] Sermon 19.3, NPNF[2] 12: 128.

[198] Sermon 49.1, NPNF[2] 12: 160.

[199] Alexandre Guillaume, *Jeûne et charité: dans l'eglise latine, des origines au XIIe siècle en particular chez saint Léon le Grand* (Rome: Pontificia Universitate Gregoriana, 1954); *Prière, jeûne et charité: des perspectives chrétiennes et une espérance pour notre temps* (Paris: S. O. S., 1985); abridged ed. (Paris: S. O. S., 1988).

[200] Ibid., 61-65.; cf. P. G. W. Glare, ed., *Oxford Latin Dictionary* (Oxford: Clarendon, 1982), 2: 1378.

[201] Guillaume, *Prière, jeûne et charité* (1985), 81-111.

[202] Ibid., 112.

[203] Ibid., 147-200.

[204] Andrew McGowan, *Ascetic Eucharists: Food and Drink in Early Christian Ritual Meals*, Oxford Early Christian Studies (Oxford: Clarendon, 1999), 140-42.

[205] Ibid., 164-66, 199-213. "Orthodox" here would refer here to adhering to accepted Christian doctrine, though often these ascetics were part of schismatic groups. The distinction here was important for the church when they attempted to mainstream various schismatics back into orthodox church life.

[206] Vööbus, 84.

[207] See discussion of the "African Code" of the Council of Carthage (A.D. 419), Canon 41, and The Council in Trullo, or Quinisext Council (A.D. 692), Canon 29.

[208] Joseph C. Dieckhaus, "The Eucharistic Fast and Frequent Communion in the West: A Canonical and Liturgical Perspective" (Licentiate in Canon Law Dissertation, Catholic University of America, 1991), 9-11.

[209] Ibid., 14.

[210] Paschal Scotti, "The Times of Fasting in the Early Church" (Licentiate in Canon Law thesis, Catholic University of America, 1995), 35-37.

[211] "Synodical Letter of the Council of Gangra," *NPNF*[2] 14: 91. While Gangra itself is not considered one of the seven ecumenical councils, its canons (along with those of Laodicea [343-81] and several other occasional councils) were accepted at Chalcedon as in continuity with apostolic tradition and binding (*NPNF*[2] 14: 59).

[212] *NPNF*[2] 14: 99-100.

[213] Ibid.: 100.

[214] Ibid.: 153. On this synod's ecumenicity, see discussion of Gangra, above.

[215] Ibid.: 155.

[216] Ibid.: 155-56. While there may be similarities to Tertullian's discussion of the Montanists' xerophagies, it appears that these are different things.

[217] Ibid.: 461-62.

[218] Ibid.: 378. For this council's authority, which is somewhat short of ecumenical status, see 356-58.

[219] Ibid.: 391.

[220] Ibid.

[221] Ibid.: 403.

[222] Ibid.: 598.

[223] Scotti, 22-24.

Chapter 4: The Development of Fasting from Monasticism Through the Reformation to the Modern Era

[1] Daniel Callam, "Fasting, Christian," in *Dictionary of the Middle Ages*, ed. Joseph R. Strayer (New York: Charles Scribner's Sons, 1985), 5: 18.

[2] Samuel Rubenson, "Asceticism: Christian Perspectives," *Encyopedia of Monasticism*, ed. William M. Johnston (Chicago: Fitzroy Dearborn, 2000), 1: 92.

[3] Αὐτὸς ἀσκῶ ἀπρόσκοπον συνείδησιν ἔχειν πρὸς τὸν θεὸν καὶ τοὺς ἀνθρώπους διὰ παντός.

[4] Callam, 5: 19.

[5] For a detailed treatment of Franciscan fasting rules, which are not examined here, see Jordan Joseph Sullivan, *Fast and Abstinence in the First Order of Saint Francis: A Historical Synopsis and a Commentary*, The Catholic University of America Canon Law Studies 374 (Washington: The Catholic University of America Press, 1957).

[6] Jordan Aumann, "Origins of Monasticism," *Monasticism: a Historical Overview*, Word and Spirit 6 (Still River, Mass.: St. Bede's, 1984), 4-10.

[7] In addition to sources cited here, see Vincent L. Wimbush, ed., *Ascetic Behavior in Greco-Roman Antiquity: A Sourcebook*, Studies in Antiquity and Christianity (Minneapolis: Fortress, 1990); Owen Chadwick, ed. and trans., *Western Asceticism*, Library of Christian Classics 12 (Philadelphia: Westminster, 1943); Alban Goodier, *An Introduction to the Study of Ascetical and Mystical Theology* (London: Burns Oates & Washbourne, 1938).

[8] Thomas O'Loughlin, "Fasting: Western Christian," *Encyclopedia of Monasticism*, 1: 470.

[9] Robert C. Gregg, trans. and ed., *Athanasius: The Life of Antony and the Letter to Marcellinus*, Classics of Western Spirituality (New York: Paulist, 1980), 7.

[10] Samuel Rubenson, "Antony, St.," in *Encyclopedia of Monasticism*, 1: 40.

[11] *Life* 7, Gregg, 36.

[12] *Life* 47, Gregg, 66-67.

[13] *Life* 5, 23, 27, Gregg, 33-34, 48, 51-52.

[14] Michael D. Peterson, "Fasting: Eastern Christian," *Encyopedia of Monasticism*, ed. William M. Johnston (Chicago: Fitzroy Dearborn, 2000), vol. 1: 469.

[15] Éphrem le Syrien, *Hymnes sur le jeûne*, trans. Dominique Cerbelaud, Spiritualité Orientale 69 (Maine-&-Loire: Abbaye de Bellefontaine, 1997).

[16] Ibid., 21, 30.

[17] O'Loughlin, 471.

[18] *John Cassian: The Conferences*, and *John Cassian: The Institutes*, trans. Boniface Ramsey, ACW 57 and 58 (New York: Paulist, 1997).

[19] *Conf.* 21.13-14, ACW 57: 729-31.

[20] *Conf.* 5.4-5, ACW 57: 183-85.

[21] Conrad Leyser, *Authority and Asceticism from Augustine to Gregory the Great*, Oxford Historical Monographs (Oxford: Clarendon, 2000), 167. Gregory went on to comment that the link between gluttony and lust is clear, because of the proximity of the stomach to the genitals (citing *Mor.* 31.45.89, CCSL 143B, 1611). This theme can be traced back to Philo, *De Agr.* (*On Husbandry*) 8.36-38, as mentioned here in the first chapter, above.

[22] *Conf.* 2.17, ACW 57: 100.

[23] For a discussion of the specifics of the disciplines, see Columba Stewart, *Cassian the Monk*, Oxford Studies in Historical Theology (Oxford: Oxford University Press, 1998), 62-76.

[24] *St. Maximus the Confessor: The Ascetic Life*, and *The Four Centuries on Charity*, trans. Polycarp Sherwood, ACW 21 (London: Longmans, Green and Co., 1955), 24, 35, 47, 57, 70; *Char.* 1.42, 79; 2.19; 3.13.

[25] Benedict, *The Holy Rule of Our Most Holy Father Saint Benedict*, ed. Benedictine Monks of St. Meinrad Archabbey (St. Meinrad, Ind.: Grail, 1956), vii-viii.

[26] *Rule* 39, Benedict, *The Rule of St. Benedict*, trans. Anthony C. Meisel and M. L. del Mastro (New York: Image/Doubleday, 1975), 80.

[27] *Rule* 40, Ibid., 81.

[28] *Rule* 41, Ibid., 81-82.

[29] *Rule* 49, Ibid., 87-88.

[30] Elizabeth A. Clark, "New Perspectives on the Origenist Controversy: Human Embodiment and Ascetic Strategies," *Forms of Devotion: Conversion, Worship, Spirituality, and Asceticism,* ed. Everett Ferguson, Recent Studies in Early Christianity: A Collection of Scholarly Essays (New York: Garland, 1999), 258-61.

[31] Vööbus, 116-19.

[32] Herbert Musurillo, "The Problem of Ascetical Fasting in the Greek Patristic Writers," *Traditio* 12 (1956): 12-13.

[33] Ibid.: 13-14.

[34] Giles Constable, *Attitudes Toward Self-Inflicted Suffering in the Middle Ages,* Stephen J. Brademas, Sr., Lecture 9 (Brookline, Mass.: Hellenic College, 1982), discusses these and numerous other examples.

[35] Constable, 7.

[36] Thomas Aquinas, *Summa Theologiæ*, trans. Samuel Parsons and Albert Pinheiro, vol. 53 (New York: Blackfriars, McGraw-Hill, 1971): 79-81.

[37] Thomas Aquinas, *Summa Theologiæ*, trans. James J. Cunningham, 57: 225-27.

[38] Ibid., 57: 65-71.

[39] Thomas Aquinas, *Summa Theologiæ*, trans. Thomas Gilby, 43: 91.

[40] Ibid.

[41] Ibid., 43: 93.

[42] Ibid., 43: 95.

[43] Ibid., 43: 99.

[44] Ibid., 43: 101.

[45] Ibid., 43: 103-5.

[46] Ibid., 43: 105-9.

[47] Ibid., 43: 111.

48 Ibid., 43: 115-17.

49 Martin Luther, "Treatise on Good Works," *Luther's Works*, ed. Jaroslav Pelikan and Helmut T. Lehmann (Philadelphia: Fortress, 1958-74), vol. 44: 74.

50 Luther, "Sermons on the Gospel of St. John," *Luther's Works* 23: 23.

51 Luther, "The Sermon on the Mount," *Luther's Works* 21: 158.

52 Ibid., 21: 25.

53 Luther, "Lectures on Titus," *Luther's Works* 29: 7.

54 Luther, "Lectures on 1 Timothy," *Luther's Works* 28: 322.

55 Ibid., 28: 323.

56 Luther, "Treatise on Good Works," *Luther's Works* 44: 74; cf. "Eight Sermons at Wittenberg: First Sermon, Mar. 9, 1522, Invocation Sunday," *Luther's Works* 51: 62.

57 Luther, "Treatise on Good Works," *Luther's Works* 44: 75; cf. "Sermon on the Mount," *Luther's Works* 21: 157-58: "For I really dare say that in what they termed 'fasting' in the papacy I never saw a genuine fast. How can I call it a fast if someone prepares a lunch of expensive fish, with the choicest spices, more and better than for two or three other meals, and washes it down with the strongest drink, and spends an hour or three at fill in his belly till it is stuffed? Yet that was the usual thing and a minor thing even among the very strictest monks. But it was the holy fathers, the bishops, the abbots, and the other prelates who were really strict in their observance, with ten and twenty courses and so much refreshment at night that several threshers could have lived on it for three days. It may well be that certain prisoners or poor and sick people were compelled to fast on account of poverty, but I know of no one who fasted for the sake of devotion, and still less now. But now these dear papists of mine have all become good Lutherans, and none of them thinks about fasting any more. Meanwhile the poor pastors on our side have to suffer hunger and trouble, and they have to observe a genuine fast every day in place of such people."

58 Luther, "Treatise on Good Works," *Luther's Works* 44: 75; "Sermon on the Mount," *Luther's Works* 21: 162.

59 Luther, "Eight Sermons at Wittenberg: First Sermon," *Luther's Works* 51: 66.

60 Luther, "Lectures on 1 Timothy," *Luther's Works* 28: 322.

61 Luther, "Treatise on Good Works," *Luther's Works* 44: 76.

62 Luther, "The Sermon on the Mount," *Luther's Works* 21: 155-56.

[63] Ibid., 21: 161.

[64] Ibid., 21: 157.

[65] Luther, "Sermon on the Mount," *Luther's Works* 21: 159.

[66] Ibid.

[67] Ibid., 21: 160.

[68] John Calvin, *Isaiah*, ed. Alister McGrath and J. I. Packer, The Crossway Classic Commentaries (Wheaton, Ill.: Crossway, 2000), 348.

[69] John Calvin, *Calvin: Institutes of the Christian Religion*, ed. John T. McNeill, trans. Ford Lewis Battles, The Library of Christian Classics 20 (Philadelphia: Westminster, 1960), 1: 611.

[70] Ibid., 1: 689-96; cf. *Institutes* 3.19.7, Ibid., 1: 838-39.

[71] Ibid., 2: 1241. According to the editor's note, in mentioning those who reject fasting, Calvin may have been referring to Zwingli.

[72] Ibid., 2: 1242.

[73] *Institutes* 4.12.17-18, Ibid., 2: 1243-44.

[74] *Institutes* 4.12.18, Ibid., 2: 1245.

[75] *Institutes* 4.12.20, Ibid., 2: 1246.

[76] *Institutes* 4.12.21, Ibid., 2: 1248.

[77] John Calvin, *A Harmony of the Gospels Matthew, Mark and Luke*, ed. David W. Torrance and Thomas F. Torrance, trans. A. W. Morrison, Calvin's New Testament Commentaries, vol. 1 (Grand Rapids: Eerdmans, 1972), 98.

[78] Ibid., 134.

[79] Ibid., 214-15.

[80] Ibid., 267.

[81] Ulrich Zwingli, *Commentary on True and False Religion*, ed. Samuel Macauley Jackson and Clarence Nevin Heller (Durham, N. C.: Labyrinth, 1981), 104.

[82] Ibid., 154.

[83] Ibid., 242, 244.

[84] Ulrich Zwingli, *The Latin Works and the Correspondence of Huldreich Zwingli, Together with Selections from His German Works*, ed. Samuel Macauley Jackson,

trans. Walter Lichtenstein, Henry Preble, and Lawrence A. McLouth, vol. 1 (New York: G. P. Putnam's Sons/Knickerbocker, 1912): 70-71.

[85] Ibid., 1: 73-79.

[86] Ibid., 1: 80.

[87] Ibid., 1: 87.

[88] Ibid., 1: 110.

[89] Ibid., 1: 123.

[90] Ulrich Zwingli, *Huldrych Zwingli Writings*, trans. E. J. Furcha, 500th Anniversary Volume ed., vol. 1 (Allison Park, Penn.: Pickwick, 1984): 70, 72.

[91] Ibid., 1: 202.

[92] John Knox, *The Works of John Knox*, ed. David Laing (New York: Ames, 1966), vol. 6: 671.

[93] Ibid., 1: 166.

[94] Ibid., 6: 388-90.

[95] Ibid., 6: 393-94.

[96] Ibid., 6: 416-22.

[97] Wayne Grudem, *Systematic Theology: An Introduction to Bible Doctrine* (Grand Rapids: Zondervan, 1994), 1190.

[98] Kenneth Ronald Davis, *Anabaptism and Asceticism: A Study in Intellectual Origins*, Studies in Anabaptist and Mennonite History 16 (Kitchener, Ont.: Herald, 1974), 129-201.

[99] This claim is made by N. van der Zijpp, "Fasting," in *The Mennonite Encyclopedia*, ed. Harold S. Bender and C. Henry Smith (Scottdale, Penn.: Mennonite, 1956), 317. Checking various indices of Mennonite writings and databases appears to validate the statement.

[100] Ibid.

[101] Ibid.

[102] Thomas Becon, *The Catechism of Thomas Becon, with Other Pieces*, ed. John Ayre, The Parker Society for the Publication of the Works of the Fathers and Early Writers of the Reformed English Church (Cambridge: University Press, 1844; reprint, 1968, Johnson Reprint), 527.

[103] Ibid., 528.

[104] Ibid., 533.

[105] Ibid., 534.

[106] Ibid., 537-38.

[107] Ibid., 545.

[108] Ibid., 547.

[109] Francis John Jayne, ed., *Anglican Pronouncements Upon Auricular Confession, Fasting Communion* (London: Simpkin, Marshall and Co., 1907[?]), 59-62.

[110] Ibid., 61.

[111] For a historical perspective and explanation of the cycles of feasts and fasts, see Vernon Staley, *The Liturgical Year: An Explanation of the Origin, History and Significance of the Festival Days and Fasting Days of the English Church* (London: A. R. Mowbray, 1907).

[112] Rhidian Jones, *The Canon Law of the Roman Catholic Church and the Church of England: A Handbook* (Edinburgh: T&T Clark, 2000), 63, 56, 122.

[113] Adalbert de Vogüé, *To Love Fasting: The Monastic Experience*, trans. Jean Baptist Hasbrouck (Petersham, Mass.: Saint Bede's, 1989), 92, citing Edward Pusey, "Tract 18: Thoughts on the Benefits of the System of Fasting Enjoined by our Church" (London: 1845).

[114] John Wesley, *The Journal of the Rev. John Wesley, A.M.*, ed. Nehemiah Curnock, Standard ed. (New York: Eaton & Mains, 1909), 1: 51.

[115] Ibid., 1: 87-88. The occasion of the letter was to defend himself from the charge that another young friend of his had died because the Wesleys taught him to fast. Wesley replied that the other man had stopped fasting a year and a half earlier, and Wesley had only begun the regular weekly practice six months earlier.

[116] Ibid., 1: 101.

[117] Ibid., 1: 188-90.

[118] Ibid., 2: 257.

[119] Ibid., 1: 184, 468.

[120] John Wesley, *The Works of John Wesley, Vol. 11: The Appeals to Men of Reason and Religion and Certain Related Open Letters*, ed. Gerald R. Cragg (Oxford: Clarendon, 1975), 62-63.

[121] Ibid., 11: 79.

[122] Wesley, *Journal of Wesley*, 3: 116, 130, 228, 432, 454; 4: 140, 147, 243, 249, 258, 299, 366, 372, 418, 423, 434; 5: 150, 223, 317, 496; 6: 7, 134, 181, 212, 222, 268, 304; 7: 423, 438, 471, 517.

[123] Ibid., 7: 51.

[124] Ibid., 4: 243.

[125] John Wesley, *The Works of John Wesley: Sermons*, ed. Albert C. Outler, Bicentennial ed. (Nashville: Abingdon, 1987), vol. 4: 94.

[126] John Wesley, *The Works of Wesley: Wesley's Standard Sermons*, ed. Edward H. Sugden, 4th annotated ed. (Grand Rapids: Francis Asbury, 1955), vol. 1: 448-49.

[127] Ibid., 1: 412-13.

[128] Ibid., 1: 420-21.

[129] Ibid., 1: 451.

[130] Ibid., 1: 455-66.

[131] Ibid., 1: 467-70.

[132] Arthur Wallis, *God's Chosen Fast* (Fort Washington, Pa.: Christian Literature Crusade, 1968), 8.

[133] Richard J. Foster, *Celebration of Discipline: The Path to Spiritual Growth*, rev. ed. (San Francisco: HarperSanFrancisco, 1988), 47 (cf. also the similar experience told in Wallis, 6). These dates should be considered within the American evangelical experience, as there are some Catholic, Orthodox and liturgical books that deal with fasting during that period. The earlier date would roughly reflect the American Civil War, because up to that time a plethora of fast-day sermons and official calls for fast days exists. The later date roughly corresponds to the beginning of a resurgence of interest in fasting as a spiritual discipline, as discussed below.

[134] For instance, Herman Arndt, *Why Did Jesus Fast?* (Cincinnati: by the author, 1922), 3, noted in his self-published work during this period that there was nothing available on fasting in the life of Christ, "which has been ignored as if it were an inscrutable mystery." He further stated, "the theologians of almost nineteen centuries seem to have entered into a conspiracy of silence on this subject" (7). In his conclusion he remarks, "Fasting has been a mystery too long for the welfare of the human race. This has caused its disuse by the majority and its abuse by those using it without intelligence" (73). Yet his work shows awareness of the Scriptures, Talmud and patristic sources on fasting in general.

[135] It is *not* being claimed here that Christian individuals or groups in various places were not fasting in meaningful ways, since that was likely happening. It would be beyond the general scope of this dissertation to try to document such local religious practices, and I have relied more upon published sources related specifically to fasting. Since there is a relative silence in these materials, this may suggest a general lack of specific attention being paid to fasting itself, although it may still have been practiced by Christians as an accompaniment to prayer and the like.

[136] de Vogüé, 69-87. Cf. also his updated comments on the book, "On Regular Fasting," *Word and Spirit: A Monastic Review* 13, *Asceticism Today* (Petersham, Mass.: St. Bede's, 1991), 110-31.

[137] Ibid., 94.

[138] Becon, 534.

[139] Léo Moulin, "Monks Fasted but Were Plump," in *On Fasting and Feasting: A Personal Collection of Favourite Writings on Food and Eating*, ed. Alan Davidson (London: Macdonald Orbis, 1988), 199-200.

[140] de Vogüé, 87-91.

[141] de Vogüé, 92, citing Edward Pusey, "Tract 18: Thoughts on the Benefits of the System of Fasting Enjoined by our Church" (London: 1845).

[142] David B. Calhoun, *Princeton Seminary: Volume 1, Faith and Learning 1812-1868* (Carlisle, Pa.: Banner of Truth, 1994), 426.

[143] Martha Lawrence. Finch, "Corporality and Orthodoxy in Early New England: Plymouth Colony, 1620-1692" (Ph. D. diss., University of California, Santa Barbara, 2000), 307-8, n. 132.

[144] For a sampling of American fast day sermons in the 17th and 18th centuries, see Richard Owen Roberts, ed., *Sanctify the Congregation: A Call to the Solemn Assembly and to Corporate Repentance* (Wheaton, Ill.: International Awakening, 1994).

[145] Gilbert Tennent, "Fasting and Prayer," in Roberts, ed., 314.

[146] Richard J. Janet, "The Decline of General Fasts in Victorian England, 1832-1857" (Ph.D. diss., University of Notre Dame, 1984), 3.

[147] Ibid., 37-48.

[148] Ibid., 55-56.

[149] Ibid., 9, 103, citing D. C. Lathbury, ed., *Gladstone Correspondence on Church and Religion* (New York: MacMillan, 1910), 2: 272-74.

[150] Janet, 8.

[151] Ibid., 247.

[152] de Vogüé, 95-101.

[153] Ibid., 101.

[154] P. R. Régamey, et. al., *Redécouverte du jeûne* (Paris: Les éditions du cerf, 1959), 136-49.

[155] Barbara Siebrunner, *Die Problematik der kirchlichen Fasten- und Abstinenzgesetzgebung: eine Untersuchung zu dem im Zuge des zweiten Vatikanischen Konzils erfolgten Wandel*, European University Studies Series 23, Theology 736 (Frankfurt am Main: Peter Lang, 2001), 152-54.

Chapter 5: Toward a Contemporary Christian Theology of Fasting

[1] Margaret R. Miles, *Fullness of Life: Historical Foundations for a New Asceticism* (Philadelphia: Westminster, 1981), 135-54.

[2] It is a bit difficult to see this as very distinct from the Augustinian approach, except that Miles stresses Augustine's emphasis on freedom from the carnal distractions of the world (perhaps owing to his neoplatonism), while she apparently sees Ignatius as more holistic.

[3] Miles, 156.

[4] Ibid.

[5] Ibid., 159.

[6] Ibid., 160.

[7] Ibid., 160-63.

[8] Archimandrite Akakios, *Fasting in the Orthodox Church: Its Theological, Pastoral, and Social Implications* (Etna, Calif.: Center for Traditionalist Orthodox Studies, 1990), 14.

[9] Ibid., citing Sergei Bulgakov, *The Orthodox Church* [no other information available].

[10] This kind of methodology can be seen in Akakios; Basil Nagosky, "The Purpose and Meaning of the Fast in the Orthodox Church" ([Masters?] thesis, Saint Vladimir's Seminary, 1959); Lazar Puhalo, "The Spiritual and Scriptural

Meaning of the Fasts," in *On Fasting: The Spiritual and Scriptural Meaning of the Orthodox Christian Fasts*, Point of Faith 4 (Dewdney, B. C.: Synaxis, 1997); George Mastrantonis, *Fasting* (www.st-anthony.org/fasting, accessed June 28 2002; available from the Greek Orthodox Website www. goarch.org; Internet); Bishop Demetri, *His Grace Bishop Demetri's Message for Great Lent 2002*, Antiochian Orthodox Christian Archdiocese of North America (accessed June 28 2002, available from www.antiochian.org/midwest/Bishop/GreatLent_2002.htm, Internet).

[11] Akakios, 43.

[12] Ibid., 45.

[13] Lazar Puhalo, "Foreward," *On Fasting: The Scriptural and Spiritual Meaning of the Orthodox Christian Fasts*, Point of Faith 4 (Dewdney, B. C.: Synaxis, 1973), 1.

[14] Akakios, 46-48; Kallistos (Timothy) Ware, *The Orthodox Church*, New ed. (New York: Penguin, 1997), 231-38; Michael Henning, "Man: 'a God by Grace?'" in *On Fasting: The Scriptural and Spiritual Meaning of the Orthodox Christian Fasts*, Point of Faith 4 (Dewdney, B. C.: Synaxis, 1997).

[15] Henning, 34-35.

[16] Ware, 236-37.

[17] Akakios, 49.

[18] Constantine Cavarnos, *Fasting and Science: A Study of the Scientific Support and Patristic Foundation for Fasting in the Orthodox Church*, trans. Bishop Chrysostomos and Hieromonk Auxentios, Monographic Supplement Series 3 (Etna, Calif.: Center for Traditionalist Orthodox Studies, 1988).

[19] Akakios, 59.

[20] Ware, 300.

[21] Akakios, 73-79; Ware, 300-301.

[22] Adalbert de Vogüé, *To Love Fasting: The Monastic Experience*, trans. Jean Baptist Hasbrouck (Petersham, Mass.: Saint Bede's, 1989); cf. George A. Maloney, *A Return to Fasting* (Pecos, N.Mex.: Dove Publications, 1974); Thomas Ryan, *Fasting Rediscovered: A Guide to Health and Wholeness for Your Body-Spirit* (New York: Paulist, 1981); Slavko Barbaric, *Fasting* (Steubenville, Ohio: Franciscan University Press, 1988).

[23] P. R. Régamey, *Redécouverte du jeûne* (Paris: Les éditions du cerf, 1959), 386-436.

[24] Alexandre Guillaume, *Prière, jeûne et charité: des perspectives chrétiennes et une espérance pour notre temps* (Paris: S. O. S., 1985).

[25] Marcellino Zalba, "Fasting," *Sacramentum Mundi: An Encyclopedia of Theology*, ed. Karl Rahner (New York: Herder and Herder, 1968), 2: 334-35.

[26] Paul VI, *Paentemini* (Apostolic Constitution), *AAS* 58 (1956): 177-98; also as cited in Zalba, "Fasting," 335.

[27] John A. Abbo and Jerome D. Hannan, *The Sacred Canons: A Concise Presentation of the Current Disciplinary Norms of the Church*, vol. 2 (St. Louis: Herder, 1952): 505-9.

[28] Peter Shannon, "The Code of Canon Law: 1918-1967," *Canon Law Postconciliar Thoughts: Renewal and Reform of Canon Law*, Concilium 28 (New York: Paulist, 1967), 49-57.

[29] For a summary of regulations and exceptions, see P. M. J. Clancy, "Fast and Abstinence," *New Catholic Encyclopedia* (New York: McGraw-Hill, 1967), 5: 847-50.

[30] Barbara Siebrunner, *Die Problematik der kirchlichen Fasten- und Abstinenzgesetzgebung: eine Untersuchung zu dem im Zuge des zweiten Vatikanischen Konzils erfolgten Wandel*, European University Studies Series 23, Theology 736 (Frankfurt am Main: Peter Lang, 2001), 100-132, 157-221.

[31] Canon Law Society of America, *Code of Canon Law: Latin-English Edition* (Washington: Canon Law Society of America, 1983), 446-47.

[32] Paul VI, "Paentemini (Apostolic Constitution)," *AAS* 58 (1956), 177-98; National Conference of Catholic Bishops, *On Penance and Abstinence: Pastoral Statement of the National Conference of Catholic Bishops* (1966).

[33] National Conference of Catholic Bishops, *On Penance and Abstinence*, 1.

[34] Ibid.

[35] Thomas Francis Anglin, *The Eucharistic Fast: An Historical Synopsis and Commentary*, The Catholic University of America Canon Law Studies 124 (Washington: Catholic University of America, 1941), 165.

[36] James Ruddy, *The Apostolic Constitution Christus Dominus: Text, Translation and Commentary, with Short Annotations on the Motu Proprio Sacram Communionem*, The Catholic University of America Canon Law Studies 390 (Washington: Catholic University of America, 1957), vii.

[37] Ibid., 1-20. Joseph C. Dieckhaus, "The Eucharistic Fast and Frequent Communion in the West: A Canonical and Liturgical Perspective" (Licentiate in Canon Law Dissertation, Catholic University of America, 1991), 54-55.

[38] Can. 919; Dieckhaus, 59-60.

[39] Paul VI and John Paul II, *Fasting and Solidarity: Pontifical Messages for Lent* (Vatican City: Pontifical Council *Cor Unum*, 1991).

[40] Ibid., 17.

[41] Ibid., 29-30.

[42] *Catechism of the Catholic Church* (Mahwah, N.J.: Paulist, 1994), 360, §1434. Cf. also §540, §1438, and §2041-2043.

[43] Monika K. Hellwig, "Penance and Reconciliation," *Commentary on the Catechism of the Catholic Church*, ed. Michael J. Walsh (Collegeville, Minn.: Liturgical, 1994), 286.

[44] This conclusion accepts the methodology of D. H. Williams, *Retrieving the Tradition and Renewing Evangelicalism: A Primer for Suspicious Protestants* (Grand Rapids: Eerdmans, 1999), and is believed to be in line with the spirit of "The Gift of Salvation" (Richard John Neuhaus, ed., *First Things* no. 79 (Jan. 1998): 20-23; Timothy George, "Evanngelicals and Catholics Together: A New Initiative," *Christianity Today* 41 (Dec. 8, 1997): 34-38), the second major statement of the Evangelicals and Catholics Together movement. This statement, signed by prominent evangelicals and Roman Catholics, affirmed that "We understand that what we here affirm is in agreement with what the Reformation traditions have meant by justification by faith alone (*sola fide*)" (21). That document itself recognizes ongoing debate over the implications of justification on several aspects of doctrine and practice, and fasting as part of penitential practice could reasonable be seen to fall into that category. Not all evangelicals are satisfied with this statement, as the following articles show: Timothy George, Thomas C. Oden, J. I. Packer, "An Open Letter About 'The Gift of Salvation,'" *Christianity Today* 42 (April 27, 1998): 9; Art Moore, "Does 'The Gift of Salvation' Sell Out the Reformation?" *Christianity Today* 42 (April 27, 1998): 17, 21; Mark A. Seifrid, "The Gift of Salvation: Its Failure to Address the Crux of Justification" (paper presented at the 50th annual conference of the Evangelical Theological Society, Orland, Fla., 1998).

[45] J. Daryl Charles, "Assessing Recent Pronouncements on Justification: Evidence from 'The Gift of Salvation' and the Catholic *Catechism*," *Pro Ecclesia* 8 (1999): 461.

46 Richard J. Foster, *Celebration of Discipline: The Path to Spiritual Growth* (San Francisco: HarperSanFrancisco, 1988); Dallas Willard, *The Spirit of the Disciplines: Understanding How God Changes Lives* (San Francisco: Harper & Row, 1988).

47 Ibid., 20-21.

48 Ibid., 22-23.

49 These include Angus Dun, *Not By Bread Alone* (New York: Harper, 1942); James Miller, *Systematic Fasting* (Apollo, Pa.: West, 1951); David R. Smith, *Fasting: A Neglected Discipline* (Fort Washington, Pa.: Christian Literature Crusade, 1954 [perhaps this is the book Foster refers to as the first published since 1861]); Arthur Wallis, *God's Chosen Fast: A Spiritual and Practical Guide to Fasting* (Fort Washington, Pa.: Christian Literature Crusade, 1968); Derek Prince, *Shaping History through Prayer and Fasting* (Old Tappan, N. J.: Revell, 1973), and *How to Fast Successfully* (Ft. Lauderdale, Fla.: CGM Publishing, 1976); Charles W. Johnson, Jr. "The Mysteries of Fasting," *Spiritual Frontiers* 5, no. 1 (1973): 44-51, and *Fasting, Longevity, and Immortality* (Turkey Hills, Pa.: Survival Publishing, 1978); Eric N. Rogers [Pseudonym], *Fasting: The Phenomenon of Self-Denial* (Nashville: Thomas Nelson, 1976); Andy Anderson, *Fasting Changed My Life* (Nashville: Broadman, 1977); Jerry Charles, *God's Guide to Fasting: A Complete and Exhaustive Biblical Encyclopedia* (Madison, N.C.: Power Press, 1977); Gordon Lindsay, *Prayer and Fasting: The Master Key to the Impossible* (Dallas: Christ for the Nations, 1977); Jerry Falwell, *Fasting: What the Bible Teaches* (Wheaton, Ill.: Tyndale, 1981); John E. Baird and Don DeWelt, *What the Bible Says About Fasting*, What the Bible Says Series (Joplin, Mo.: College Press, 1984); Bob and Michael W. Benson, *Disciplines for the Inner Life* (Waco, Tex.: Word, 1985); Wesley L. Duewel, *Mighty Prevailing Prayer* (Grand Rapids: Francis Asbury, 1990); Bill Bright, *The Coming Revival: America's Call to Fast, Pray, and 'Seek God's Face'* (Orlando: NewLife Publications, 1995); Ian Newberry, *Available for God: A Study of the Biblical Teaching and the Practice of Fasting*, trans. Peter Coleman (Carlisle: OM/Paternoster, 1996); Elmer L. Towns, *Fasting for Spiritual Breakthrough: A Guide to Nine Biblical Fasts* (Ventura, Calif.: Regal, 1996); John Piper, *A Hunger for God: Desiring God Through Fasting and Prayer* (Wheaton, Ill.: Crossway, 1997); Ronnie W. Floyd, *The Power of Prayer and Fasting: 10 Secrets of Spiritual Strength* (Nashville: Broadman & Holman, 1997.

50 William Loftin Hargrave, "Fasting in the Early Church: Being a Study of Fasting Based Upon References to the Subject in the Old and New Testaments, and Upon the Writings of Some of the Ante-Nicene Fathers" (S. T. M. thesis, University of the South, 1952); David Eddle Briggs, "Biblical Teaching on

Fasting" (Th. M. thesis, Dallas Theological Seminary, 1953); Wayne Barton, "Toward an Understanding of Fasting in the New Testament" (Th. D. diss., New Orleans Baptist Theological Seminary, 1954); Frederick Gordon Moore, "The New Testament Concept, Practice, and Significance of Fasting: Its Historical Background and Present Implications" (B. D. thesis, Western Conservative Baptist Theological Seminary, 1955); Frederic R. Dinkins, "The Biblical Practice and Doctrine of Fasting" (Th. M. thesis, Columbia Theological Seminary, 1966); James W. McAfee, "The Practice of Fasting" (Th. M. thesis, Dallas Theological Seminary, 1973); Donald Vinson Winter, "Fasting: A Biblical and Practical Approach" (M. A. thesis, Columbia Bible College Graduate School of Bible and Missions, 1976); Thomas Wilson Jacob, "The Meaning and Importance of Fasting in the Teaching of Jesus" (M. A. thesis, Wheaton College, 1976); Stanley D. Nairn, "Identification and Purposes of Fasting" (M. Div. thesis, Grace Theological Seminary, 1976); William Lee Johnson, "Motivations for Fasting in Early Christianity" (Th. M. thesis, Southern Baptist Theological Seminary, 1978); Gary D. Dehnke, "Fasting: Practice and Function in the New Testament and in the Early Church" (M. Div. thesis, Concordia Theological Seminary, 1983); Daniel Edward Wickwire, "The Role of Prayer and Fasting in Binding and Loosing with Special Reference to the Problem of Reaching the Unreached People of the World Today" (Masters thesis, The Columbia Graduate School of Bible and Missions, Columbia, S. C., 1983); R. D. Chatham, *Fasting: A Biblical Historical Study* (South Plainfield, N.J.: Bridge Publishing, 1987); Charles W. Quinley, "Not By Bread Alone: A Study in the Christian Discipline of Fasting" (D. Min. diss., Asbury Theological Seminary, 1989).

[51] Thomas H. Felter, "The Relevance of the New Testament Treatment of Fasting to Modern Life" (M. A. thesis, Wheaton College, 1960); Keith Main, *Prayer and Fasting: A Study in the Devotional Life of the Early Church* (New York: Carlton, 1971); Marion Michael Fink, Jr., "The Responses in the New Testament to the Practice of Fasting" (Ph.D. diss, The Southern Baptist Theological Seminary, 1974).

[52] See esp. Willard, 130-150. Foster's work does not deal specifically with tradition in any section, but is permeated with quotations and evidence of interaction.

[53] Foster, 56-61.

[54] Willard, 5.

[55] Foster, 6-11.

[56] "Spiritual Disciplines and Means of Grace: Contrast or Continuum? An Interview with Dallas Willard," *Modern Reformation*, July/Aug 2002, 42.

[57] This is especially seen in the temptation narratives in Matt 4:1-4 and Luke 4:1-4, and the response to the fasting question in the synoptic Gospels that discusses the bridegroom in Matt 9:14-15, Mark 2:18-20, and Luke 5:33-35.

[58] Kent D. Berghuis, "Fasting and the Nature of the Age" (paper presented at the ETS annual meeting, Boston, 1999).

[59] Michael S. Horton, *Covenant and Eschatology: The Divine Drama* (Louisville: Westminster John Knox, 2002), 223.

[60] Dallas Willard, "Christ-Centered Piety," in *Where Shall My Wond'ring Soul Begin? The Landscape of Evangelical Piety and Thought*, ed. Mark A. Noll and Ronald F. Thiemann (Grand Rapids: Eerdmans, 2000), 27-35.

[61] This combines several elements mentioned by Doriani's discussion of deriving doctrine from narrative (161-212). Remembering Christ recalls the redemptive acts of God in history. Imitating Christ illustrates his point that "the 'imitation of Christ' motif uses narrative to guide behavior" (201): "Whether explicit (his prayers) or implicit (his fellowship with sinners), Jesus' life generally sets patterns for kingdom life. Those who imitate him also become patterns for righteousness" (206). Anticipating Christ is an example of what O'Collins and Kendall, 7, 31, refer to as "The principle of eschatological provisionality."

[62] Horton, 224.

[63] Main, 43.

[64] Cf. 1 Cor 11:26; Matt 26:29; Mark 14:25; Luke 22:18.

[65] William Isley, "Fasting: The Discipline for the in-between Time" (paper presented at the National Spiritual Formation Conference, Dallas, 2001), 8.

[66] Willem VanGemeren, *The Progress of Redemption: The Story of Salvation from Creation to the New Jerusalem* (Grand Rapids: Baker, 1988), 161.

[67] In many Protestant environments, Christmas and Easter alone stand out as specifically Christian holidays. American evangelicals are more likely to follow the Hallmark calendar than the Christian one.

[68] "Spiritual Disciplines and Means of Grace: Contrast or Continuum? An Interview with Dallas Willard," 41-42.

[69] Herman Ridderbos, *Paul: An Outline of His Theology*, trans. John Richard De Witt (Grand Rapids: Eerdmans, 1975), 265.

[70] It is interesting to note the balance in this context, as Jesus also commends John the Baptist, who "came neither eating nor drinking" (Matt 11:18). The real focus here is on those who rejected the witness of them both.

[71] Isley, 7.

[72] Horton, 271.

[73] *About Fasting* 2.7.

[74] John Piper, *A Hunger for God: Desiring God through Prayer and Fasting* (Wheaton, Ill.: Crossway, 1997), 83-96.

[75] Isley, 9.

[76] Willard, *Spirit of the Disciplines*, 152.

[77] Veronika E. Grimm, *From Feasting to Fasting, the Evolution of a Sin: Attitudes to Food in Late Antiquity* (London: Routledge, 1996).

[78] Ibid., 23.

[79] Ibid., 64.

[80] Ibid., 60-61.

[81] Ibid., 63. Rom 7:24-25 (NASB) in full reads, "Wretched man that I am! Who will set me free from the body of this death? *Thanks be to God through Jesus Christ our Lord!* So then, on the one hand I myself with my mind am serving the law of God, but on the other, with my flesh the law of sin." (The italicized sentence is omitted by Grimm.)

[82] The book's jacket illustration, which pictures "The Temptation of St. Hilarion" by Dominique Papety, aptly illustrates the basic thesis of Grimm's book. A beautiful, nearly nude woman with a table full of wine and luscious foods appears before the emaciated, pale saint. His arms reach out in desperate refusal while he looks up to the sky, his meager rations at his side.

[83] Miles, 158.

[84] Samuel Rubenson, "Asceticism: Christian Perspectives," in *Encyclopedia of Monasticism*, ed. William M. Johnston (Chicago: Fitzroy Dearborn, 2000), 93.

[85] Teresa M. Shaw, *The Burden of the Flesh: Fasting and Sexuality in Early Christianity* (Minneapolis, Minn.: Fortress, 1998).

[86] Ibid., 25.

[87] For instance, in contrast to Shaw's comments above, labor and hierarchy might arguably be seen as part of the unfallen state in Gen 2:15-25. It should be remembered that Shaw is doing an analysis of early Christian texts, so these themes may have been present in some ancient references even if analysis of the biblical texts does not seem to justify them.

[88] Shaw, 27-64.

[89] Caroline Walker Bynum finds a similar emphasis in her study of medieval women and food rituals. She argues "that medieval efforts to discipline and manipulate the body should be interpreted more as elaborate changes rung upon the *possibilities* provided by fleshliness than as flights from physicality" (*Holy Feast and Holy Fast: The Religious Significance of Food to Medieval Women* [Berkely, Calif.: University of California, 1987], 6). For Bynum, fasting is a way of using food to control the self through renunciation. This theme of control of the body in fasting and chastity, particularly against outside, antagonistic forces is also discussed by Gail Paterson Corrington, "The Defense of the Body and the Discourse of Appetite: Continence and Control in the Greco-Roman World," *Semeia* 57 (1992): 65-74. The extreme asceticism and literalism in the spirituality of the medieval women Bynum examined "were not, at the deepest level, masochism or dualism but, rather, efforts to gain power and to give meaning" (Bynum, 208). While her study has a decidedly feminist interest, at least this shows that Christian fasting and ascetic practices do not have to be viewed through the negative lens of an inherent Christian rejection of the physical body. Christians have tried to engage the body in spirituality through history, through ways that are sometimes commendable and other times insupportable.

[90] Mary Timothy Prokes, *Toward a Theology of the Body* (Grand Rapids: Eerdmans, 1996), 25.

[91] Samuel M Powell, and Michael E. Lodahl, ed., *Embodied Holiness: Toward a Corporate Theology of Spiritual Growth* (Downers Grove, Ill.: InterVarsity, 1999), 8.

[92] The intricacies of such a study of biblical anthropology can be seen in Robert Jewett, *Paul's Anthropological Terms: A Study of Their Use in Conflict Settings*, ed. Otto Michel and Martin Hengel, Arbeiten zur Geschichte des antiken Judentums und des Urchristentums 10 (Leiden: Brill, 1971). After an exhaustive study of several key terms, he concludes that the terms themselves are not used by Paul with regular, technical meanings, but more typically in polemical contexts. The result is that the terms themselves cannot really be used to develop a consistent anthropology, but rather need to be more carefully related to the contexts in which they are found (cf. 447). A sound (if older and more constrained) view is that of Ridderbos, who speaks of "body" and "flesh" in pauline anthropology denoting "approximately the earthly human life with the inclusion of death," and notes the more inward terms as constituent (but often overlapping or synonymous) terms as members of the self (Ridderbos, 114-26). For more recent treatments of biblical theological anthropology, see John W. Cooper, *Body, Soul and Life Everlasting: Biblical Anthropology and the Monism-Dualism Debate*, updated ed. (Grand Rapids: Eerdmans, 2000); David E. Aune

and John McCarthy, eds., *The Whole and Divided Self: The Bible and Theological Anthropology* (New York: Crossroad Herder, 1997).

[93] Horton, 243.

[94] Willard, *Spirit of the Disciplines*, 175.

[95] Ibid., 158-60.

[96] Ibid., 175-76.

[97] Gal 5:19-21: "Now the deeds of the flesh are evident, which are: immorality, impurity, sensuality, idolatry, sorcery, enmities, strife, jealousy, outbursts of anger, disputes, dissensions, factions, envyings, drunkenness, carousings, and things like these, of which I forewarn you just as I have forewarned you that those who practice such things shall not inherit the kingdom of God" (NASB).

[98] Perhaps it should also be noted that references to religious fasting in Islam, especially related to Ramadan, greatly outnumber references to Christian fasting.

[99] Pitirim Sorokin, *The Crisis of Our Age* (Oxford: Oneworld, 1992; reprint, 1941 ed.).

[100] Harold O. J. Brown, *The Sensate Culture: Western Civilization between Chaos and Transformation* (Dallas: Word, 1996); Kent D. Berghuis, "Pitirim Sorokin as Cultural Physician: His Diagnosis, Prognosis and Prescription," (Paper presented at the 1997 ETS meeting, Santa Clara, Calif., 1997).

[101] Miles, 159.

[102] Frederica Mathewes-Green, "To Hell on a Cream Puff," *Christianity Today* 39 (1995): 44.

[103] Ibid.

[104] This interpretation is in line with the majority of critical commentators on this passage (see statements to that effect in William Hendriksen, *New Testament Commentary: Exposition of Philippians* [Grand Rapids: Baker, 1962], 178, who lists Alford, Barclay, Barnes, Braune, Beare, Ellicott, Erdman, Johnstone, Kennedy, Laurin, Lightfoot, Meyer, Michael, and Rainy as supporting his opinion that sensualists, or antinomians, are in view; cf. also Gordon D. Fee, *Paul's Letter to the Philippians*, NICNT [Grand Rapids: Eerdmans, 1995], 369-72; Moisés Silva, *Philippians*, The Wycliffe Exegetical Commentary [Chicago: Moody, 1988], 208-9). Since Paul has been addressing the problem of Judaizers and circumcision in the previous context, there is a minority view that sees Phil 3:18-19 as referring to them (Homer A. Kent, Jr., *Philippians*, The Expositor's Bible Commentary, vol. 11 [Grand Rapids: Zondervan, 1978], 147, lists Lenski, Müller, and Barth as in favor of this

interpretation, although Kent himself believes the adversaries to be antinomians; Markus Bockmuehl, *The Epistle to the Philippians*, BNTC [Peabody, Mass.: 1998], 231, who also prefers the antinomian interpretation, says the Judaizer interpretation goes back as early as Ambrosiaster and is found later in Erasmus and Bengel, however, "the immediate context suggests no other connection with Jewish Christians; Paul never equates Judaizing dietary observance with idolatry; and the respective terms are used nowhere else in this allusive sense. What is more, the Jewish-Christian proselytizers of 3.2-11 seem on the face of it most unlikely to subscribe to the moral laxity condemned in the 'enemies of the cross' of 2.18-19. A closer parallel exists with the Jewish apostates who in 3 Macc. 7.11 have abandoned faithfulness to the commandments of God 'for the sake of the belly', and with 'the servants of their belly' in *Gen. Wisd.* 17.5 [cf. 14.6; 15.7; also Sir. 37.5]." Cf. John Calvin, *The Epistles of Paul the Apostle to the Galatians, Ephesians, Philippians and Colossians*, trans. T. H. L. Parker, Calvin's Commentaries, vol. 11, ed. David W. Torrance and Thomas F. Torrance [Grand Rapids: Eerdmans, 1972], 281-82; Gerald Hawthorne, *Philippians*, WBC 43 [Waco, Tex.: Word, 1983], 166; Peter O'Brien, *The Epistle to the Philippians: A Commentary on the Greek Text*, NIGCT [Grand Rapids: Eerdmans, 1991], 454; Jeremy Moiser, "The Meaning of *koilia* in Philippians 3:19," *ExpTim* 108 [1997]: 365-66, following J. Behm, κοιλία, *TDNT* 3: 186). The language of this passage is similar to Rom 16:17-18, and so the interpretation adopted would likely be the same for both.

[105] Kathleen Dugan, "Fasting for Life: The Place of Fasting in the Christian Tradition," *JAAR* 63, no. 3 (1995): 543.

[106] An oblate can be a layman who does not take vows, but lives periodically under the rules of the community.

[107] Dennis L. Okholm, "Being Stuffed and Being Filled," in *Limning the Psyche: Explorations in Christian Psychology*, ed. Robert C. Roberts and Mark R. Talbot (Grand Rapids: Eerdmans, 1997), 329-35.

[108] Bernard J. Tyrrell, *Christotherapy II: The Fasting and Feasting Heart* (New York: Paulist, 1982).

[109] Christine J. Gardner, "Hungry for God: Why More and More Christians Are Fasting for Revival," *Christianity Today* 43 (April 5, 1999): 32-38.

[110] Editorial, "Not a Fast Fix: It's Hard to Fast, and Even Harder to Do It for the Right Reasons," *Christianity Today* 43 (April 5, 1999): 30-31.

[111] Dugan: 547.

[112] Ibid.: 548.

[113] Evangelicals frequently associate terms like "consecrated" and "sanctified" with a commitment of life to God, and this language suggests that the act of presenting the body to God is a sacred thing.

[114] As in Curtis C. Mitchell, "The Practice of Fasting in the New Testament," *Bibliotheca Sacra* 147, no. 588 (1990): 169.

[115] The comprehensive list of biblical fasting passages in the Appendix has been marked to highlight the fact that the majority of the instances of fasting in the Bible clearly refer to corporate contexts.

[116] Cf. the corporate contexts of Judg 20:26; 1 Sam 7:6, 31:13; 2 Sam 1:12; 2 Chr 20:3; Ezra 8:21-23; Neh 9:1; Esth 4:3, 16, 9:31.

[117] This could of course include the sum of individuals who fast on various occasions, not requiring corporate contexts *per se*. Yet, the fact that groups of Pharisees were associated in Jewish fasting practices, and that the disciples of John were treated as a group in their fasting, would suggest that there would at the least be a kind of corporate awareness of the need of the members of the group to fast.

[118] As discussed above in chapter 2, Paul's fastings here were likely something less than intentional, religious fasts. Rather, he willingly entered into situations where he would be forced to forego food for the sake of the ministry, and the word "fasting" could apply to such an activity for Paul. The point being made here is that it was the sake of the ministry (a corporate context) that impelled him into these fastings.

[119] Foster, v.

[120] Cf. Eph 4:1-6. Additionally, the Roman Catholic Church has officially recognized something of its spiritual bond to all those who profess Christ in Vatican II, *Lumen Gentium*, "Dogmatic Constitution on the Church" (Austin Flannery, ed., *Vatican Council II: Volume 1, The Conciliar and Post Conciliar Documents* [Northport, N.Y.: Costello, 1996], 366-67): "The Church knows that she is joined in many ways to the baptized who are honored by the name of Christian, but who do not however profess the Catholic faith in its entirety or have not preserved unity or communion under the successor of Peter. For there are many who hold sacred scripture in honor as a rule of faith and of life, who have a sincere religious zeal, who lovingly believe in God the Father Almighty and in Christ, the Son of God and the Saviour, who are sealed by baptism which units them to Christ, and who indeed recognize and receive other sacraments in their own Churches or ecclesiastical communities.... these Christians are indeed in some real way joined to us in the Holy Spirit for, by his gifts and graces his sanctifying power is also active in them and he has strengthened some of them even to the shedding of their blood."

[121] Peter Gunning, *The Paschal or Lent Fast: Apostolical and Perpetual*, new ed. (Oxford: John Henry Parker, 1845), 110-15.

Appendix 1: Basil's Sermons *About Fasting* (Sermon 1)

[1] PG 31:163-98; *Thesaurus Linguae Graecae*, CD ROM #E (University of California, Irvine, 1999). Italics have been added to a few texts that cite biblical passages. It as been replicated in the online version of this book here: http://www.bible.org/page.php?page_id=5178

[2] PG 31. 1507-10.

[3] Reginald Pole, *A Treatie of Iustification* (Lovanii: Ioannem Foulerum, 1569; reprint, Farnborough: Gregg, 1967), 48-57.

[4] Ps 80:4 (LXX; 81:3 in English); LXX has ἡμῶν; cf. also Lev 23:24.

[5] Indicating a direct application of a typological interpretation for the liturgical reading of the Psalm just cited.

[6] Phrases from Isa 58:4, 6.

[7] A loose citation of Matt 6:16-17.

[8] Matt 6:17.

[9] Synonyms for "anointed" and "washed" signify an intensification, or spiritualization of terms. The outward act is a ritual purification of the body for spiritual purposes.

[10] Matt 6:16.

[11] Or "hypocrite."

[12] Perhaps this is a self-deprecating play on his own name, "and an idiot might put on the face of Basil"? The i¹diw‾thj could be someone untrained in religion, an inquirer, as 1 Cor 14:16 (L&N).

[13] Lit. "beneficence" or "good deeds;" but Lampe cites passage here as alms; cf. Matt 6:2.

[14] Lev 16:29, 23:27.

[15] Gen 2:17.

[16] Matt 9:12.

[17] Or "penance."

[18] Gen 3:17-18.

[19] Lampe, 597; refers specifically killing animals for eating.

[20] Luke 16:20-31; perhaps the connection of fasting to Lazarus is his poverty and desire to eat the crumbs from the rich man's table.

[21] Quote from Gen 9:3; reference to wine, 9:20-21.

[22] Gen 9:20-21.

[23] Exod 24:18; Deut 9:9.

[24] Exod 32:6.

[25] Gen 25:30-34.

[26] 1 Kgs (LXX)/1 Sam (Eng) 1:13-16.

[27] Judg 13:4.

[28] Judg 13:14.

[29] Fasting is personified in several of these sentences.

[30] 3/1 Kgs 19:8-13.

[31] 3/1 Kgs 17:19-23? Perhaps the reference to the fasting in the story of Elijah raising the widow's son has to do with the miraculous divine provision of flour and oil when they had none.

[32] 3/1 Kgs 17:1. Perhaps the fasting is the miraculous provision of food by the ravens in the following verses.

[33] 3/1 Kgs 17:1.

[34] Apparently a reference to his leaving the place of comfort for austerity.

[35] 4/2 Kgs 4:38-41; This does not appear to refer to 4:42-44 as PG 31.172.

[36] Can mean "undefiled," but context suggests a technical, physical term; reference to "Greeks" follows Pole, who cites a textual variant not mentioned in PG.

[37] Dan 1: 8-16.

[38] LXX, Song of the Three Youths, 46-50; Eng., [Dan 13:] 23-27 (RSV).

[39] Unclear if "desire" refers to choice foods here, or what verb should be supplied; Pole has "of God specially beloved."

[40] Dan 10:2 refers to abstaining from choice foods, eating only bread and drinking water; perhaps Basil got the reference in Dan 1:12 about water mixed into this story; also, the chronology is not consistent with the story of the lions' den (Daniel 6), but it is not clear what Basil had in mind here.

[41] Dan 6: 21.

[42] I.e., the household help, or slaves, won't quit or run away.

[43] Exod 20:10.

[44] Apparently the length of the upcoming Lenten fast in Basil's day.

[45] There appears to be a play on words throughout here on the stench of childbirth and interest (both from tovko"), which goes on to children in the next line, as well as snakes and debt (ojfi" is a snake, but the form is very much like ojfeilw, to "owe").

[46] Lampe, 578.

[47] Luke 16:19-25.

[48] Luke 16:24.

[49] The water refers to abstinence from wine during the Lenten season. PG 31.177, n. 43.

[50] Apparently a reference to gout ruining the feet, and so requiring someone else to run errands.

[51] Heb 11:38a, 37b (textual order inverted).

[52] Luke 16:21, 23.

[53] Matt 3:4.

[54] Matt 11:11.

[55] 2 Cor 11:27, 12:2.

[56] Matt 4:2.

[57] Luke 24:43.

[58] Gal 5:17.

[59] 2 Cor 4:16.

[60] 2 Cor 12:10.

[61] Exod 34:28; Deut 9:18, 10:10.

[62] Jonah 3:4-10.

[63] Heb 3:17.

[64] Num 14:37.

[65] Ps 104:37, LXX.

[66] Exod 16:3; cf. Acts 7:39

[67] Ps 77:25.

[68] Mark 9:29, with Byz. Mss, as KJV.

[69] Jer 5:8.

[70] Cf. Rom 1:26.

[71] 1 Cor 7:5, Byz. mss.

[72] Isa 58:6; cf. also previous quote above, 1.1.

[73] Isa 58:4.

[74] Allusion to Isa 51:21, or 29:9.

[75] Ps 63:2 LXX (64:1, Eng.).

[76] Or, "he is torn apart"; this term can be used as a cursing expression, "split you!" (LSJ).

[77] LSJ notes this as a proverbial saying.

[78] John 14:23.

[79] The change from a festival to a fast day.

Appendix 1: Basil's Sermons *About Fasting* (Sermon 1)

[1] Isa 40:1-2; LXX reads καρδιαν instead of ὦτα as here; LXX includes ἱερεῖς, though the MT does not, which is why the reference to priests does not appear in English versions. The usual Eng. rendering of παρακαλεῖτε as "comfort" does not fit the force of the context of Basil's sermon here, as he uses this text as a justification for his priestly exhortation, drawing a parallel to a coach or army commander.

[2] Eph 6:12.

[3] Shine, as if from the use of oil (LSJ).

[4] The proclamation is the beginning of Lent, and this passage demonstrates that Basil assumes the practice to be empire-wide.

[5] Fasting appears to be personified here, although it is not always clearly discernible when to translate the feminine pronoun that refers to fasting with the English personal pronoun or the more generic "it."

[6] This appears to allude to Matt 6:16, where the hypocrites put on a gloomy face when they fast. Basil seems to be suggesting that if the rich do not humble themselves by fasting, then they will really have something to be gloomy about as a judgment from God.

[7] 2 Tim 2:3, 5.

[8] 1 Cor 9:25.

[9] 1 Thess 5:8; Eph 6:14-17; cf. also Wis Sol 5:17-20.

[10] Cf. 1 Sam 17:5-7 which uses similar terms to describe Goliath, the giant enemy of David.

[11] Cf. Matt 6:16-17; Basil turns Jesus' reference to hypocrites to Jewish fasting.

[12] Gal 5:17.

[13] Gal 5:17.

[14] Or possibly suggesting the present, "let's now be crowned with self-control."

[15] Referring to feasting before fast days (Carnival).

[16] Difficult sentence; possibly a reference to the medical practice of attempting to conceal circumcision (LSJ, Louw-Nida). In that case, perhaps Basil is suggesting either the shame of drunkenness trying to conceal itself, or possibly a reference to drunkenness as not fitting for the gospel dispensation.

[17] 1 Cor 6:10.

[18] Job 3:18.

[19] Cf. Exod 34:28.

[20] Cf. 1 Sam/Kgs 1:11, LXX; the Hebrew (hence English) does not mention drinking. Last phrase is similar Judg 13:14, as PG 193 cites, but that actually refers to Samson's mother. It is closer to Judg 13:6.

[21] Judg 15:16, 16:3, 14:6, 16:21-25.

[22] 1 Kgs 17:1.

[23] Cf. 1 Kgs 18:30-40.

[24] Fasting again appears to be personified through some of these sentences (cf. note 5 above). Also, "receive" is the verb supplied in the following sentences.

[25] The picture is that of being on a slippery mountaintop.

[26] Matt 6:16-17.

[27] Isa 58:5, LXX (English translations follow the Hebrew, which puts the sentence in question form).

[28] 2 Cor 6:16.

[29] Cf. 1 Cor 3:16.

[30] Cf. the emphasis on doing righteous deeds, including fasting, in secret, in Matt 6:4, 6, 18.

[31] Prov 10:3.

[32] Ps 36:25.

[33] Gen 42:2, 43:2; this could possibly allude to the fact that the children of Israel eventually ended up in slavery after going to Egypt for literal food, and the spiritual food Basil refers to does not result in slavery, but in spiritual freedom.

[34] Amos 8:11.

[35] Prov 9:2.

[36] Heb 5:14.

[37] Cf. Jesus' reference to the sons of the bride chamber not fasting when the bridegroom is present in Matt 9:15, Mark 2:19, and Luke 5:34. Basil alludes here to the eschatological day of being in Christ's presence, when the fulfillment of the purpose of fasting is enjoyed.

Appendix 2: Fasting in Scripture

[1] Kent Berghuis, "Teaching Biblical Fasting" (paper presented at the ETS annual meeting, Orland, Fla., 1998), 11-15; "A Biblical Perspective on Fasting," BSac 158, no. 629 (2001): 97-103.

[2] From the Hebrew root צוֹם and Greek words related to νηστεύω.

[3] As in the KJV; the NASB translates νήστεις (acc. pl. masc. from the adjective νῆστις) in Matt 15:32 as "hungry," perhaps implying that it was not an intentional fast but merely the lack of food; yet the NASB inconsistently translates the same word as "fasting" in Mark 8:3.

[4] This verse is well-attested in the Byzantine witnesses, but omitted from Vaticanus, the original hand of Sinaiticus, and a number of other manuscripts. For this reason, and because it was likely assimilated to the parallel in Mark, the omission was assigned an {A} rating in The Greek New Testament, United Bible Societies, 4th ed. (UBS[4]).

[5] This verse ends with "prayer" (προσευχή) in Vaticanus, the original hand of Sinaiticus, and several minor witnesses. But a corrector of Sinaiticus, 𝔓45[vid], and a large number of later uncials and minuscules add "and fasting" (καὶ νηστείά). Recognizing scribal tendencies the UBS[4] assigned the omission an {A} rating, and they refer the reader to 1 Cor 7:5.

[6] The fact that τοῦτο δὲ τὸ γένος is neuter would suggest that Jesus was referring back to the unclean spirit (τὸ δαιμόνιον) which had just come out of the boy.

[7] The reference to fasting is omitted in Sinaiticus, the original hand of Alexandrinus, Vaticanus, 𝔓74, and several other witnesses, while being found in most of the Byzantine and a number of Western manuscripts. Previous editions of the UBS Greek NT gave the reading that lacked the reference to fasting a {D} rating; the {B} rating in the UBS[4] seems a little optimistic.

[8] This was probably not an intentional fast. But because of the storm, the likelihood of seasickness and the extreme conditions on the vessel, the crew could not find a good time to eat.

[9] The reference to "fasting" in this verse is omitted by almost all of the Alexandrian and Western witnesses, with the Byzantine including it. The UBS[4] assigns the omission a certainty of {A}, apparently seeing this textual addition as informing Mark 9:29 and Matt 17:21, as suggested by footnote 25 on Mark 9:29.

[10] The NASB translates νηστείαις "hunger" and "without food," respectively.